David H. Walker (ed.)

Global Infectious Diseases

Prevention, Control, and Eradication

With a Foreword
by Thomas N. James

Springer-Verlag Wien New York

Prof. David H. Walker
Department of Pathology, University of Texas Medical Branch,
Galveston, U.S.A.

Printed in Austria by Ferdinand Berger & Söhne, A-3580 Horn

Printed on acid-free paper

Product Liability: The publisher can give no guarantee for information about drug dosage and application thereof contained in this book. In every individual case the respective user must check its accuracy by consulting other pharmaceutical literature. The use of registered names, trademarks, etc. in this publication does not imply, even in the absence of a specific statement, that such names are exempt from the relevant protective laws and regulations and therefore free for general use.

With 33 Figures

ISBN 3-211-82329-8 Springer-Verlag Wien-New York
ISBN 0-387-82329-8 Springer-Verlag New York-Wien

Dedicated to my wife, Marjorie,
and my sons, Jesse and Andrew, with love.

Acknowledgments

I would like to acknowledge the foresight and support of The University of Texas Medical Branch at Galveston, the President, Thomas N. James, M.D. and the Vice President for Research, K. Lemone Yielding, M.D. for initiating the concept of the "Centennial Symposium on Tropical Medicine". This concept evolved to an interactive consideration of global infectious diseases and the directions for their control in the twenty-first century. The information that was discussed brought forth the nation's leading thinkers whose ideas have been contributed as book chapters in their specialized fields. I would also acknowledge Ms. Rose Herndon and Ms. Carol Lehr for their assistance in organizing the Symposium and in the preparation of this book.

Foreword

Introducing a book on global infectious diseases is a daunting challenge. Modern developments in molecular research, newly available opportunities for earth-orbiting, satellite-based surveillance as a means of predicting certain regional epidemics, and the introduction of remarkable new antibiotics which can cure some awesome problems such as river-blindness would each have astonished even the most jaded reader only a few decades ago. Just the same, even with these laudable advances, malaria is still with us and both poliomyelitis and tuberculosis are growing worldwide problems.

As a holdover from my own medical school days, I must confess to an affection for the older term of "tropical medicine" and its historic context, in preference to the more popular present name which is the title of this book. A century or two ago the motives to study tropical medicine were obvious: nations having enormous amounts of maritime trade with distant lands established colonial empires where health in the colonies was a concern for both the natives and the colonists. It is unsurprising that the great institutes for such studies sprang up in London, Amsterdam, Hamburg, New York and New Orleans, but few of these centers and other similar ones have continued to flourish or even to survive, perhaps because the days of empires have gone. If that is so, this book will serve to remind us that we are still in the biblical sense our brothers' keepers, that the health of any affects the health of all, and that most diseases (including tropical ones) ignore geographic boundaries.

At The University of Texas Medical Branch and its home on Galveston Island, we are the heirs of a historic legacy on this subject, since malaria and yellow fever at one time were devastating scourges here. Eradication of both of these local medical problems does not absolve us of a need to find ways to accomplish the same thing in places still afflicted. Three chapters in this book are contributions from our faculty, where a formal program addressing a number of aspects of tropical medicine has now been organized.

There is a long list of tropical diseases, which today include AIDS as well as the resurgence of scarlet fever with its sequel of rheumatic heart disease, but two tropical diseases particularly illustrate the magnitude of our challenge. The first is malaria, still one of the leading causes of death for the whole world and diagnosed in several thousand cases brought to the United States from endemic areas every year. There are entire philanthropic foundations dedicated to diseases which involve only a tiny fraction of as many examples of illness and death as malaria does. It warrants far more attention. The second is Chagas' disease, one of the most common causes of congestive heart failure and sudden death in the entire world. New migrants to the United States from endemic areas not only sometimes have either dormant or active forms of Chagas' cardiomyopathy, but there is a serious concern that many blood donors in our urban centers are potential transmitters of the trypanosome.

It is not my responsibility to recite such a litany for those likely to read this book, for you are especially familiar already with what we face. Citizens of the United States increasingly travel throughout the world and stay for longer periods than in days when travel was less easily done. Conversely, individuals of other countries increasingly come to the United States as tourists, family visitors, students, merchants, diplomats, reporters and the like, some to stay days or weeks and others for much longer times. To this we may add the growing number of immigrants from distant (and ecologically different) lands. But whether they are our own returning home or foreigners coming to visit or to live here, all are potential carriers of the illnesses which comprise the subject of this book.

As has been dramatically illustrated by recent world events, the global "village" is here to stay, and with it comes a wider and ultimately ubiquitous distribution of global pestilence. Those who dedicate their efforts to addressing ways to deal successfully with this challenge will help everyone, including you and me.

Thomas N. James, M.D., M.A.C.P.
President
The University of Texas
Medical Branch at Galveston

Contents

Contributors

Frederick A. Murphy, D.V.M., Ph.D., Director, Center for Infectious Diseases, Centers for Disease Control, Atlanta, GA

Colonel Thomas P. Monath, M.D., USAMRIID, Fort Detrick, Frederick, MD

Franz von Lichtenberg, M.D., Brigham and Women's Hospital, Harvard Medical School, Boston, MA

*Alan G. Barbour, M.D.,*University of Texas Health Science Center, San Antonio, TX

Ralph T. Bryan, M.D., Centers for Disease Control, Atlanta, GA

Richard L. Guerrant, M.D., University of Virginia Medical School, Charlottesville, VA

June E. Osborn, M.D., School of Public Health, University of Michigan, Ann Arbor, MI

Louis V. Kirchhoff, M.D., University of Iowa College of Medicine, Iowa City, IA

Stanley M. Lemon, M.D., University of North Carolina, Chapel Hill, NC

Michael R. McGinnis, Ph.D., University of Texas Medical Branch, Galveston, TX

David H. Walker, M.D., University of Texas Medical Branch, Galveston, TX

Eric A. Ottesen, M.D., National Institutes of Health, Bethesda, MD

Carter L. Diggs, M.D., Ph.D., Atlantic Resources Corporation, Consultant for the Agency for International Development, Washington, DC

Thomas N. James, M.D., President, The University of Texas Medical Branch, Galveston, TX

D. A. Henderson, M.D., M.P.H., Associate Director for Life Sciences, Office of Science and Technology Policy, Executive Office of the President, Washington, DC

Infectious Diseases in Developing Countries: An Introduction to the Major Problems in Global Medicine

David H. Walker[1] and **Frederick A. Murphy**[2]

[1] Department of Pathology, The University of Texas Medical Branch, Galveston, Texas
[2] School of Veterinary Medicine, University of California, Davis, California

Advances in contemporary molecular biology and immunology have carried the problems of viral, bacterial, fungal, rickettsial, protozoal, and helminthic diseases into the mainstream of biomedical science. Amazing new tools developed via recombinant-DNA and other technologies offer great opportunities for progress in alleviating the suffering and social stagnation which are the consequences, in part, of the burden of infectious diseases among populations of developing countries.

When one examines the health status of populations of various countries, there are striking differences, beyond the simple differences between the haves and the have nots. The reasons for these differences, of course, include economic realities, but they also derive from differences in educational status, natural resources, and social and political infrastructural factors. It is often difficult in this regard to distinguish causes and effects – poor health leads to poverty and vice versa. There are wide choices open to policymakers in developing countries and donor countries in regard to approaches to be taken to deal with the overwhelming problems. Priority might be given to population control, or to agricultural (food and fiber) development, or to economic development, or to the climate for political and social self-determination. Clearly, the health problems of various populations of developing countries are not equally addressable under each of these points of emphasis – but, in each case it seems clear that improvement of the health of children and adults can provide a great incentive in affecting the success of other programs. For example, the reduction of mortality of children has a major positive effect on population planning, educational development, and economic development, and it certainly has a major positive effect on socio-political stability.

There are two counterforces that seem to be confounding the promise of contemporary molecular biology and immunology to affect the health of various populations in developing countries. One is what seems to be a failure of public will to support necessary redirection and expansion of resources in the developing world. Clearly, we must do a better job in reaching out to the public in developed countries and convince that public of the worthiness of our enterprise. The second what seems to be a failure of public trust in science and scientific technology. The practitioners of modern biotechnology have been accused of humanistic shortcomings – "they are only concerned with the glamour of their science." Clearly, this is not the case, but we must do a better job in reaching out to the public to project our true motivations. Only then will the message that we have incredibly powerful new technologies to bring to bear on specific problems be a welcome message.

This volume addresses the question, "What are the most feasible approaches to control infectious diseases of principal concern in the developing world?" Twelve infectious disease areas have been chosen for emphasis and to generate general principles: malaria, schistosomiasis, AIDS, arboviral diseases, diarrheal diseases, viral hepatitis, fungal diseases, filariasis, rickettsioses, borrelioses, cysticercosis, and Chagas' disease were chosen not only for their medical and economic importance, but also for their varied ecologic and epidemiologic dimensions. This array of diseases offers the possibilities for consideration of various different approaches to control.

The emphasis of this volume on control distinguishes it from that of other books on tropical diseases. It should be clearly understood that the choice of topics does not imply that other diseases are unimportant. Inclusion of malaria (300 million cases annually and at least a million deaths), schistosomiasis (200–300 million cases), filariasis (90 million with lymphatic filariasis and 30 million with onchocerciasis), and diarrheal diseases (nearly a billion episodes per year in children in developing countries with 4.5 million childhood diarrhea deaths annually), of course, are surprises to no one. For many other diseases, the morbidity and mortality are unknown and not necessarily because the diseases are not important. Often the clinical diagnoses are difficult, requisite diagnostic tools are lacking, and reporting systems are inadequate. Other disease categories such as measles, whooping cough, pneumonia, tetanus, and leprosy have major adverse impact on morbidity and mortality of persons living in tropical areas. However, the goal of this work is not to be encyclopedic, but rather to focus on the potential for control.

Eradication may be considered an ultimate goal. Smallpox was a major human scourge that has now been eradicated (as will be recounted and analyzed by Dr. Henderson in Chapter 14). Eradication requires permanently breaking a link in the chain of events that maintain an infection. However, in most cases control is the practical goal; control can yield the salutary effects of dampening disease impact. For a particular infectious disease, control might be best effected through eliminating its intermediate host (e.g., snails), arthropod vector (e.g., mosquitoes, fleas, ticks, lice, chiggers, flies, triatomid bugs), or through vaccination, water purification, sewage treatment, food hygiene, veterinary disease control, education of the population regarding personal and behavioral preventive measures, and medical diagnosis and treatment of the infected human reservoir. In some instances, improved economic conditions might have important effects upon allowing progress to occur (e.g., money for government water and sewage projects or for individuals to purchase window screens to keep insects from entering the home or to purchase shoes that would minimize hookworm or traumatic implantation of fungi). What are the prospects for selecting diseases for successful eradication? What are the possibilities for favorable impact in ameliorating the condition of developing countries where infectious diseases are a prime reason that the population is unhealthy? The answers to these and similar questions are important keys to a more favorable condition of mankind.

Reference

1. The U.S. Capacity to Address Tropical Infectious Disease Problems (1987) Board on Science and Technology for International Development, Office of International Affairs, National Research Council and the Institute of Medicine National Academy of Sciences. Washington, D.C., National Academy Press

The Challenge: Biotechnology Transfer to Public Health. Examples from Arbovirology

Thomas P. Monath

Virology Division, U. S. Army Medical Research Institute of Infectious Diseases, Fort Detrick, Frederick, Maryland, U.S.A.

Introduction

Infectious diseases remain the preeminent health problems in the developing world, and immunization the most effective approach to controlling them. Recombinant DNA technology has provided a plethora of new approaches for the development of vaccines. The priorities for development of new vaccines and delivery methods have been redefined by the Children's Vaccine Initiative. Among the diseases targeted for vaccine improvement or development are three arbovirus infections, dengue, Japanese encephalitis, and yellow fever. The burden of disease caused by these mosquito-borne viruses, the current status of classical vaccines, and progress toward development of genetically-engineered vaccines are reviewed. Since 1984, the World Health Organization has promulgated research leading toward the development of molecular approaches to vaccines against these flaviviruses. Considerable headway has been made in the understanding of genome variation, the identification of protective epitopes, and in cloning and expression of relevant proteins in vaccinia and baculovirus systems. In addition, the development of full-length complementary DNA clones which yield infectious RNA transcripts is being pursued as a means of producing stable, attenuated and chimeric flavivirus vaccines. However, progress in molecular biology reveals a widening gap between our ability to devise new products and our ability to manufacture them at low cost and utilize them for the prevention of disease in the developing world. The high costs of research and development may preclude the use of new vaccines in the Third World; economic and political solutions needed to overcome this obstacle must keep pace with technical innovation. Moreover, biotechnology provides a countervailing force to the funding of research and the pursuit of careers in field biology, epidemiology, hygiene, and other traditional disciplines which are required to define the changing determinants of disease ecology, delineate targets for prevention, formulate public health policy, and evaluate the results of prevention programs. Yellow fever provides an example of a disease which is poorly controlled despite the availability of an effective vaccine.

The advent of molecular biology has revolutionized traditional approaches to the diagnosis, treatment, and prevention of diseases affecting plants and animals. Tracing the major accomplishments of a century of progress in the struggle against infectious diseases illustrates how biotechnology has provided fundamentally novel strategies for their control. The explosion of knowledge in molecular biology is now being applied to these problems by many groups engaged in research, including the pharmaceutical industry. This revolution has been accompanied by a predicament, however. A widening gap is revealed between our ability to devise new products and our ability to utilize them for the prevention and control of disease, especially in the developing world. Narrowing the gap between discovery and production of new technologies and their practical deployment will be one of the cardinal challenges of public health in the 21st Century.

Biotechnology had its origins during most of our lifetimes. I was a toddler of 3 years when Avery, MacLeod, and McCarty at the Rockefeller Institute identified DNA as the genetic material of prokaryotic cells. I was 12 years old, and just uncovering the mysteries of my first chemistry set, when Watson, Crick, Franklin, and Wilkins described the three-dimensional structure of DNA. I had reached medical school when Arber, Meselson and others developed site-specific restriction endonucleases and Nirenberg and his colleagues elucidated the genetic code for the synthesis of proteins. I was a young medical officer at the Centers for Disease Control (CDC), when Temin and Baltimore described reverse transcriptase and Boyer developed DNA cloning techniques. My hair was just beginning to gray in the mid-1970's, when Milstein and Kohler fused antibody-producing lymphocytes with myeloma cells to produce monoclonal antibodies and Sanger and Gilbert developed DNA sequencing techniques. The pace of technology then really exploded as I finally admitted I might be reaching middle age. In 1980, the U.S. Supreme Court ruled that microorganisms are patentable, opening the floodgates of research using recombinant DNA in the biotechnology industry. Within two years, the first diagnostic kit using monoclonal antibodies and the first genetically engineered pharmaceutical product (human insulin) were licensed by the Food and Drug Administration (FDA). In 1982, the first recombinant human vaccine – hepatitis B surface antigen expressed in eukaryotic cells – was described and, shortly thereafter, successfully tested in clinical trials. Also in 1982, Paoletti initiated the exploitation of vaccinia virus as a live vector of foreign genes, now being applied to a wide array of viruses, bacteria, and protozoa. By 1985, this technology was considered one of the most promising expression systems for recombinant vaccines. Vaccinia recombinants are now in field use against fox rabies, vaccinia-vectored vaccines against hepatitis B and human immunodeficiency virus (HIV) have been tested in humans, and trials of a rinderpest recombinant vaccine are planned in Africa. In 1985, Saiki and colleagues described an enzymatic process for amplifying specific DNA sequences in vitro – the polymerase chain reaction – a technique which has revolutionized approaches to gene mapping, sequencing, and the development of sensitive diagnostic assays. In 1988, the first patent was issued for a genetically engineered (transgenic) animal. Work is now underway to exploit this technology to the control of infectious diseases, including the generation of disease-resistant animals and incompetent vectors. Within the next few years, technological approaches which are anticipated to produce major breakthroughs include the development of many new vaccines; wide application of therapeutic human monoclonal antibodies and immunological tissue targeting of drugs; new adjuvants, immunostimulators and delivery systems for drugs and vaccines; computerized modeling for drug and vaccine design; and molecularly targeted antiviral drugs, to mention only a few. The challenge for public health will be how to harness these sophisticated approaches to confront disease, especially in the developing world where infectious diseases will be preeminent for the foreseeable future. The challenge requires that economic and political solutions follow the scientific breakthroughs.

One index of progress in the application of biotechnology to medicine is the annual survey of products in development conducted by the Pharmaceutical Manufacturers Association (PMA). Since 1986, when these surveys were initiated, the number of biotechnology and genetic engineering patents issued has increased nearly 60%. More than half of the products are medicines or vaccines. As of March, 1990, there were 11 biotechnology products licensed for general use, 32 in final stages of FDA approval, and 72 undergoing clinical trials (Table 1). Among these are 3 licensed and 14 experimental vaccines, all but one against infectious diseases, including hepatitis B, *Hemophilus influenzae* type b, HIV, herpes viruses, and malaria (Table 2). However, this relatively short list does not accurately reflect the rapidly expanding worldwide scope of efforts within university and government laboratories on vaccine development, much of it directed at new approaches through biotechnology. In fact, the proliferation of new live vectors and candidate vaccines often makes it difficult to select the most advantageous approach for clinical development.

The most important health problems of the developing world continue to be the infectious diseases, and immunization is the most effective and cost-efficient means of protecting populations against them. However, despite an array of new vaccines in various stages of development, only a handful are in practical use in the developing world, and these old vaccines are not the children of biotechnology. Only six vaccines are currently in routine use for childhood immunization (Table 3), and vaccine coverage is still less than hoped for (1). It is estimated that without an accelerated rate of coverage, 30 million children will die of vaccine-preventable diseases in the 1990s (2). The toll from diseases against which vaccines are not yet deployed is even more staggering: 20 million deaths from malaria in this de-

Table 1. Biotechnology Products Approved or in Clinical Development as of March, 1990 (Source: Pharmaceutical Manufacturers Association)

Product type	Indication	No. products: clinical trials	No. products: licensed
Colony Stimulating Factors	Cancer, AIDS	7	
Superoxide dismutases	Reperfusion injury	2	
Erythropoietin	Anemias	2	1
Factor VIII	Hemophilia	2	
Growth Factors	Wound healing	7	
Growth Hormone	Growth failure	4	2
Interferons	Cancer, infectious diseases	8	2
Interleukins	Cancer, AIDS	10	
Monoclonal antibodies	Cancer, transplantation, infectious diseases	37	1
CD4's	AIDS	4	
Tumor Necrosis Factor	Cancer	3	
Vaccines	Infectious diseases, cancer	14	3
Other		4	2
Total		104	11

cade, 40 million from diarrheal diseases, and 40 million from acute respiratory disease. Nevertheless, there is optimism that the global vaccination programs can be strengthened and that new vaccines against these infectious diseases can be brought into use.

Since 1984, the development of new vaccines and improvement of existing technologies have been actively promoted and funded by two programs administered by WHO and UNDP. In the *Program for Vaccine Development*, five targets are being addressed by individual Steering Committees under the overall guidance of a Scientific Advisory Group of Experts (SAGE). The targets include two arbovirus diseases – dengue and Japanese encephalitis; as well as hepatitis A and poliomyelitis; tuberculosis; acute viral respiratory infections; and encapsulated bacteria (3). The program attempts to coordinate research efforts world-wide, promote information-sharing, focus research on the most promising technologies, and provide limited direct funding of new research, with the hope that the results will attract other resources. The underlying principle guiding the efforts of SAGE and the individual Steering Committees is the commitment to more fully characterize disease agents at the molecular level, delineate the antigens responsible for induction of immunity, elucidate the basis for protective host im-

Table 2. Biotechnology Vaccines, Approved and in Clinical Trials, as of March, 1990[1]

Indication	In clinical trial	Approved
Hepatitis B	4	2
AIDS	3	
Herpes 2	2	
Malaria	4	
Hemophilus B		1
Melanoma	1	

[1] Source: Pharmaceutical Manufacturers Association

Table 3. Vaccines Included in the WHO Expanded Program of Immunization, 1991

1. BCG
2. Diphtheria
3. Pertussis
4. Tetanus
5. Poliomyelitis
6. Measles

munity, and develop and evaluate vaccine candidates. New approaches for the use of infectious clone technology and live vectors of foreign genes seem particularly promising as efficient and cost-effective means of inducing long-lasting immunity (4).

The second WHO *Program on Transdisease Vaccinology* is addressing the important issues of adjuvants and novel approaches to antigen presentation and delivery, including the use of live vectors, microencapsulated antigens, and oral administration of vaccines classically delivered by syringe and needle. One of the most important obstacles to the use of vaccines in developing countries is the requirement for multiple inoculations and repeated interactions between the population and the health care delivery system. Controlled-release technologies are being explored which show promise of multivalent immunization with a single inoculation.

In 1986, the Institute of Medicine sponsored a study on *New Vaccine Development, Establishing Priorities* (5) and identified 29 vaccine candidates for development against 19 diseases not currently incorporated in the WHO Expanded Programme of Immunization (Table 4). The new vaccines included 1) improved existing products, generally derived by changing from tissue-based manufacture to cell cultures; 2) new vaccines produced

Table 4. Diseases of Importance in Developing Countries Targeted for Vaccine Development, Institute of Medicine, 1986

Disease/Pathogen	Improve existing	New, classical	Biotechnology
Yellow fever	+		
Dengue			+
Japanese encephalitis	+		
E. coli (ETEC)		+	+
Hemophilus B			+
Hepatitis A		+	+
Hepatitis B			+
Leprosy		+	
Neisseria meningitidis			+
Parainfluenza			+
Malaria			+
Rabies		+	+
Respiratory syncytial virus		+	+
Rotavirus		+	
Salmonella typhi			+
Shigella			+
Streptococcus A			+
Vibrio cholerae		+	+

by classical approaches; and 3) new vaccines produced by biotechnology. Vaccines for 14 of the 19 target diseases affecting developing countries would be the result of genetic engineering or other biotechnological approaches. Three of the target diseases, for which significant health benefits would accrue by implementing vaccination programs, were arthropod-borne viruses – yellow fever, dengue, and Japanese encephalitis.

In 1990, WHO, UNICEF, UNDP, and the Rockefeller Foundation announced its new global *Children's Vaccine Initiative* (CVI), which has as its goal the development and implementation of new, multivalent vaccines for the protection of the world's children against the major killer diseases. Many of the vaccines required are yet to be developed or licensed (e.g., against toxin-producing *E. coli,* hepatitis A, respiratory syncytial virus, groups A and B streptococci, rotavirus, dengue, malaria, typhoid, parainfluenza, and pneumococcal meningitis). In addition to the vaccines themselves, new strategies for delivery are envisioned, including microencapsulated antigens for mucosal and parenteral presentation. The technological objectives thus include: 1) immunization with the minimal number of injections; 2) immunization at the earliest point in life, possibly at birth; 3) high thermostability; 4) provision of lifelong immunity; and 5) cost within reach of programs for universal immunization. In the United States, the CVI is coordinated by the National Vaccine Program of the Department of Health and Human Services and implemented in part by DHHS agencies, the Centers for Disease Control, National Institutes of Health, and Food and Drug Administration. Priorities for new funding for the National Vaccine Program have been defined by these agencies, and the target diseases are similar, in general, to those already identified by WHO and the IOM report.

To illustrate and extend some of the aspects of these initiatives, I have selected several examples from arbovirology which serve as specific paradigms to explore the general theme of vaccines from biotechnology and the implementation of vaccination strategies in the developing world. The examples selected – dengue, Japanese encephalitis, and yellow fever, – represent diseases which have also been targeted by WHO, the IOM, or the CVI for new or improved vaccine development. All three diseases are caused by members of the family Flaviviridae. Significant progress has been made in recent years on the molecular biology of this group of viruses and on approaches toward production of recombinant vaccines.

Dengue and Dengue Hemorrhagic Fever/Dengue Shock Syndrome (DHF/DSS)

Dengue is widely credited as the most important vector-borne viral infection of humans, because of its worldwide distribution, high morbidity and cost associated with epidemics, the great difficulty in successful application of mosquito control as an alternate strategy to vaccination, and the occurrence of severe and potentially lethal disease – DHF/DSS – in a subset of those infected. The current global situation is characterized by an expanding geographic distribution of the disease, by an increasing incidence of DHF/DSS in Southeast Asia, and by the emergence of DHF/DSS in previously unaffected regions, principally the Americas and Pacific island nations. This changing pattern is attributable to expanding urbanization and the attendant increased distribution and population density of the vector, *Aedes aegypti*; to the reinfestation of South and Central America by *Ae. aegypti*; to the senescence of effective vector control programs; and to increasing air travel with introduction of dengue virus strains and serotypes to new and receptive areas. Figure 1 shows the present distribution of dengue and areas receptive to dengue by virtue of being infested with *Ae. aegypti*. Over 2 billion people reside in these areas, and millions are affected by dengue fever annually (6). Morbidity estimates are available only for the severe form, DHF/DSS. These data indicate an increasing incidence, with over 250,000 cases reported annually in recent years, principally in Southeast Asia (Table 5). However, within the last decade, epidemic DHF/DSS

Table 5. Global Incidence of Dengue Hemorrhagic Fever[1]

Time period	No. years	Cases	Mean cases/year
1956–1980	25	715,283	29,803
1981–1985	5	687,522	137,504
1986–1990[2]	5	1,338,461	267,692
Totals		2,741,266	78,322

[1] Gubler DJ (1991) Virus Info Exch Newsl 8: 2–3
[2] 1989–90 data provisional

appeared in a number of countries for the first time, notably Sri Lanka, and several countries in the New World – Cuba, Venezuela, and Brazil. The epidemiological pattern of DHF/DSS in the Americas in the 1980s resembles the emergence of this disease in Southeast Asia in the early 1960s and predicts an increasing incidence of severe disease in this hemisphere in the future.

The approach to dengue immunization is greatly complicated by the occurrence of 4 serotypes, which do not provide cross-protective immunity. Instead, heterologous immunity appears to underlie the pathogenesis of DHF/DSS, presumably by non-neutralizing antibody-mediated enhancement of dengue virus replication in Fc-receptor-bearing monocyte-macrophages. In addition, cross-reactive cytotoxic T cells target infected cells during secondary infection, with release of precursors of the coagulation cascade and vasoactive mediators of shock. For these reasons, primary immunization with a dengue vaccine must meet certain unique criteria: 1) simultaneous induction of immunity to all 4 dengue serotypes; and 2) induction of long-lasting immunity which does not wane from levels which are protective to levels which enhance virus replication.

The preparation of inactivated, whole virion dengue vaccines is generally accepted as impractical because of low virus yields in cell culture. Attempts to produce live, attenuated vaccines in mouse brain were begun in the 1940s by Sabin and Schlesinger, but the modern era began in the 1970s with efforts by the Walter Reed Army Institute of Research to produce vaccines in cell culture substrates acceptable by current regulatory standards. The first of these vaccines to be tested in humans was a temperature-sensitive, small plaque variant of dengue virus type 2 (7). During the 1980s, candidate vaccines with similar characteristics against all 4 serotypes were tested in humans. The results, summarized in Table 6, were disappointing. Either preimmunization with yellow fever 17D was required (dengue-2, Pr159/S1), or the vaccine demonstrated overattenuation (dengue-4, H241 and Carib 341750), or it caused unmodified illness (dengue-1, 45AZ5 and dengue 3, CH53489). In vitro and in vivo laboratory markers of attenuation were found to be unreliable predictors of clinical response. Therefore,

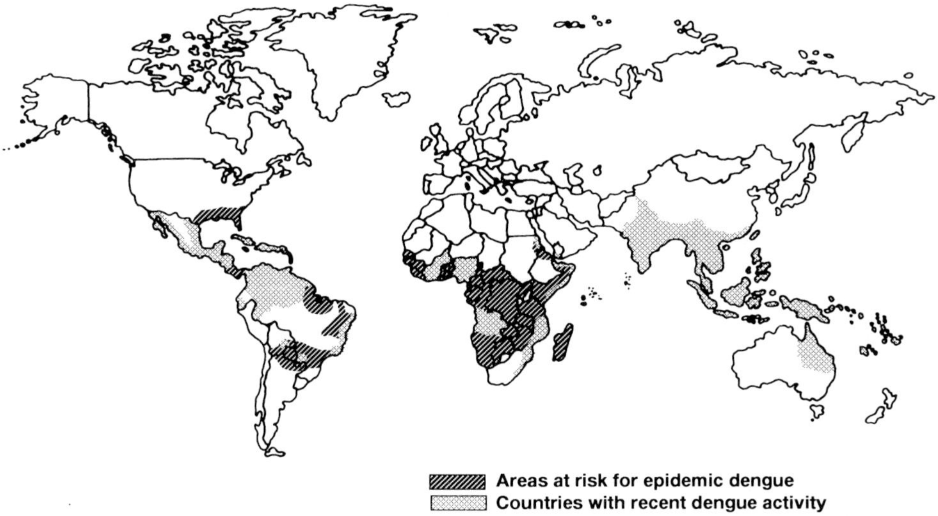

Fig. 1. World distribution of dengue and of areas at risk of epidemics by virtue of infestation by the principal vector, *Aedes aegypti.* Modified from Gubler (6), with permission

present efforts at finding candidate vaccines are directed at testing decreasing cell culture passage levels of selected virus strains in small groups of human volunteers.

A parallel effort at development of live vaccines has been undertaken in Thailand by Bhamarapravati and colleagues, with support provided by WHO. Candidate vaccines against all 4 dengue have been tested in flavivirus-naïve and JE-immune humans alone and in various simultaneous combinations, including a trivalent (dengue 1, 2, 4) vaccine (8, 9). The results have been encouraging and indicate 90–100% immunogenicity, apparently without significant side-effects. A number of problems remain to be overcome, however. The dengue type 1 candidate requires a high dose for adequate immunization, creating a problem for cost-effective production. It is still uncertain what the effect of preexisting dengue immunity, either acquired by active infection or by passive maternal transfer, will have on immunogenicity and reactogenicity of the live vaccine.

Since 1984, the WHO Steering Committee on Dengue and Japanese Encephalitis has sought alternative approaches to immunization through biotechnology. The response of the scientific community has been magnificent, and progress in flavivirus molecular biology is so extensive as to defy concise summarization. Only relevant highlights can be presented here [see Brandt (10) for a partial review]. Efforts have been directed at 1) cloning and sequencing representative strains of each dengue serotype and definition of genetic variation among geographic dengue virus strains; 2) defining the protective epitopes of dengue viruses, including both B-cell and helper T-cell activities; 3) expression of relevant subunit proteins in

Table 6. Status of Clinical Trials of Live, Attenuated Dengue Vaccines, Walter Reed Army Institute of Research, 1991[1]

Serotype	Strain	No. vaccinated by YF immune status	Seroconversion rate (%)	Clinical response	Conclusion
DEN-1	45AZ5	2 (I)[2]	100	Dengue fever	Not attenuated
DEN-2	PR159/S1	70 (I)	90	mild symptoms	Requires YF immunity
		28 (N)	62	mild symptoms	
DEN-3	CH53489	2 (I)	100	Dengue fever	Not attenuated
DEN-4	H241	5 (I)	40	mild symptoms	Over-attenuated
	Carib 341750	8 (N)	65	minimal symptoms	Further tests at lower passage

[1] Eckels K (1990) pers. comm.
[2] *I* previously immunized with yellow fever 17D; *N* not immunized

various expression vectors; 4) cloning genes for protective epitopes into recombinant live vectors; and 5) generation of dengue virus infectious clones.

Flaviviruses contain a single-strand positive-sense RNA genome about 11 kilobases long (11, 12). There is a single long open reading frame of about 10 kilobases which encodes 3 structural and 7 nonstructural proteins (Fig. 2). The structural proteins, encoded at the 5'-terminus, include a capsid protein (C) associated with the RNA genome; a glycosylated prM protein which is proteolytically cleaved to form a small membrane (M) subunit of the virion envelope; and a major glycosylated envelope (E) protein. The E glycoprotein comprises the surface projections of the whole virion and is involved in major biological functions such as attachment to cells and induction of humoral and cellular immunity. The nonstructural proteins have important enzymatic functions in post-translational proteolytic cleavage and RNA transcription.

Studies employing monoclonal antibodies, active immunization with purified or expressed proteins, and synthetic peptides have demonstrated protective epitopes on at least 3 glycoproteins, including two structural proteins [the intracellular precursor to the membrane protein (prM) and the envelope (E) glycoprotein] and a large glycosylated nonstructural protein (NS1). However, the individual amino acid sequences constituting protective epitopes have not yet been completely defined. Protection of animals by antibodies to the E glycoprotein is clearly correlated with virus neutralization, but antibodies to prM and NS1 protect without directly neutralizing virus. The protection afforded by antibodies to NS1 appears to be mediated by complement-dependent lysis of infected cells. Since NS1 is not a struc-

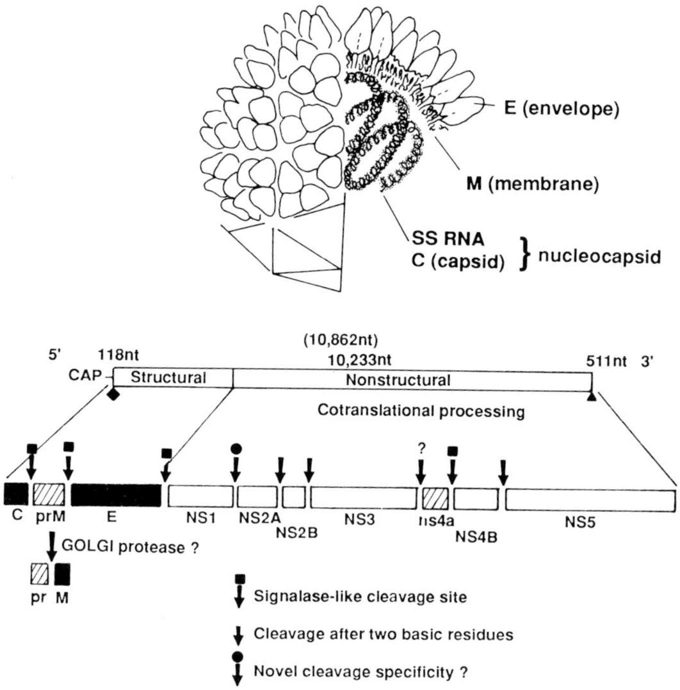

Fig. 2. Structure of the flavivirus virion, showing the organization of the genome, coding assignments of the structural and nonstructural polypeptides, and enzymatic cleavage sites for posttranslational processing. The data shown were first described by Rice et al. (11)

tural component of the virus, it is an attractive target for vaccine development. Antibodies to this protein would not bind to virions or engage the immune enhancement phenomenon. However, a body of evidence is accumulating that effective subunit vaccines derived from expression vectors should probably include at least 4 proteins, prM, E, NS1, and NS2a, both because this provides multiple antigens relevant to protection and because of the complex interdependency of individual proteins in their functional expression. The production of authentic NS1 appears to depend on the presence of the downstream (NS2a) sequences, and, similarly, functional assembly and conformation of the E protein appears to depend on prM and possibly on NS1(13, 14). Development of successful recombinant flavivirus vaccines thus depends on native presentation of viral proteins, and prokaryotic expression systems or synthetic peptides may have limited usefulness. Moreover, it appears from studies with synthetic peptides that both B and T-cell responses are strongly dependent on MHC haplotype. Thus, incorporation of multiple epitopes subserving protection in a recombinant vaccine may be important to avoid variation in immune responses of an outbred (human) population.

Considerable effort has been made to investigate vaccinia and baculovirus expression of dengue proteins as approaches to vaccine development (13–15). Recombinant vaccinia virus has received the most attention, because of the potential advantages of a live vector in the induction of both humoral and cellular immunity. The molecular strategy includes construction of plasmids for homologous recombination of flavivirus gene sequences and a vaccinia promoter into the nonessential thymidine kinase gene locus of vaccinia virus. Recombinant constructs containing genes for individual or multiple flavivirus proteins have been investigated, with variable success in immunizing and protecting laboratory animals (Table 7). In early experiments, neither binding nor neutralizing antibodies to the dengue type 4 E glycoprotein were detected in animals receiving vaccinia or baculovirus expressing this protein, probably because the proteins were synthesized intracellularly and were not secreted in an extracellular form. Recently, Mason et al. (16) demonstrated that a vaccinia construct of Japanese encephalitis (JE) virus containing genes for prM through NS2a secreted particles into the supernatant fluid with characteristics of the slowly sedimenting hemagglutinin (SHA) produced by wild-type virions. The SHA particles represent empty envelopes with the M and E proteins in a conformationally native, immunogenic configuration. It appears that deletion of the capsid (C) protein but retention of NS1 were essential to secretion of SHA particles. Mice immunized with this vaccinia construct produced high titers of neutralizing antibodies and were solidly protected against a high dose of JE virus.

Table 7. Immunization of Mice and Monkeys with Recombinant Baculovirus-Infected Cell Lysates and Vaccinia Recombinants Expressing Dengue Proteins[a]

Expression system	Dengue genes	Antibody response, mice	Survival, mice (%)	Protection, monkeys (%)
Baculovirus	C-M-E-NS1-NS2a	NS1	100	33
	RSVG-E[b]		100	33
	Control		0	0
Vaccinia	C-M-E-NS1-NS2a	NS1	97	0
	C-M-E		100	
	E		100 (ill)	
	RSVG-E		100 (ill)	
	NS1-NS2a	NS1	100	
	NS1-15%NS2a	weak NS1	67	
	Control		16	

[a] From Bray et al (1989) J Virol 63: 2853; Zhang et al (1988) J Virol 62: 3027

[b] Dengue animo-terminal signal sequence replaced with respiratory syncytial virus glycoprotein sequence

It is still uncertain whether vaccinia or baculovirus will provide a suitable approach to dengue immunization. Live vaccinia vectors which secrete particulate antigen may offer the advantage of long-lasting immunity, but this remains to be tested, and at present, the durability of immunization cannot be predicted. The potential disadvantages of vaccinia, including neurologic and dermatologic accidents and unchecked replication in immunologically-deficient hosts, are well-known and not specific to dengue vaccines. The possibility that replication of the vector might be restricted by preexisting immunity to expressed dengue antigens deserves investigation. Baculovirus expression offers the possibility of efficient production of large quantities of expressed protein, but methods for purification from infected cells or for inducing secretion of dengue particulate antigens will have to be worked out. Preliminary studies suggest that deletion of the carboxy-terminus of the E glycoprotein gene produces a truncated protein missing the anchor sequence and that this form is secreted from infected cells (17, 18), providing another approach to improved expression of flavivirus proteins.

A most promising advance, which follows on similar work with polio and yellow fever viruses, is the successful cloning of full-length complementary DNA (cDNA) of dengue type 4 by C-J. Lai and his associates at NIH (19). RNA prepared by in vitro transcription was used to transfect cells, with recovery of infectious progeny virus identical to the parental virus. This accomplishment sets the stage for the preparation of well-characterized dengue vaccines using infectious clone technology. The use of cDNA avoids the high rate of mutation associated with RNA virus passage and permits discrete engineering of the dengue viral genome. The cDNA clone can be manipulated by site-directed mutagenesis or by deletion of coding regions, with the objective of inducing an attenuated phenotype or even a vaccine lacking determinants engaged in immune enhancement. It also provides a cassette system for insertion of foreign genes, including those of heterologous dengue serotypes, to make chimeric vaccines inducing broad protection. Although this approach has advantages over the empirical development of live vaccines, it has the same inherent difficulties mentioned earlier: lack of markers of attenuation short of human testing and the uncertain safety and immunogenicity in persons with preexisting immunity.

It is reasonable to predict that the pressures exerted on health authorities in the Americas by the threat of DHF/DSS will lead to deployment of the live, attenuated dengue vaccines years in advance of successful development of a genetically-engineered product. If the live vaccines prove to be effective, it may be more difficult to pursue the expensive course of full development of a second-generation recombinant vaccine. Nevertheless, the long-range view must consider the need to incorporate dengue antigens in vaccines administered to infants with maternal antibodies, limiting the use of traditional live vaccines. The ultimate goal of a rationally-designed, multivalent, recombinant dengue vaccine will require a full exploration of the molecular determinants of dengue virulence, immune enhancement, and immunological protection.

In addition to the three approaches to molecular dengue vaccines described – vaccinia-vectoring, baculovirus-expression, and infectious clones – other laboratories are exploring alternative uses of biotechnology. These approaches include the use of synthetic peptides, chimeric molecules of hepatitis core protein and dengue sequences, anti-idiotypic antibodies, other recombinant live vectors, such as BCG and avian poxviruses. The embarrassment of riches afforded by molecular biology may complicate the search for the optimal vaccine, as it is often difficult to sort out the relative advantages and disadvantages of the multiple candidates. Another problem illustrated by the current effort on dengue vaccines, and molecular vaccine research in general, is the gap between laboratory research and clinical development. Vaccine research is being conducted in laboratories with little understanding of the process of vaccine development. There are relatively few institutions with expertise and infrastructure capable of the transition to clinical development of a product for human use, and they are not readily accessible to most laboratories engaged in research on molecular vaccines. Innovative solutions to this problem are required and may require fundamental changes in our national research institutions.

Japanese Encephalitis

Japanese encephalitis, another mosquito-borne flavivirus disease, causes an estimated 30,000 cases of central nervous system (CNS) infection annually in areas of Asia inhabited by 2.5 billion people (5). Surveillance and reporting in many areas are insensitive, however. Children under 15 years are principally affected; approximately 25% of the cases are fatal, and a high proportion – perhaps 50% – of the survivors have neuropsychiatric sequelae. In temperate regions of Asia, the disease often appears in intense summertime epidemics, with thousands of cases and attack rates of 10–100/100,000 population. In some areas, such as northern Thailand, the lifetime risk of acquiring JE infection approaches 100%. Fortunately, most infections are inapparent. Various estimates indicate that 1 encephalitis case occurs per 20 to 400 infections. It follows that the annual number of infections in Asia is between 600,000 and 12 million. In addition to the burden of human disease, JE causes encephalitis in horses and stillbirth and reduced fertility in swine. Since pigs are the principal amplifying viremic host in the epidemic transmission cycle, immunization of swine has a potential role in the protection of human populations.

Classical JE vaccines prepared from infected weanling mouse brain were first developed in the Soviet Union and in Japan in the 1940s. The crude vaccines were purified in Japan by precipitation steps and ultracentrifugation, and the purified product came into routine use in schoolchildren in 1966. The vaccine contains no detectable myelin basic protein and has not been associated with allergic encephalitis despite the administration of nearly 600 million doses. Similar vaccines are produced in Taiwan, South Korea, and to a limited extent in Vietnam and India. Safety and efficacy of the two-dose primary immunization schedule of the mouse-brain vaccine was proven in a field trial conducted in Thailand in 1985 (20). Although widely used in several affluent Asian countries, with a decline in disease incidence attributable in part to vaccination, the mouse-brain vaccine has the disadvantages of high cost ($2.30/dose or $4.60 for the recommended two-dose primary series) and the requirement for repeated booster inoculations. As an alternative to the expensive tissue-based vaccine, the Chinese developed an inactivated primary hamster cell culture vaccine, widely used for immunization of children under 10 years of age. Annual production is given as 100 million doses. The cost of this product is unknown, but since yields are low (6.0–7.0 logs/ml), the cost per dose is probably relatively high. Most countries in Southeast Asia and the Indian subcontinent currently have no vaccination policy, and these populations remain susceptible to endemic and epidemic disease.

Because of the high cost of killed vaccines and the need for repeated inoculations to induce and maintain immunity, alternative vaccines are required. Several candidate live, attenuated JE vaccines have been produced in China and tested in humans. All are derived from the same parent, designated SA14, by sequential passages in a variety of hosts. Vaccines for human use are prepared in primary hamster kidney cells. One live vaccine, designated SA14-5-3, has been given to more than 5 million children, but was found to immunize fewer than 80%. A more promising vaccine, designated SA14-14-2, proved safe and highly immunogenic in human trials in China (21). At the Walter Reed Army Institute of Research, the SA14-14-2 vaccine was passed in an acceptable substrate (primary canine kidney), shown to retain all phenotypic markers of the original vaccine, and to be free from adventitious agents (22). Because of the obvious benefits of an inexpensive live vaccine for use in China and other developing countries, further development of SA14-14-2 is being pursued in China and the U.S. In fact, the CDC has recently identified this vaccine as a priority for new funding under the National Vaccine Program.

The live attenuated SA14-14-2 vaccine and its virulent parent have been genetically characterized in United States by Dennis Trent's group at CDC, Fort Collins. The vaccine and parent are separated by 121 passages, with biological cloning in a variety of host systems. The vaccine differed from parent virus by a total of 45 nucleotides resulting in 15 amino acid substitutions (Fig. 3), with the highest rate of change in the amino-terminal half of the E glycoprotein, including a change at position 107 in the highly conserved region which presumably subserves fusion during virus uncoating (23). While the specific attenuating mutations have not yet been defined, these studies provide a basis for the future genetic manipulation of JE infectious clones and selection of coding regions for producing chimeric viruses.

The WHO Programme on Vaccine Development has promulgated molecular approaches to new JE vaccines. The approaches used to date are essentially identical to those described for dengue and include vaccinia and baculovirus expression of single or multiple viral proteins. The complete nucleotide sequence of JE virus was described by Sumiyoshi

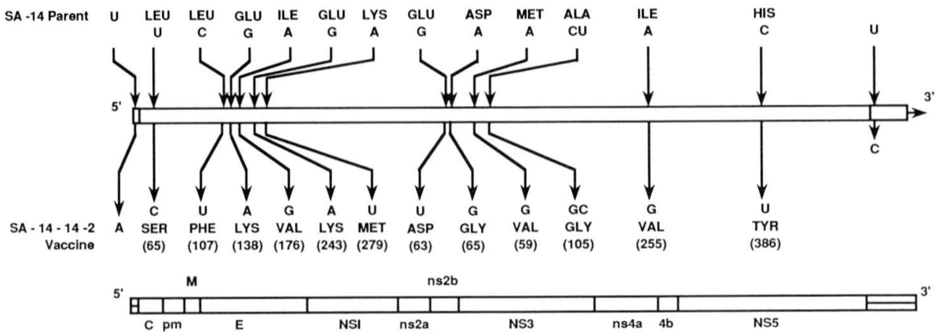

Fig. 3. Identification of the nucleotide and amino acid differences between the virulent parent (SA-14) and the live, attenuated Japanese encephalitis vaccine (SA14-14-2) derived therefrom; modified from Nitayaphan et al (23), with permission. Since reversion to virulence has not been demonstrated, it is likely than there is more than one change responsible for attenuation. Multiple changes in the amino-terminal half of the E glycoprotein are likely candidates because of the functional importance of this region

et al. in 1987 (24). Several groups have now successfully expressed the E glycoprotein in vaccinia and baculovirus systems, demonstrating neutralizing antibodies and protective immunity in mice. I have already mentioned the work of Mason, showing the highest degree of protection by a vaccinia recombinant having the prM-E-NS1-NS2a sequences and secreting SHA-like particles from infected cells (16). This vaccine candidate is being tested as a veterinary vaccine candidate in horses and pigs at USDA's Plum Island Animal Research Laboratory and is a promising candidate for a human vaccine.

A major obstacle to the success of global immunization is the requirement for multiple inoculations of inactivated antigens, such as DPT and polio. This problem may extend to many recombinant subunit and synthetic immunogens currently under investigation.The need to inoculate the same child multiple times during the first year of life greatly increases costs and represents the central impediment to complete immunization. One promising approach to overcome this obstacle is the use of controlled-release technology. Microspheres composed of biocompatible and biodegradable polymers of lactide and glycolide – the same material used to manufacture resorbable sutures – have been intensively studied as a way of long-term delivery of drugs and hormones and are now being explored for vaccine delivery (25). Antigen embedded in microspheres is released at a rate which can be controlled by manipulating the size of the microsphere and the ratio of lactide to glycolide in the copolymer. Increasing the proportion of lactide in the copolymer results in higher stability and prolonged time to release of the entrapped antigen. By using a mixture of copolymers in a single parenteral inoculation, it is possible achieve a "pulsed" release of antigen mimicking the effect of multiple inoculations spaced weeks or even months apart. Such formulations are under active study as a means of delivering the 3-dose tetanus toxoid series in a single inoculum.

The inactivated JE vaccines currently in use must be administered to children in a series of at least three inoculations – a primary series of two inoculations and a booster dose at 12 months. Preliminary studies have been conducted on the development of a microcapsule system, which would achieve programmed release of JE vaccine with a single injection (Tice, T.R., unpublished data, 1985). In these experiments mice received a mixture of unencapsulated vaccine and microspheres programmed to release vaccine antigen at 2–3 weeks (microspheres polymer containing 50:50 ratio of lactide:glycolide) and 6–8 weeks after inoculation (65:35 ratio of lactide:glycolide). The results indicated that a single inoculation of the controlled-release formulation achieved immunization equivalent to three separate injections of equivalent doses of vaccine. If similar results can be achieved in humans, significant improvements in vaccine coverage could be achieved at reduced cost.

Yellow Fever

Official reporting of yellow fever belies the epidemiological importance of this disease. In South America, 100–300 cases of jungle yellow fever are reported annually. Since approximately 90% of the reported cases are fatal, surveillance detects only the most severe cases and underestimates the true incidence by at least fivefold.

However, the most pressing problem in South America is not the control of jungle yellow fever. In the late 1970's Brazil and Bolivia were reinvaded by the urban vector, *Ae. aegypti.* This reinfestation rapidly involved other countries of South America and was followed by explosive epidemics of dengue fever (Fig. 4). The reintroduction of *Ae. aegypti* greatly complicates the strategy for yellow fever vaccination in the continent. In Brazil alone, over 121 million people inhabit *Ae. aegypti*-infested coastal areas and are at risk of the introduction and spread of urban yellow fever for the first time in over 50 years. Because of the absence of the urban vector for many years, this large coastal population of Brazil has never been immunized. Similar considerations now apply to urban populations in coastal Peru and Ecuador. Public health authorities are now faced with a difficult decision. Should the immunological barrier to the urbanization of yellow fever be extended to the susceptible coastal populations? The logistical and economic problems in providing vaccine coverage to a population 8–10 times larger than that inhabiting the jungle areas are staggering.

In Africa, the annual incidence of yellow fever has been highly variable, reflecting periodic, spectacular epidemics. The incidence has increased dramatically since 1986, due principally to a period of sustained epidemic activity in Nigeria (Fig. 5), where 1000–3000 cases have been reported each year. However, the official reports represent only a small fraction of the true incidence, as shown repeatedly by direct epidemiological investigation

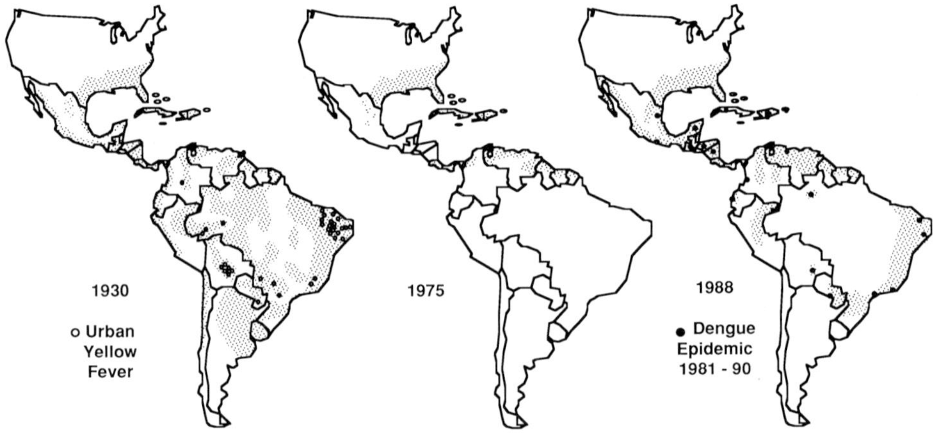

Fig. 4. Changes in the distribution of *Aedes aegypti* as a result of efforts between 1947 and 1974 to eradicate the mosquito and dissolution of vector control thereafter. Prior to the eradication effort, urban yellow fever epidemics were commonplace in South America. In the 1980s large outbreaks of *Ae. aegypti*-borne dengue fever have occurred, illustrating the renewed risk of urban yellow fever in the Americas. Reproduced from Monath TP (1991) Yellow fever: *Victor, Victoria.* Conqueror, Conquest? Am J Trop Med Hyg with permission

of epidemics. In 1986 and 1987, for example, only 2% of the cases and 3% of the deaths were officially recorded (26, 27).

Yellow fever in Africa comes to light only during major epidemics. In fact the disease burden of endemic disease is probably much greater than that attributable to epidemics. In Nigeria, for example, serosurvey data indicate an annual incidence of endemic disease with jaundice to be 1.1–2.4 per 1,000 and yellow fever death at 0.2–0.5 per 1,000 – approximately 20-fold lower than the incidence during epidemics and far below the threshold of detection by the existing passive surveillance system. Extrapolation to the total population at risk gives a nationwide annual total of 163,642 jaundice cases and 32,728 deaths due to endemic yellow fever (28). Many factors contribute to the lack of recognition of endemic yellow fever, including the difficulty in distinguishing the disease from other causes of jaundice; the widely-held belief that jaundice is best treated by traditional herbalists rather than western medicine; occurrence of the disease in remote, rural areas; and lack of death registries.

Because the disease goes unrecognized during the relatively long intervals between epidemics, many African countries have established a policy of emergency control rather than preventive immunization. This policy is flawed by the absence of surveillance, late recognition of epidemics, and logistical difficulty of mounting an effective mass immunization campaign in the face of an epidemic. The result has often been that only a small proportion of the affected population is immunized before the epidemic has run its natural course. The advent of the Expanded Program of Immunization in 1974, which provides an effective cold-chain for delivery, makes possible the inclusion of the thermolabile yellow fever vaccine in national

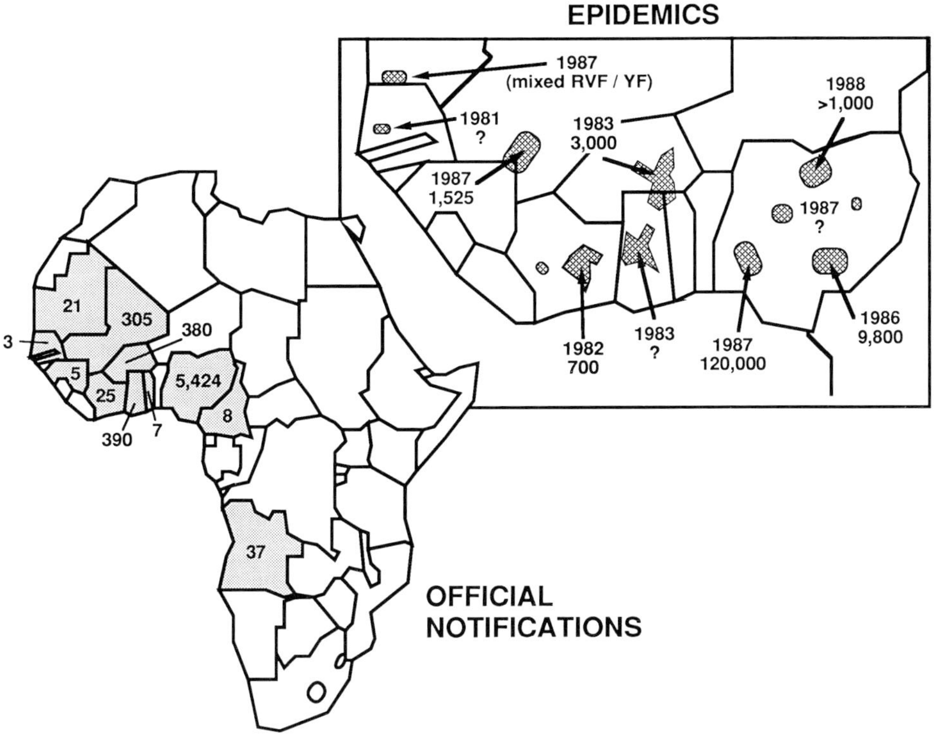

Fig. 5. Incidence of yellow fever reflected by official notification to the World Health Organization, and location and estimated morbidity associated with epidemics, Africa, 1980–1988. Reproduced from Monath TP (1991) Yellow fever: *Victor, Victoria*. Conqueror, Conquest? Am J Trop Med Hyg

programs of childhood immunization. Eight African countries have recently incorporated yellow fever vaccine in their EPI, and this year, Nigeria has been added to the list. Because of Nigeria's large size and population (currently 116 million, expected to reach 154 million by the end of the decade, and representing nearly 60% of the entire population in the yellow fever endemic zone in West Africa), the allocation of scarce resources to the inclusion of yellow fever vaccine in the EPI must be carefully considered. A recent analysis of the cost-effectiveness of yellow fever vaccination strategies in Nigeria indicates that routine vaccination of infants alone, as part of the EPI, would eliminate the risk of epidemics within 20–30 years (28). Endemic yellow fever morbidity would decline from 130 cases/100,000 population to 51 cases/100,000 over a time horizon of 35 years. The cost of the program per death prevented is $158 in the early phase of the program, and falls to $76 as cumulative immunity increases. Prevention of endemic disease would thus be cost-effective at ratios comparable to other diseases currently targeted by the EPI.

If it has been difficult to implement an effective policy for utilization of the present yellow fever vaccine, is it reasonable to suggest biotechnological innovations? The current vaccine is produced in embryonated eggs by the same technology developed 53 years ago. There are currently production facilities in 11 countries, but nearly all of the vaccine available for use in developing countries is produced in Brazil and Senegal and sold at modest cost: US$ 0.18–0.20/dose. It is important to note that the cost of adding this vaccine in countries with an operating EPI should not be much more than the cost of the vaccine alone, since yellow fever and measles vaccines can be mixed and given in combination to children >9 months of age. The vaccine induces neutralizing antibodies in >90–95% of those vaccinated, and immunity is probably life-long. Over 200 million vaccinations have been given, and there have been only 18 recorded serious reactions, all in the form of postvaccinal encephalitis, with one death. Any new yellow fever vaccine would have to beat this remarkable record of achievement!

In 1981, the first of several meetings was held by WHO/PAHO to discuss the desirability and feasibility of modernizing yellow fever vaccine production. A number of problems with the present vaccine were considered.

1. The limited capacity for production and scale-up. Current stocks worldwide approximate 25 million doses, enough to vaccinate only the population of Sao Paulo, Brazil.

2. The instability of the vaccine to heat, even in its lyophilized state, increasing the logistical problems associated with vaccine delivery;

3. The contamination of many vaccines with avian leukosis virus, clearly an unacceptable aspect by modern standards, although no effects on human health have been noted.

4. The residual neurovirulence of the vaccine that limits its use in young infants. Monkeys inoculated intracerebrally develop inflammatory pathological changes in brain tissue, and clinical signs of severe encephalitis occurring in up to 10% are acceptable for vaccine to pass neurovirulence testing. Eighteen cases of encephalitis following inoculation of 17D vaccine have been reported, all but four cases in infants less than 4 months old. Since the danger to young infants was recognized in the 1950s and immunization practices were modified to exclude infants under 9 or 12 months from vaccination in the 1960s, denominator data are inadequate to assess fully the incidence of this complication. On the basis of the limited available data, the risk of postvaccinal encephalitis in fact may be significant for young infants, ranging from 0.06–0.97% (20).

A special concern is the age at which infants would receive 17D vaccine in the EPI. The current practice in most countries is to administer live measles vaccine to infants more than 9 months old, an age considered safe for use of 17D vaccine. This strategy has been questioned because increasing urbanization has lowered the age at which children are affected by epidemic measles, so that vaccination at an earlier age is desirable (29). The Edmonston-Zagreb vaccine may be effective as early as 4 months (30) and is currently being introduced in some programs for infants 6 months old. Because measles may be the last vaccine given to infants in the EPI schedule, yellow fever vaccination must be given at the same window of opportunity to be economical. If encephalitis complicates administration of 17D to young infants, the annual immunization of millions of infants less than 6 months old in the EPI may uncover an unacceptably high incidence of untoward reactions.

5. The heterogeneity of the strains used for vaccine production and of the virion populations contained in these strains. At least two distinct substrains of 17D (17DD and 17D-204) are used by different vaccine manufacturers and can be distinguished by monoclonal antibodies and RNA fingerprinting (31). All existing vaccines in turn represent uncloned mixtures of virions with variable biological properties. Plaque variants within 17D vaccine have markedly different virulence for mice and ability to replicate in human macrophages (32). The heterogeneity of uncloned virus can produce dramatic changes in the dominant population under selective pressures, but these pressures are not predictable and are host-dependent.

There has been one fatal case of 17D vaccine encephalitis, a 3-year old girl in the United States in 1965. The brain isolate differed from the vaccine by RNA fingerprinting and lethality for adult mice by the intranasal route (Barrett ADT, Monath TP, Miller BR, unpublished data, 1988). This suggested that a virus variant, possibly one already contained in the heterogenous mixture of 17D vaccine, selectively invaded the central nervous system producing fatal encephalitis. This possibility was supported by other studies using monoclonal antibodies, that detected a variant within commercial 17D vaccine with antigenic and neurovirulence characteristics of wild-type, parental (Asibi) virus (33).

Previous considerations for improving the present yellow fever vaccines focussed on the development of 17D virus in cell culture rather than embryonated eggs and on the addition of stabilizers to improve resistance to heat. Although this approach would resolve some problems with the vaccine, others would remain, particularly those of vaccine heterogeneity, genetic stability and neurovirulence. However, molecular approaches are now being explored, which may resolve these issues. In 1985, Rice and colleagues reported the entire gene sequence of 17D vaccine (11) and, in 1987, of the parental Asibi strain (34). Of the 32 amino acid differences that evolved during 230 passages in the development of 17D vaccine, it is still uncertain which change or changes are responsible for loss of virulence. To address this question, Rice's group has constructed full-length cDNA templates of 17D and Asibi viruses, which yield infectious RNA transcripts (35). These infectious clones can be used to map individual nucleotide changes with respect to their phenotypic characteristics in animal models, including those responsible for neurotropism. This goal has considerable practical interest, since elimination of the remaining neurotropic properties of 17D vaccine might permit its use with Edmonston-Zagreb measles vaccine in young infants in the EPI. Moreover, the use of recombinant 17D viral DNA as the starting material for live vaccine production may provide a better approach than the present seed-lot system for stabilizing the yellow fever vaccine genome.

The availability of a full-length yellow fever infectious clone also provides the opportunity for inserting foreign genes containing protective epitopes on the E and NS1 proteins of other flaviviruses, such as dengue or JE, into the 17D backbone. At the WHO meeting in 1990, the Steering Committee recommended that, prior to the construction of chimeric infectious cDNA vaccines, proof of concept should be achieved by developing a new 17D yellow fever vaccine derived from the infectious clone. Accordingly, studies have been initiated as a collaborative effort between Rice's group, the Instituto Oswaldo Cruz in Rio de Janiero, and the U.S. Army Medical Research Institute of Infectious Diseases.

The new vaccine would be derived in a straightforward manner by transfection of an approved cell culture substrate and passage of the progeny virus to embryonated eggs to prepare a new primary seed. This, in turn, would be used to prepare secondary seed and vaccine lots using the standard manufacturing process in eggs. Quality controls, including monkey neurovirulence tests, would be performed as required by WHO standards, and the new vaccine would ultimately be tested in humans. A preliminary study of progeny virus from cell cultures transfected with RNA transcripts from the full length 17D cDNA demonstrated acceptable characteristics of attenuation in monkeys. The unique aspect of this work was the likelihood that the proof of concept – the development of a new vaccine derived from cDNA – could be accomplished with very limited resources, probably less than $1 million.

However, the ultimate development of an improved yellow fever vaccine presents a very different set of problems. The objectives would be much more complex and might include:

- High-yield production in an cell culture substrate in lieu of egg-derived tissue;
- Deletion or substitution of gene(s) responsible for neurovirulence and the extensive biological characterization of such a vaccine in non-human primates and ultimately in humans (including infants); and
- Construction of chimeric vaccines incorporating foreign epitopes conferring multivalent heterologous immunity – for example against dengue viruses – as well as homologous protection, and the biological and clinical evaluation of such vaccmes.

The resources required for the research and development for such a vaccine might be conservatively estimated at $5–10 million, an amount which would purchase 25–50 million doses – 1–2 year's requirements – of standard 17D vaccine for the entire world! There would be no commercial incentive to develop such a vaccine, and the vaccine development costs could not be passed back to the consumer, since that would defeat the purpose of its application in the developing world.

This example illustrates a problem common to other new vaccines anticipated for inclusion in the Children's Vaccine Initiative. Although the technological basis for vaccine development is within grasp, the economics and ability to coordinate efforts among industry, the research community, foundations, national governments, and international agencies are much less clear. In general, vaccines are the neglected stepchildren of the pharmaceutical industry. The economic incentives of vaccine development are limited, and liability and patentability problems well-known (36). One possible solution is to redirect funding from international aid programs to vaccine development through contractual agreements with the biotechnology industry. This represents a departure from past policies, which have funnelled aid resources into needy programs in the developing world itself. Many countries may resist the notion that international aid programs should divert funds to private industry in the developed world, and strong political and nationalistic forces strongly favor the development of biotechnology in the developing countries themselves. This issue has yet to be fully aired, and I suspect it will be the focus of considerable debate.

If the technical problems of vaccine development are yielding to biotechnology, the obstacles to utilization of vaccines in general and of new vaccines in particular have their roots in politics and economics and are much less easily solved. It is clear that the development of a vaccine is not in itself an answer to a public health need. In the case of yellow fever, a tissue-based vaccine developed over 50 years ago meets nearly all the criteria for an ideal intervention but has not been effectively utilized. Vaccine development must be followed by a clear strategy for its application and implementation of a public health policy. As illustrated by the case of yellow fever, disease identification and definition is deficient throughout much of the area affected. Only a small fraction of the cases are recognized and reported. The true requirements for vaccine are not clear, and consequently, effective health policies are not formulated. Surveillance and disease definition were the essential first steps in developing the strategy for vaccine implementation and for convincing governments of the need for childhood immunization in the EPI (1, 29). Data from sentinel sites and other surveillance mechanisms formed the underpinning of the programs aimed at tetanus, poliomyelitis, and measles. Similar mechanisms have not been implemented for most of the diseases targeted for new vaccine development. The clinical diagnosis of diseases such as yellow fever, dengue, rotavirus, respiratory syncytial virus, typhoid, shigella, enterotoxic *E. coli* and others is inherently much more difficult than for tetanus, polio, and measles. Laboratory-based epidemiological studies are required to provide the empirical data to convince governments of the need for preventive immunization and are essential for monitoring the value of immunization strategies. However, little priority is currently given to such surveillance or field research efforts by national authorities or international funding agencies.

The biotechnological revolution has captured the imagination of scientists around the world. The ability to explore and understand biological systems at the most fundamental level is an extraordinarily powerful intellectual lure. Moreover, strong economic incentives have been created by an expanding biotechnology industry. Today, molecular biology is the unitary focus of most undergraduate and graduate students in the biological sciences. Awards of government research grants are largely predicated upon innovative applications of molecular techniques, even in subject areas as far afield as epidemiology. In the developing world, students and young scientists are following the track of modern science, encouraged by their governments, which view this development as a matter of national pride, and by efforts of international agencies to strengthen scientific infrastructures in areas most afflicted by disease, famine, and other problems potentially addressable by biotechnology.

Despite its tremendous potential, it is also true that biotechnology provides a countervailing force to the pursuit of careers in field biology, epidemiology, hygiene, and other traditional disciplines. This is true in the developed world and also – perhaps with more serious consequences – in many developing countries. The accelerated pace and progress of biotechnology in the developed world is accompanied by an increasing flow of physicians and scientific talent out of the developing world – the well-known "brain drain". The gap is widening between developed and developing countries in the opportunities for education, monetary rewards, and personal scientific achievement, and it is exacerbated by the deteriorating economic situation and unchecked population growth in the developing world, particularly Africa (37).

The new opportunities for the prevention and control of infectious diseases that arise with technological breakthroughs in vaccines, diagnostic tests, and therapies, are outpacing the ability to evaluate and apply them in the areas most affected by disease. The targets for new approaches often remain ill-defined, by virtue of inadequate disease surveillance, absence of accessible laboratory diagnosis, and lack of reliable data on disease incidence – problems that can be addressed only by field and epidemiological studies. New viral hemorrhagic fevers and arbovirus diseases continue to emerge in tropical areas of the world, yet the laboratories, medical virologists and entomologists working in this area have fared poorly in the competition for resources with molecular biology and may be in danger of extinction. The first task in developing a health policy – that of identifying and defining the major health problems – is too often forgotten, and there are fewer trained people and resources available to undertake this task. The problems are not static. The emergence of new diseases demands effective surveillance and field investigation. Changing demographic patterns, urbanization, ecologic and climatic perturbations, and expanding human population groups with immunodeficiency disease make the problem of disease definition an ever-moving target. Thus, a parallel challenge to the transitioning of the new tools for disease prevention from biotechnology must be the strengthening of the public health infrastructure, including traditional disciplines such as medical microbiology and virology, epidemiology, and medical ecology.

References

1. Henderson RH, Keja J (1989) Global control of vaccine-preventable diseases: how progress can be evaluated. Rev Infect Dis 11: 649
2. Nakajima H (1990) Epidemiology and the future of the world. PAHO Epidemiol Bull 11 :1
3. Bektimirov T, Lambert P-H, Torrigiani G (1990) Vaccine development perspectives of the World Health Organization. J Med Virol 31: 62
4. Anon (1990) Potential use of live viral and bacterial vectors for vaccines. WHO Meeting, Geneva, 19-22 June, 1989. Vaccine 8: 425
5. Institute of Medicine (1986) New Vaccine Development: Establishing Priorities. Vol II. Diseases of Importance in Developing Countries. Washington D.C., National Academy Press, 432 pp
6. Gubler DJ (1991) Dengue hemorrhagic fever: a global update. Virus Info Exch Newsletter 8: 2
7. Scott R McN, Eckels KH, Bancroft WH, Summers PL, McCown JM, Anderson JH, Russell PK (1983) Dengue 2 vaccine: dose-response in volunteers in relation to yellow fever immune status. J Infect Dis 148: 1055
8. Bhamarapratavi N, Yoksan S, Chayaniyayothin T, Angsubphakorn S, Bunyratvej A (1987) Immunization with a live attenuated dengue-2-virus candidate vaccine (16681-PDK 53): clinical, immunological and biological responses in adult volunteers. Bull WHO 65: 189
9. Bhamarapratavi N, Yoksan S (1989) Study of bivalent dengue vaccine in volunteers. Lancet 1: 770
10. Brandt WE (1990) Development of dengue and Japanese encephalitis vaccines. J Infect Dis 162: 577
11. Rice CM, Lenches EM, Eddy SR, Shin SJ, Sheets RL, Strauss JH (1985) Nucleotide sequence of yellow fever virus: implications for flavivirus gene expression and evolution. Science 229: 726
12. Chambers TJ, Hahn CS, Galler R, Rice CM (1990) Flavivirus genome organization, expression and replication. Ann Rev Microbiol 44: 649
13. Bray M, Zhao B, Markoff L, Eckels KH, Chanock RM, Lai C-J (1989) Mice immunized with recombinant vaccinia virus expressing dengue 4 virus structural proteins with or without nonstructural protein NS1 are protected against fatal dengue encephalitis. J Virol 63: 2853
14. Zhang Y-M, Hayes EP, McCarty TC, Dubois DR, Summers PL, Eckels KH, Chanock RM, Lai C-J (1988) Immunization of mice with dengue structural proteins and nonstructural protein NSl expressed by baculovirus recombinant induces resistance to dengue virus encephalitis. J Virol 62: 3027
15. Falgout B, Bray M, Schlesinger J, Lai C-J (1990) Immunization of mice with recombinant vaccinia virus expressing dengue virus nonstructural protein NSl protects against lethal dengue encephalitis. J Virol 64: 4356
16. Mason PW, Pincus S, Foumier MJ, Mason TL, Shope RE, Paoletti E (1991) Japanese encephalitis virus-vaccinia recombinants produce particulate forms of the structural membrane proteins and induce high levels of protection against lethal JEV infection. Virology 180: 294
17. Men R, Bray M, Lai C-J (1991) Carboxy-terminally truncated dengue virus envelope glycoproteins expressed on the cell surface and secreted extracellularly exhibit increased immunogenicity in mice. J Virol 65: 1400
18. Deubel V, Bordier M, Megret F, Gentry MK, Schlesinger JJ, Girard M (1991) Processing, secretion, and immunoreactivity of carboxy terminally truncated dengue-2 virus envelope proteins expressed in insect cells by recombinant baculoviruses. Virology 180: 442
19. Lai C-J, Zhao Z, Hori H, Bray M (1991) Infectious RNA transcribed from stably cloned full-length cDNA of dengue type 4 virus. Proc Natl Acad Sci (USA) (in press)
20. Hoke CH, Nisalak A, Sangawhipa N, Jatanasen S, Laorakapongse T, Innis BL, Kotchasenee S, Gingrich JB, Latendresse J, Fukai K, Burke DS (1988) Protection against Japanese encephalitis by inactivated vaccines. N Engl J Med 319: 608
21. Xin YY, Ming ZG, Peng GY, Jian A, Min LH (1988) Safety of a live-attenuated Japanese encephalitis virus vaccine (SA14-14-2) for children. Am J Trop Med Hyg 39: 214

22. Eckels KH, Yong-Xin Y, Dubois DR, Marchette NJ, Trent DW, Johnson AJ (1988) Japanese encephalitis virus live-attenuated vaccine, Chinese strain SA14-14-2; adaptation to primary canine kidney cell cultures and preparation of a vaccine for human use. Vaccine 6: 513
23. Nitayaphan S, Grant JA, Chang G-J, Trent DW (1990) Nucleotide sequence of the virulent SA-14 strain of Japanese encephalitis virus and its attenuated vaccine derivative, SA-14-14-2. Virology 177: 541
24. Sumiyoshi H, Mori C, Fuke I, Morita K, Kuhara S, Kondou J, Kikuchi Y, Nagamatu H, Igarashi A (1987) Complete nucleotide sequence of the Japanese encephalitis virus genome RNA. Virology 161: 497
25. Tice TR, Cowsar DR (1984) Biodegradable controlled release parenteral systems. Pharmacol Technol J 8: 26
26. DeCock KM, Monath TP, Nasidi A, Tukei PM, Enriquez J, Lichfield P, Craven RB, Fabiyi A, Okafor BC, Ravaonjanahary C, Sorungbe A (1988) Epidemic yellow fever in eastern Nigeria, 1986. Lancet 1: 630
27. Nasidi A, Monath TP, DeCock K, Tomori O, Cordellier R, Olaleye OD, Harry TO, Adeniyi JA, Sorungbe AO, Ajose-Coker AO, van Der Laan G, Oyediran ABO (1989) Urban yellow fever epidemic in westem Nigeria, 1987. Trans R Soc Trop Med Hyg 83: 401
28. Monath, TP, Nasidi A.Should yellow fever vaccine be a part of the Expanded Programme of Immunization in Africa? A cost-effectiveness analysis for Nigeria. Bull. WHO (submitted)
29. Hall AJ, Greenwood BM, Whittle H (1990) Modern Vaccines. Practice in developing countries. Lancet 335: 774
30. Khanum S, Uddin N, Garelick , Mann G, Tomkins A (1987) Comparison of Edmonston-Zagreb and Schwarz strains of measles vacine given by aerosol or subcutaneous injection. Lancet 1: 150
31. Monath TP, Kinney RM, Schlesinger JJ, Brandriss MW, Bres P (1983) Ontogeny of yellow fever 17D vaccine: RNA olgonucleotide fingerprint and monoclonal antibody analysis of vaccines produced worldwide. J Gen Virol 64: 627
32. Liprandi F (1981) Isolation of plaque variants differing in virulence from the 17D strain of yellow fever virus. J Gen Virol 56: 363
33. Gould EA, Buckley A, Cane PA, Higgs S, Cammack N (1989) Use of a monoclonal antibody specific for wild-type yellow fever virus to identify a wild-type antigenic variant in 17D vaccine pools. J Gen Virol 70: 1889
34. Hahn CS, Dalrymple JM, Strauss JH, Rice CM (1987) Comparison of the virulent Asibi strain of yellow fever virus with the 17D vaccine strain derived from it. Proc Natl Acad Sci (USA) 84: 2019
35. Rice CM, Grakoui A, Galler R, Chambers TJ (1989) Transcription of infectious virus RNA from full-length cDNA templates produced by in vitro ligation. New Biology 1: 285
36. Robbins A, Freeman P (1988) Obstacles to developing vaccines for the Third World. Sci Am 259: 126
37. Bloom BR, Cerami A (eds) (1989) Biomedical science and the third world. Under the volcano. Ann NY Acad Sci 569: 1

AIDS: The Uses and Limitations of Science

June E. Osborn

University of Michigan School of Public Health and National Commission on AIDS

Introduction

We are at the mark of an historic anniversary: it was on June 5, 1981, that the Morbidity and Mortality Weekly Reports published a brief summary of five unusual cases of *Pneumocystis carinii* pneumonia (PCP) occurring in a cluster in previously healthy young men (1). Since PCP had almost always occurred in the context of immune suppression, that clue had been pursued, and indeed their immune systems turned out to be profoundly suppressed. As we now know, that was the faint trumpet that heralded the arrival of a vast pandemic caused by a human retrovirus that had not been recognized before.

In retrospect, the human immunodeficiency-virus (or HIV-1) had probably maintained itself through sexual and/or vertical transmission in isolated enclaves of humanity for decades or even centuries. While the first serologic evidence of HIV-1 infection only dates back to 1959 (2), there is reason to believe – from molecular genetic analysis – that the virus is much older than that in evolutionary terms (3); and its capacity for vertical transmission and sustained asymptomatic infection make it quite reasonable to suppose that it had survived in relative isolation for a long while. But in the second half of the twentieth century, the accelerating pace of urbanization and global travel offered the sexually transmitted virus a vast new panorama of opportunity, and it quickly circled the globe.

Now, ten years after first recognition of AIDS – and eight years after identification of the human immunodeficiency virus – there is no corner of the earth that does not have its seminal dose of the new retrovirus. The World Health Organization estimates that by the end of the century, thirty million people will be infected with HIV; and those projections do not incorporate the recent, ominous news that Asia, with one-third of the human population, is suddenly – possibly widely – involved.

In the United States, which was the epicenter of the pandemic at the outset, nearly 180,000 people have been diagnosed with AIDS, of whom

110,000 have already died; and there is little question that at least one million more are already infected. Finally, it is estimated by the U.S. Public Health Service that new infections are occurring at a yearly rate conservatively set at 45,000, but the upper limit of their estimate is over *200,000 new infections per year* (4)!

In this chapter I can only try to touch the highlights of what has been learned in the past decade – for we know more about HIV in 1991 than about any other pathogen of man. Of necessity some of the discussion will be cursory, since there is a lot of ground to cover and it is important to try to grasp the full picture of this human tragedy. The new virus is now a fact of life, a powerful pathogen that will be with us forever and will continue to pose threats and challenges for generations to come.

A Brief History of the AIDS Pandemic

After the June 5, 1981 "announcement" of the five cases from Los Angeles, there followed quickly a report of Kaposi's sarcoma in several immunosuppressed young men in New York (5). At about the same time, a scattering of reports began to appear in the clinical literature describing rather prominent, persistent but nondescript lymphadenopathy in still other men – all of whom, as it turned out, had led a lifestyle characterized by many homosexual partners. Initially, and sadly, the first public reactions firmly identified the new syndromes with gay men, and homophobia overtook common sense – for there has never been a sexually transmitted disease that conformed to such biases. Soon, however, there were cases that should have alerted everyone to the universality of risk: it became evident that in a number of areas of the United States, acquired immunosuppression and resultant opportunistic infections were occurring in heterosexual users of intravenous drugs – and their sexual partners – and in people from the West Indies who were avowedly heterosexual.

Throughout 1982 the evidence made it increasingly clear that a new disease entity – ultimately dubbed "AIDS" – was spreading primarily or exclusively by sexual and blood-borne routes. Then in 1983, the first recognized cases in hemophiliacs, transfusion recipients and children born to infected mothers essentially completed the final list of known modes of spread. Subsequently, a few clear instances of transmission through breast feeding added one additional route – but the frequency and importance of that occurrence is still unclear, and it is generally agreed that such transmission is probably so infrequent that considerations of nutrition should be overriding when potential malnutrition is at issue.

In any event, by 1983 the full range of epidemiologic detail was laid out, and soon the discovery of what we now call human immunodeficiency virus-1 was made in France (6) and in two labs in the United States (7, 8). By 1984 the group of investigators in Gallo's lab had developed the technology not only to cultivate HIV but also to amplify its growth so that serologic testing for antibody could be done on a large-scale basis. With remarkable rapidity, this led, by May of 1985, to systematic screening of the U.S. blood supply. That is another date that should be celebrated, for with the advent of testing of donated blood, a wide avenue of future dissemination of HIV was effectively blocked. Before that occurred, however, several thousand people had been infected through blood and plasma infusions – a tragedy the results of which are still being felt as people transfused before 1985 continue to become ill. But mercifully, subsequent transmission by that route has been extremely rare, and the U.S. blood supply has never been safer.

From that point onward – and thanks to accumulating data about modes of spread that do not work – we knew very early in the epidemic what we needed to know to prevent further spread of HIV. Once the blood supply was secured, behavioral choice was an element in almost all remaining routes of transmission, which meant that knowledgable people could – at least theoretically – avoid the virus. Indeed, in communities of gay men where the incidence of new infections had been as high as 18% per year in the dreadful first years after 1981, by the mid-1980s that figure had dropped to zero (9), clearly reflecting the efficacy of education concerning high risk behavior. Those data were of special interest in that they resoundingly confirmed the remarkably limited modes of spread of the virus – no new infections were occurring even among people who by that time were spending most of their non-working hours caring for dying friends. That dramatic demonstration of the effectiveness of AIDS education is nearly unparalleled in the annals of health education, but it makes it all the more tragic to know that when such intervention was possible, it did not happen widely. It is sad to say that, instead of promptly aborting the dreadful progression of HIV through systematic AIDS education, we in the United States missed a major chance and are now in the throes of a massive epidemic that is still unchecked.

The pace of the epidemic in the rest of the world has been equally brisk, although in western Europe the potential to interrupt spread through education has been better realized than it has here. I will not attempt a detailed discussion, but a cursory overview may be helpful. There is no question that the major epicenters of the pandemic at the outset were the United States, parts of the Caribbean and probably Brazil. However, almost simultaneously there were cases diagnosed in Australia, Canada and several countries in western Europe. While early cases of AIDS in most of those areas again showed a preponderance of gay men and/or intravenous drug users, at least some instances of heterosexual spread were noted everywhere, and their proportion was steadily increasing.

Then as the decade of the eighties progressed, countries in Central and East Africa began to experience the full-scale nightmare of heterosexual spread, augmented but not fully explained by co-occurrence with other sexually transmitted diseases. Another distinctive but closely related retrovirus called HIV-2 was discovered in West Africa (10), which area seemed initially to have been less affected by HIV-1. There was a brief burst of optimism stemming from the hope that HIV-2 might be nonpathogenic and might even prove to be a vaccine candidate to protect against HIV-1;

but those hopes were dashed by subsequent events. While HIV-2 may be even slower than HIV-1 to express itself in full-scale immunosuppression of the host, it clearly does cause AIDS, and it does not protect against HIV-1. Indeed, at present the Ivory Coast is in the throes of a particularly intense epidemic marked by widespread infection with both HIV-1 and HIV-2, neither of which appears to be innocuous.

On the African continent, HIV-1 in particular has spread with special vigor along trucking routes and in the context of local wars – and southern Africa now is fully caught up in the spreading tragedy, with increasing numbers of overt AIDS cases in Zimbabwe, Namibia and South Africa.

One particularly dreadful feature of AIDS is its devastation of families – in a literal sense it is a disease of the dying family; but children born before their mother's infection are spared, as are two-thirds of those born afterwards. The result is a particularly horrendous dynamic: that of AIDS orphans, of whom it is estimated that there are already over one million in Africa (11). That effect has been seen in the United States as well and will become more important as heterosexual AIDS advances everywhere.

Asia's epidemiologic picture is superficially different for the moment: in fact, during the first few years of the AIDS epidemic, it seemed that Asia had been spared, surely reflecting the fact that the virus was introduced into that part of the world slightly later. Unhappily, as has happened so often in this first decade of AIDS, the Asian perception of being somehow exempt from this new plague led to considerable inattention, and preventive opportunities were lost through the becalming belief that events in the rest of the world wouldn't happen there. But in the past two or three years, that illusion has been destroyed by explosive spread of HIV-1 in Thailand and southeast Asia, fueled by both heterosexual spread and intravenous drug use. It is now clear as well that substantial epidemics are underway in south China and in India, and there is reason to be very concerned that they represent much larger conflagrations that have smoldered for years unattended because of denial.

As Eastern Europe opened to the west in the late 1980s, it too was relatively uninvolved, but the rate of viral spread assures that those countries will not be exempt either. Indeed, there is not a country in the world, now, that does not have HIV, and therefore trouble. Thus, by the end of the first decade, it is evident that HIV-1 is here to stay: it is like the advent of nuclear weapons, in that the world will never be the same. The rejection and disbelief that has characterized public reaction in the first decade is terribly dangerous, for the adequacy with which we react now will have enormous impact on the future of our children's children – and here in the United States, we have not done very well so far!

Epidemiology: Modes of Transmission

Before reviewing some of the fundamental virology and pathogenesis of HIV disease, let me reiterate what we know about transmission of the virus, for it provides a firm basis for guidance about how we should be responding. As noted earlier, only sex, blood, or birth to an infected mother can transmit the virus of AIDS. Even needlestick injury straight out of the vein of a person with AIDS is remarkably inefficient – estimated at no more than 4 transmissions per thousand exposures (12). In fact, for a while it was a bit puzzling that injecting drug use was so remarkably efficient in contrast to needlesticks – but it was soon learned that, among intravenous drug users, sharing of injection apparatus usually involved pulling back on the syringe to flush the last bit of drug into the blood stream, so that in fact substantial quantities of blood were likely to be involved.

Not only is it known what modes of transmission *do* work – better yet, we know with remarkable certainty what does *not* work. Careful studies have followed family members who tended their dying loved ones for months without precautions, wiping up secretions and sharing toothbrushes, razors, utensils and fond embraces. Not one instance of viral transmission has occurred in such settings (13). There was even a study done in Haiti in dreadfully impoverished surroundings, where older siblings were the caretakers of younger children with AIDS – and those caretakers remained uniformly uninfected while parents and congenitally infected infants sickened and died (14). In point of fact, HIV is a terribly difficult virus to transmit. Were the public to grasp fully the real-life importance of that set of findings, much of the ugly panic and discriminatory response that has characterized reaction to people with HIV infection could abate, and the rest of the dreadful problems of AIDS could be addressed more easily.

The possibility that insects might spread the virus was raised early and kept alive by alarmists and publicists in the face of data that flatly contradicted such a mode of transmission (15). Indeed, it took an act of faith to keep talking about mosquito-borne infection when children beyond the newborn period were entirely spared in heavily infested areas until the age of onset of sexual activity. And yet, even today, the latent worry is in the public mind. Such misinformation is doubly dangerous, for it fuels fear and at the same time sets up a kind of perceptual static that allows people to avoid the real behavioral messages we need to convey.

So the vast majority of possible routes of spread of HIV simply do not work. On the other hand, it is important to note that all kinds of sexual routes do work; there is variation, to be sure, but in the instance of sexual spread, the issue is one of relative efficiency – and inefficiency is a very weak reed to lean on when it comes to sex.

As noted before, the early recognition that homosexual men were the earliest infected led to a remarkable assumption that only homosexual sex would transmit the virus. That was patently false even from the outset, for the heterosexual partners of intravenous drug users were becoming infected even if they themselves did not inject drugs; and in much of the world, heterosexual spread was the dominant mode from the beginning.

As studies began to yield solid data, it became evident that anal receptive intercourse was much more "efficient" than other kinds of sexual intercourse (16). Even then, the self-delusion of public thinking played a dangerous role, for there is accumulating evidence that heterosexual anal intercourse carries high risk (17) and is in fact quite a prevalent behavior – in many countries and cultures it is quietly acknowledged as a poor person's means of contraception. Here is a context in which preventive education might make considerable difference, and yet in many areas (especially in the United States) it is forbidden to mention anal intercourse in school- or community-based prevention programs on the grounds that it would "promote homosexuality."

Emphasizing that AIDS is a sexually transmitted disease has had mixed results as well – for it has prompted some politicians to harken back to the "good old days" and to urge that we revert to what are often referred to as "tried-and-true public health measures" such as mandatory testing, mandatory contact tracing and even quarantine. I have often wondered just *what* people thought was "tried-and-true." After all, it was penicillin – not public health stratagems – that stopped syphilis (18) (and of course that was only a temporary lull in that battle, for syphilis is making a dramatic comeback in the 1990s[19]). The rest of the sexually transmitted diseases had exploded in the 1970s, despite intensified efforts to apply so-called standard procedures; and by 1980 routine premarital serologic testing for syphilis had been dropped in most of the states as being an ineffective public health measure that was exceptionally wasteful of resources.

In fact, there are few more worrisome "catch-phrases" in the present confused debate than the call to treat AIDS "just like any other sexually transmitted disease!" Nowhere have we failed more dramatically in public health than in the control of sexually transmitted diseases. What is more, with its eleven-year incubation period, uniform expressivity and lethal outcome, AIDS is not just like the rest. Far from using earlier STD efforts as a model, it should be hoped that what is learned from thoughtful dealing with the AIDS epidemic will help in grappling with other STDs.

Virology, Immunology and Pathogenesis

The good news in the epidemic thus far has been in the realm of biomedical science. I have reviewed the progress made in epidemiology, which should not be undervalued. But I want to take a few minutes to add some detail about the virology, immunology and pathogenesis of HIV, for those are remarkably well understood also. As you know, HIV is a member of the lentivirus subgroup of retroviruses and shares with that group a reverse transcription mechanism during initial infection that results in creation, from an RNA template, of complete viral genetic information in the form of double-stranded DNA that is then integrated into the host cell DNA (20). The genomic organization is remarkably complex compared to most of the other retroviruses and includes sequences that up- and down-regulate viral expression in ways that may ultimately submit to intervention (21). Those points are directly relevant to clinical concerns, for the intimate nature of the interweaving of infecting viral genetic information with that of the host cell makes cure very unlikely; whereas the rapidly increasing insights into control mechanisms do make it imaginable that someone could someday learn to control "on" and "off" switches in a way that might infinitely defer viral expression and disease progression.

The form of the virus at the initiation of infection may be important and may explain, in part, the distinctive fragility of the virion that one can infer by its difficulty of transmission. It seems likely that *cell-associated virus* is the dominant state for transmission, and as in other cell-associated viral infections, that probably requires excellent physiologic preservation of the transmitting cell.

Such reliance on vital cells is not invariable, however, as was sadly demonstrated by the failure of fractionation procedures to remove HIV from fraction VIII and fraction IX concentrates of plasma, used in treatment of two of the most frequent forms of hemophilia. The residual HIV following fractionation and pooling of material from literally thousands of donors per batch resulted in infection of more than fifty percent of persons with severe hemophilia in the early years of the epidemic.

It is still something of a mystery that HIV could survive that fractionation, but it clearly is an exception to the more usual situation. The usual reliance of HIV on cell association is generally accepted, and it has important implications for vaccine development, since classic viral neutralization almost certainly cannot occur in such circumstances, and immune mediated cellular cytotoxicity may well be necessary for a fully effective protective response.

HIV has a number of other features worthy of mention, and these too are shared with some of the other lentiviruses. The remarkably protracted "incubation period" – now estimated to be at least eleven years on the average (22) – is fairly characteristic of the group, as is the fact that the virus is not truly latent during those clinically silent years but rather is steadily productive at a low level (23). Worse yet, the antigenic variation that had been observed in such lentivirus infections as equine infectious anemia is a very prominent property of HIV. The extent of that variation in important sites on the *env* gene sequence is of sufficient magnitude that early immune responses to the virus in a given host can be rendered irrelevant by subsequent antigenic changes (24).

There is another property of the virus which has fewer precedents and that is what may best be called *biologic variation* – that is, virus recovered from one site and/or at one stage of infection has strikingly different host-range and virulence properties from an isolate recovered from the same host at another stage (25). In addition, simultaneous isolates from macrophages, lymphocytes and neural tissue have been found to differ quite markedly in their Iytic effect on cells in culture and in their cellular tropism (26). In short, the biologic propensities of HIV are worrisomely pliable.

Immunologic and pathogenetic features of HIV infection are no less intriguing. Antibodies to various components of the virion can be demonstrated fairly soon after infection – usually within two to three months – which of course facilitates ELISA and other screening tests. Western blot confirmation of those test results reveals characteristic bands of antibody reaction with various surface and core viral antigens, which confirmation is necessary for diagnostic purposes since false positives can occur with disturbing frequency on initial screening alone (27). The phenomenon of false positives is of particular importance in low-prevalence populations (28), and the immense, negative impact of seropositivity on a person's entire existence makes caution in diagnosis absolutely essential.

In general, the humoral responses to HIV antigens are sustained throughout the long years preceding overt HIV disease and only occasionally diminish to the point of disappearance in profoundly ill AIDS patients. Thus, antibodies are reliable as diagnostic indicators of infection. Considerable effort has been devoted to extend their usefulness to prognosis, but no particular antibodies have been consistently associated with protective immunity. In fact, thus far there is no reason to propose that there is such a thing as truly protective immunity – at least not durably so – during human HIV infection. As to indicators of progression, diminution of antibodies to the viral protein, p24, coupled with reappearance of that antigen in the blood seem to be one of the most reliable correlates of impending onset of symptomatic HIV disease.

Much less can be said about cellular immunity in HIV infection. A variety of cellular immune responses to HIV have been reported (29), and such phenomena as cytotoxic T lymphocyte reactions are being monitored in vaccine work (30), but the idea that these might play a role in protection is largely inferential. Primate models of analogous infection with the simian immunodeficiency virus seem to offer particular promise in analyzing important features of host response to these retrovirus infections (31); no attempt will be made to describe that work here.

But back to a description of HIV pathogenesis: the course of infection is marked by an initial viremia which recedes with the appearance of antibodies (32). There then follows a long interval – measured in years – in which immunologic evidence of infection is the sole indicator of future trouble and during which virus is quite difficult to isolate. During that seemingly quiescent period, however, there appears to be a steady attrition of CD4 lymphocytes (33), which ultimately results in a final symptomatic stage, starting ten or eleven years after initial infection, in which CD4 cells have declined to the point where opportunistic infections and certain tumors occur.

In addition to the well-recognized effects on the immune system, the central nervous system is invaded by HIV quite regularly, possibly transported there by macrophages (34). The exact nature of the infection in brain tissue is still not clear, but it is generally agreed that viral nucleic acids and gene products are confined to microglial cells rather than neurons within the brain (35). CNS invasion seems to occur early and can be demonstrated with such a high frequency that it may be a uniform characteristic of HIV disease (36) – as is suggested by the high rate of occurrence of AIDS dementia and other neurologic syndromes once full-scale disease expression occurs (37). It is important to note, however, that the presence of HIV in the central nervous system during the long asymptomatic interval appears to be without clinical consequence. An increasing number of large prospective studies have shown that there is no significant evidence of malfunction on neurologic or psychomotor testing until overt HIV disease is underway (38–40).

Finally, as the consequences of deepening immune deficiency begin to be expressed, the titer and/or ease of virus recovery from plasma and lymphocytes again increases (41), and it has been proposed that people with overt HIV disease become more infectious during this late, symptomatic stage of infection (42). In the context of biologic variation (mentioned previously) it has also been suggested that the circulating virus in these long-infected patients may be more virulent as well as more abundant (43). Some of the seeming inconsistences and contradictions in transmission studies may be explained by such phenomena, but the data are not definitive.

In summary, the pathogenesis of HIV disease involves constant presence of virus in plasma and lymphocytes, with peak titers at the beginning and end of the progression, invasion of CD4 cells resulting in a steady erosion of their numbers over a period of years, and asymptomatic early infection of the CNS which takes on clinical significance only at the time that other manifestations of HIV disease become apparent.

Clinical Manifestations and Natural History

The clinical manifestations of this progression vary widely, but their general pattern follows the theme described above. There may be an "acute syndrome" a few weeks after initial infection (44); when that occurs, it closely resembles infectious mononucleosis and in the context of known high risk behavior or exposure can be a useful presumptive clue to early diagnosis of HIV infection (45). More commonly, there is no recognizable symptomatology for many years in adults. As noted before, the mean interval between initial infection and onset of overt AIDS is now thought to be at least 10 or 11 years (22), and there are numbers of people who remain clinically well more than 13 years after first demonstration of positive HIV serology (46). As immune capacity is steadily eroded, the earliest clinical harbingers of trouble may be oral candidiasis or severe herpes simplex, and when Kaposi's sarcoma occurs it often precedes opportunistic infections by a year or more.

The litany of opportunistic microorganisms that then besets a person with HIV disease is familiar now, but rather curious in its selectivity. *Pneumocystis carinii* and cytomegalovirus are major offenders, and toxoplasma and *Mycobacterium* species – either tuberculosis or the avium intracellulare subgroup – are also prominent. Cryptococcus, cryptosporidia, EB virus, varicella zoster, and many others add to the list of miseries. Their manifestations include pneumonia, chronic meningitis, brain abscess, gastrointestinal infections, and peripheral neuropathies, and in nearly one-third of patients with AIDS, cytomegalovirus retinitis threatens or causes blindness (47).

There are many tumors that can complicate the clinical picture as well; the topic of Kaposi's sarcoma alone is truly fascinating, for it almost seems to defy categorization between tumor and non-tumor, and a number of investigators – notably Gallo and his group – are pursuing leads that may have great relevance for fundamental understanding of oncogenesis *per se* (48).

Initially it was thought that the syndromes comprising AIDS all reflected infectious or neoplastic consequences of progressive immune suppression. However it is now evident that a number of manifestations of illness seem to relate directly to HIV infection itself. Of particular interest in that regard is the occurrence of strikingly severe tissue wasting, sometimes as the major or even the sole manifestation of HIV disease (49). This wasting syndrome – evocatively referred to by the Ugandans as "slim disease" – has been incompletely explained thus far. The possible role of tumor necrosis factor has been suggested (50), and intrinsic as well as extrinsic bowel disease is a possibility, since cells of the gastrointestinal tract seem capable of supporting viral replication (51), and chronic diarrhea is certainly a common manifestation, often without a convincing enteric pathogen as causal agent. Finally, as indicated previously, when HIV disease reaches an overt stage, AIDS dementia and a variety of other central nervous system manifestations mediated by HIV itself may be prominent factors in clinical presentation and care (37), and indeed the great majority of people with AIDS at autopsy have striking loss of CNS tissue and other gross evidence of brain involvement (52).

In summary, then, this awesome array of ills combines to constitute the syndrome called AIDS – surely one of the most dreadful afflictions of humankind. The horror of the syndrome is enhanced by its usual occurrence in the prime of life – and once HIV disease begins, in the absence of treatment, its course is inexorable over a period of months, usually terminating with one or more bouts of *Pneumocystis carinii* pneumonia or a similarly deadly infection. It is sobering to note that, ten years into the epidemic, AIDS is moving quickly from sixth to third on the list of causes of years-of-productive-life-lost in the United States (53).

Treatment and Prognosis

When clinicians first faced this nightmare in the early eighties, the bizarre collection of microbes and symptoms seemed overwhelming; but with research and clinical experience, remarkable progress occurred, so that the outlook for a person newly diagnosed with AIDS is somewhat less bleak – if access to treatment can be obtained. The antiviral drug zidovudine (54) – or AZT, as it is more popularly called – was introduced in 1987. It was initially given at needlessly high doses, resulting in major toxicity that limited its usefulness. With additional experience it has been found that no more than 25% of earlier dosage is needed to achieve antiviral effect (55), which has allowed more people – but not all – to tolerate it. AZT, in combination with aggressive treatment for PCP, has clearly extended the life expectancy of people with AIDS by at least two years (56), and it is no longer rare for people to live four or five years after diagnosis. It is also characteristic, however, for the beneficial effects of AZT to wane rapidly after one-and-a-half or two years of therapy (57).

After these initial steps in progress – reported in 1987 – additional increments occurred. It was found that the *Pneumocystis carinii* pneumonia that so often resulted in early death could be deferred by prophylactic treatment with aerosolized pentamidine (58) and, subsequently, with other prophylactic strategies (59). That improvement alone has bought many months of increased survival for people with HIV disease, and indeed many European clinicians feel that PCP prophylaxis is largely responsible for the significant improvement in AIDS prognosis.

In 1989 another step was taken in managing HIV disease, in that it was reported that AZT taken as soon as CD4 cells dropped below 500 – approximately half of normal – could forestall the onset of overt disease (60). That finding was the basis for the recommendation that all people at risk should henceforth seek testing so that they could know their status and be treated at the earliest moment (61). Sadly, that abstract recommendation does not jibe with the current state of clinical care in the United States. Increasingly, a plurality of people with HIV infection do not even have access to primary care, and there are few places outside of specialized centers that are prepared to give the kind of careful followup implicit in that recommendation. A recent finding added further uncertainty, in that it suggested that, while AIDS-specific diseases might be delayed by such "early intervention", the ultimate duration to death might not be significantly shortened. Thus, in the opinion of a number of AIDS clinicians and researchers, the question of early AZT treatment of asymptomatic people with HIV is still up in the air. However, there is no question that early diagnosis and careful clinical follow-up can significantly extend and improve their lives.

Short-term prospects for dramatic improvements in antiviral therapy are not bright. Two drugs – DDI and DDC – that share mechanisms of action with AZT are currently under study and may improve the picture modestly, in that they do not seem to have cross-resistance, their toxicity may be somewhat lower, and combination strategies may be possible (62, 63). However, despite diligent searches, no radical "breakthrough" drugs appear imminent.

Treatment of opportunistic infections offers considerable room for progress, as evidenced by the addition of gangcyclovir for cytomegalovirus disease (64) and fluconazole for fungal infections (65). It should not be surprising, however, to learn that almost all of the infections that plague people with AIDS must be treated indefinitely (66) – reinforcing the old maxim that there is no antimicrobial agent that is fully effective in the absence of an intact host immune response.

Vaccine Status

Where do we stand with vaccine research? Well, we are just barely off the drawing board – if that. The intrinsic problems are daunting, as you will have inferred from earlier discussion. Virtually all of our successful vaccines were either developed in imitation of natural, protective immunity or at least were correlated empirically with protective markers after the fact. In the instance of HIV, there does not seem to be naturally protective immunity to start with, so even vaccine design is difficult. The phenomena of antigenic variation and possible biologic variation complicate matters further, and in brief, I think it would be safe to say that we are years away from a general use vaccine that would be of help (67).

Even if an excellent vaccine were in hand tomorrow, however, it would not help much with our present problem. The recrudescence of measles should warn us about excessive reliance on a vaccine strategy; furthermore, as noted earlier, proper deployment of AIDS education can teach people to avoid risk – and there will never be as good a vaccine as that. Indeed, education will be *the* vaccine for AIDS for at least a decade to come; but just as a vaccine is of no use in its bottle, so education about HIV is of no use unless it is delivered clearly and reiteratively and in the language of the intended listener.

Current Status of the Epidemic

So where does all that leave us currently? It is worth stating the dreadful statistics of AIDS and HIV. Only ten years after the first case descriptions, there have been nearly 180,000 Americans diagnosed with AIDS. An additional million or more people are infected with HIV. Our health care system is staggering under the weight of about 70,000 surviving persons living with AIDS, and yet it is estimated that at least 600,000 – nearly ten times as many – should be in programs of early intervention and care due to CD4 cell counts dropping into the dangerous range (68).

The predominance of gay and bisexual men and intravenous drug users still characterizes the distribution of AIDS cases, but HIV seroprevalence studies show a steady trend toward equality of the sexes – with women the most rapidly increasing category and children following close behind (69). The concentration of AIDS in urban communities is less dramatic, now, and small towns and rural America are rapidly being swept up by the tide of advancing HIV (70) – for, contrary to popular presumption, sex and drugs are everywhere and rural America chose the dangerous path of denial for a long time.

In short, we are in deep trouble. Were there not a single additional instance of HIV infection, we would have our work cut out for us for the decade to come. But instead, it is estimated that new infections are occurring at a rate of between 45,000 and 200,000 a year! In the year 2000 it has been projected that there will be 98,000 *new* cases of AIDS (71) – and that is really awful, since those are people who got infected last week. We will not be able to bring this terrible cascade of events to a halt until the universality of risk is recognized.

Summary and Conclusions

In this chapter, with its focus on infectious diseases and microbiology, I will not go deeply into the kinds of problems we now are grappling with in the arena of public policy concerning AIDS. I hope you will bear with me, however, if I touch lightly on some of the most pressing matters at hand, particularly in the context of prevention and of care for persons living with HIV and AIDS.

First, prevention: as I tried to indicate, this is an arena in which we should be able to do best, for the sharply restricted transmission of HIV allows us to use education and specific interventions such as condom use and interruption of the injecting-drug-use conduit of viral spread. And yet we are doing poorly. Take the matter of public education: it is unrealistic to hope that public service announcements alone will stem the tide, and yet it is crucial that the public at least understand that there is a tide to be stemmed and that we must do so quickly. Opinion surveys and public polls suggest that most adults – and for that matter, many adolescents – have absorbed parts of the message about how HIV is transmitted; but if the questions are appropriately probing, it turns out that far fewer know or believe that other exposures are *not* hazardous (72, 73). That creates a substrate of potential for public panic that undercuts efforts to deal with the epidemic and fuels an explosive environment in which dreadful discrimination against sick people can and does occur. Paradoxically, it also facilitates a degree of denial that allows people to be inattentive about their own risk behaviors, past or present.

Besides public education, there are a number of other preventive measures that are currently underutilized. In particular, HIV counseling and testing strategies have been badly misused. So often testing has been invoked in threatening tones or contexts that people are frightened to seek to know their status; and the testing centers often deal off-handedly with negative test results, rather than recognizing that it is counselling *in the context of testing* that can best provide a ring of educated seronegatives around possible sources of future transmission (74). It is in that context of HIV counseling and testing that our best hope lies, in fact, for interruption of cycles of spread. The optimal way to deploy this strategy is with provision made for confidentiality or anonymity if needed.

We have not done this well. It is often hard for someone to get tested, and social dynamics have been so threatening that anonymity remains a major prerequisite for many to seek to know their status in the first place. Name-reporting of seropositives is increasingly frequent as state legislatures react – but in my view it is of questionable benefit to public health and is profoundly threatening to the people we want to attract and educate. We must keep in mind that, in most parts of the United States, some of the risk behaviors perceived to dominate in HIV transmission are illegal; and the health consequences of HIV are well enough feared by self-insured employers and insurance companies alike that the very act of *seeking* testing can have adverse effects, regardless of the test result.

Finally, in the realm of prevention, advocacy of condom use and intervention with illicit drug users require urgent attention, for they are almost the sole available strategies and weapons we have to fight with at the HIV "front." Condom use does not assure perfect protection – only abstinence can do that – but condoms can decrease risk of transmission by at least an order of magnitude when properly deployed (75).

Similarly, needle exchange or bleach instruction interventions are clearly stop-gap strategies that are far less desirable than would be drug treatment; yet there is not a major city in this country where poor people can get treatment for substance addiction without weeks or months on waiting lists, and meanwhile they are at constant risk for HIV transmission while addicted (76). It is a sad fact that our approach to the appalling epidemic of illicit substance use that so threatens the future of our children and our nation has been almost entirely punitive and legalistic, with almost no attention paid to public health. We have declared a war on drugs with no accommodations made for the prisoners of that war!

The other area of policy I want to mention is health care access and financing for persons living with AIDS. First, the only things new about the tremendous problems facing us in caring for over a million young Americans with a chronic and lethal disease are the virus and the particular features of the awful diseases it spawns – all the other difficulties that beset us reflect a crumbling health care system, and diligent efforts to cope and to solve them thoughtfully will be of benefit not only to people with HIV disease but to our elderly and chronically ill as well. Health care access is limited or nonexistent for nearly 40,000,000 Americans who lack adequate health insurance, and their needs could be met far better with a continuum of care options than with their current dependence on expensive tertiary care institutions.

In the same context, we have much remedial work to do. The people at greatest risk for HIV lack access even to primary care, and in the specific setting of illicit drug use – with its special importance to epidemic dynamics – even primary care must be linked to access to treatment of substance addiction as the underlying problem (77).

In closing, if all of this seems daunting, it is critical that we meet these challenges nonetheless. It is sometimes said that AIDS is "just one disease" – that, after a strenuous decade, we have done enough about AIDS and in fairness should turn our attention to other diseases. I have dealt with several parts of the rebuttal: AIDS research is so fundamental that its spinoffs are broadly valuable. The health care needs of people with AIDS are congruent with those of millions of others in terms of access, financing and delivery. But most important of all, AIDS is preventable by means of avoidance, and yet it is in no sense under control. HIV represents an expanding threat for which no end is in sight, and cure and vaccine are, at best, on the far horizon. It is truly like the day after Hiroshima: the world changed with the emergence of HIV and will never be the same again. We have been acting as if it were happening to others – and yet there are no others. We must unite as a human family and help!

References

1. Centers for Disease Control (1981) *Pneumocystis* pneumonia – Los Angeles. MMWR 30: 250–252
2. Huminer D, Pitlik SD (1988) Further evidence for the existence of AIDS in the pre-AIDS era. Rev Infect Dis 10: 1061
3. Temin HM (1989) Is HIV unique or merely different? J Acquir Immune Defic Syndr 2: 1–9
4. Centers for Disease Control (1990) Estimates of HIV prevalence and projected AIDS cases: Summary of a workshop, October 31–November 1, 1989. MMWR 39: 110–119
5. Centers for Disease Control (1981) Kaposi's sarcoma and *Pneumocystis* pneumonia among homosexual men – New York City and California. MMWR 30: 305–308
6. Barre-Sinoussi F, Chermann JC, Rey F, Nugeyre MT, Chamaret S, Gruest J, Dauguet C, Axler-Blin C, Vezinet-Brun F, Rouzioux C, Rozenbaum W, Montagnier L (1983) Isolation of a T-lymphotropic retrovirus from a patient at risk for acquired immune deficiency syndrome (AIDS). Science 220: 868–871
7. Gallo RC, Salahuddin SZ, Popovic M, Shearer GM, Kaplan M, Haynes BF, Palker TJ, Redfield R, Oleske J, Safai B, White G, Foster P, Markham DP (1984) Frequent detection and isolation of cytopathic retroviruses (HTLV-III) from patients with AIDS and at risk for AIDS. Science 224: 500–503.
8. Levy JA, Hoffman AD, Kramer SM, Landis JA, Shimabukuro JM (1984) Isolation of lymphocytopathic retroviruses from San Francisco patients with AIDS. Science 225: 840–842
9. Winkelstein WJ, Samuel M, Padian NS, Wiley JA, Lang W, Anderson RE, Levy JE (1987) The San Francisco men's health study: III. Reduction in human immunodeficiency virus transmission among homosexual/bisexual men, 1982–86. Am J Public Health 76: 685–687
10. Clavel F, Mansinho K, Shamaret S, Gutard D, Favier V, et al (1987) Human immunodeficiency virus type 2 infection associated with AIDS in West Africa. N Engl J Med 316: 1180–1185
11. Kiereini E (1990) AIDS in Africa. Plenary presentation at Sixth International AIDS Meeting, San Francisco
12. Marcus R, CDC Cooperative Needlestick Surveillance Group (1988) Surveillance of health care workers exposed to blood from patients infected with the human immunodeficiency virus. N Engl J Med 319: 1118–1123
13. Friedland GH, Klein RS (1987) Transmission of the human immunodeficiency virus. N Engl J Med 317: 1125–1135.
14. Pape JW, Stanback ME, Pamphile M, Boncy M, Deschamps MH, Verdier R-I, Beaulieu M-E, Blattner W, Liautaud B, Johnson WD (1990) Prevalence of HIV infection and high-risk activities in Haiti. J Acquir Immune Defic Syndr 3: 995–1001
15. Miike L (September 1987) Do insects transmit AIDS? (Office of Technology Assessment, Staff Paper 1)
16. Reviewed in: Osborn JE (1988) The AIDS epidemic: Six years. Ann Rev Public Health 9: 551–583
17. Voeller B (1990) Heterosexual anal intercourse: An AIDS risk factor. In: Voeller B, Reinisch JM, Gottlieb M (eds) AIDS and sex: an integrated biomedical and biobehavioral approach. The Kinsey Institute Series, Oxford University Press, pp 276–310
18. Brandt AM (1988) The syphilis epidemic and its relation to AIDS. Science 239: 375–380
19. Rolfs RT, Nakashima AK (1990) Epidemiology of primary and secondary syphilis in the United States, 1981 through 1989. JAMA 264: 1432–1437
20. McCune JM (1991) HIV-1: The infective process in vivo. Cell 64: 351–363

21. Steffy K, Wong-Staal F (1991) Genetic regulation of human immunodeficiency virus. Microbiol Rev 55: 193–205
22. Lifson AR, Buchbinder SP, Sheppard HW, Mawle AC, Wilber JC, Stanley M, Hart CE, Hessol NA, Holmberg SD (1991) Long-term human immunodeficiency virus infection in asymptomatic homosexual and bisexual men with normal CD4+ lymphocyte counts: Immunologic and virologic characteristics. J Infect Dis 163: 959–965
23. Ho DD, Moudgh T, Alam M (1989) Quantitation of human immunodeficiency virus type 1 in the blood of infected persons. N Eng J Med 321: 1621–1625
24. Nowak MA, May RM, Anderson RM (1990) The evolutionary dynamics of HIV-1 quasispecies and the development of immunodeficiency disease. AIDS 4: 1095–1103
25. Cloyd MW, Moore BE (1990) Spectrum of biological properties of human immunodeficiency virus (HIV-1) isolates. Virology 174: 103–116
26. Cheng-Mayer C, Quiroga M, Tung JW, Dina D, Levy JA (1990) Viral determinants of human immunodeficiency virus type 1 T-cell or macrophage tropism, cytopathogenicity, and CD4 antigen modulation. J Virol 64: 4390–4398
27. Centers for Disease Control (1988) Update: Serologic testing for antibody to human immunodeficiency virus. MMWR 36: 833–840
28. Cleary PD, Barry JM, Mayer KH, Brandt AM, Goston L, Fineberg HV (1987) Compulsory premarital screening for the human immunodeficiency virus: Technical and public health considerations. JAMA 258: 1757–1762
29. Katzenstein DA, Sawyer LA, Quinnan GV (1988) Issues in the evalution of AIDS vaccines. AIDS 2: 151–155
30. Autran B, Plata F, Debre P (1991) MHC-restricted cytotoxicity against HIV. J Acquir Immune Defic Syndr 4: 361–367
31. Palca J (1990) A reliable animal model for AIDS. Science 248: 1078
32. Daar ES, Moudgil T, Meyer RD, Ho DD (1991) Transient high levels of viremia in patients with primary human immunodeficiency virus type 1 infection. N Engl J Med 324: 961–964
33. Masur H, Ognibene FP, Yarchoan R, Shelhamer JH, Baird BF, Travis W, Suffredini AF, Deyton L, Kovacs JA, Falloon J, Davey R, Polis M, Metcalf M, Baseler M, Wesley R, Gill VJ, Fauci AS, Lane HC (1989) CD4 counts as predictors of opportunistic pneumonias in human immunodeficiency virus (HIV) infection. Ann Intern Med 111: 223–231
34. Pulliam L, Herndier BG, Tang NM, McGrath MS (1991) Human immunodeficiency virus-infected macrophages produce soluble factors that cause histological and neurochemical alterations in cultured human brains. J Clin Invest 87: 503–512
35. Jordan CA, Wakins BA, Kufta C, Dubois-Dalcq M (1991) Infection of brain microglial cells by human immunodeficiency virus type 1 is CD4 dependent. J Virol 65: 736–742
36. Marshall DW, Brey RL, Butzin CA, Lucey DR, Abbadessa SM, Boswell RN (1991) CSF changes in a longitudinal study of 124 neurologically normal HIV-1-infected U.S. Air Force personnel. J Acquir Immune Defic Syndr 4: 777–781
37. Bridge TP, Ingraham JL (1990) Central nervous system effects of human immunodeficiency virus type 1. Ann Rev Med 41: 159–168
38. Franzblau A, Letz R, Hershman D, Mason P, Wallace JI, Bekesi JG (1991) Quantitative neurologic and neurobehavioral testing of persons infected with human immunodeficiency virus-1. Arch Neurol (in press)
39. Selnes OA, Miller E, McArthur J, Bordon B, Munoz A, Sheridan K, Fox R, Saah AJ, Multicenter AIDS Cohort Study (1990) HIV-1 infection: No evidence of cognitive decline during the asymptomatic stages. Neurology 40: 204–208
40. Miller EN, Selnes OE, McArthur JC, Satz P, Becker JT, Cohen BA, Sheridan K, Machado AM, Van Gorp WG, Visischer B (1990) Neuropsychological performance in HIV-1-infected homosexual men: The Multicenter AIDS Cohort Study (MACS). Neurology 40: 197–203
41. Baltimore D, Feinberg MB (1989) HIV revealed: Toward a natural history of the infection. N Engl J Med 321: 1673–1675
42. Saag MS, Crain MJ, Deker WD, Campbell-Hill S, Robinson S, Brown WE, Leuther M, Whitley RJ, Hahn BH, Shaw GM (1991) High-level viremia in adults and children infected with human immunodeficiency virus: Relation to disease stage and CD4+ lymphocyte levels. J Infect Dis 164: 72–80

43. Levy JA (1990) Changing concepts in HIV infection: Challenges for the 1990s. AIDS 4: 1051–1058
44. Clark SJ, Saag MS, Decker WD, Campbell-Hill S, Roberson JL, Veldkamp PJ, Kappes JC, Hahn BH, Shaw GM (1991) High titers of cytopathic virus in plasma of patients with symptomatic primary HIV-1 infection. N Engl J Med 324: 954–960
45. Tindall B, Cooper DA (1991) Primary AIDS infection: Host responses and intervention strategies. AIDS 5: 1–14
46. Biggar RJ, International Registry of Seroconverters (1990) AIDS incubation in 1891 seroconverters from different exposure groups. AIDS 4: 1059–1066
47. Jacobson MA, Mills J (1988) Serious cytomegalovirus disease in the acquired immunodeficiency syndrome (AIDS). Ann Intern Med 108: 585–594
48. Gallo R (1991) Kaposi's sarcoma: A special tumor of AIDS. In: Virus hunting. Basic Books pp 260–275
49. Simpson DM, Bender AN, Farraye J, Mendelson SG, Wolfe DE (1990) Human immunodeficiency virus wasting syndrome may represent a treatable myopathy. Neurology 40: 535–538
50. Matsuyama T, Hamamoto Y, Soma G-I, Mizuno D, Yamamoto N, Kobayashi N (1989) Cytocidal effect of tumor necrosis factor on cells chronically infected with human immunodeficiency virus (HIV): Enhancement of HIV replication. J Virol 63: 2504–2509
51. Greenson JK, Belitsos PC, Yardley JH, Bartlett JG (1991)AIDS enteropathy: Occult enteric infections and duodenal mucosal alterations in chronic diarrhea. Ann Intern Med 114: 366–372
52. Navia BA, Cho E-S, Petito CK, Price RW (1986) The AIDS dementia complex: II. Neuropathology. Ann Neurol 19: 525–535
53. Centers for Disease Control (1991) Update: YPLL before age 65 – U.S. 1988 and 1989. MMWR 40: 60–62
54. Richman DD (1991) Antiviral therapy of HIV infection. Ann Rev Med 42: 69–90
55. Fischl MA, Parker CB, Pettinelli C, et al (1990) A randomized controlled trial of a reduced daily dose of zidovudine in patients with the acquired immunodeficiency syndrome. N Engl J Med 323: 1009–1014
56. Moore RD, Hidalgo J, Sugland BW, Chaisson RE (1991) Zidovudine and the natural history of the acquired imunodeficiency syndrome. N Engl J Med 324: 1412–1416
57. Fischl MA, Richman DD, Causey DM, Grieco MH, Bryson Y, Mildvan D, Laskin OL, Groopman JE, Volberding PA, Schooley RT, Jackson GG, Durack DT, Andrews JC, Nusinoff-Lehrman S, Barry DW, AZT Collaborative Working Group (1989) Prolonged zidovudine therapy in patients with AIDS and advanced AIDS-related complex. JAMA 262: 2405–2410
58. Hirschel B, Lazzarin A, Chopard P, Opravil M, Furrer H-J, Ruttimann S, Vernazza P, Chave JP, Ancarani F, Gabriel V, Heald A, King R, Malinverni R, Martin J-L, Mermillod B, Nicod L, Simoni L, Vivirito MC, Zerboni R, C3-Swiss Group for Clinical Studies on AIDS (1991) A controlled study of inhaled pentamidine for primary prevention of *Pneumocystis carinii* pneumonia. N Engl J Med 324: 1079–1083
59. Medina I, Mills J, Leoung G, Hopewell PC, Lee B, Modin G, Benowitz N, Wofsy CB (1990) Oral therapy for *Pneumocystis carinii* pneumonia in the acquired immunodeficiency syndrome. N Engl J Med 323: 776–782
60. Volberding PA, Lagakos SW, Koch MA, Pettinelli C, Myers MW, Booth DK, Balfour HH, Reichman RC, Bartlett JA, Hirsch MS, Murphy RL, Hardy D, Soeiro R, Fischl MA, Bartlett JG, Merigan TC, Hyslop NE, Richman DD, Valentine FT, Coreythe L, AIDS Clinical Trials Group of NIAID (1990) Zidovudine in asymptomatic human immunodeficiency virus infection. A controlled trial in persons with fewer than 500 CD4-positive cells per cubic millimeter. N Engl J Med 322: 941–949
61. Centers for Disease Control (1990) Guidelines for prophylaxis against *Pneumocystis carinii* pneumonia for persons infected with human immunodeficiency virus. MMWR 38: 1–9
62. Lambert JS, Seidlin M, Reichman RC, Plank CS, Laverty M, Morse GD, Knupp C, McLaren C, Pettinelli C, Valentine FT, Dolin R (1990) 2',3'-dideoxyinosine (ddI) in patients with the acquired immunodeficiency syndrome or AIDS-related complex. N Engl J Med 322: 1333–1340

63. Hirsch MS (1990) Chemotherapy of human immunodeficiency virus infections: Current practice and future prospects. J Infect Dis 161: 845–857
64. Drew WL, Miner RC, Busch DF, Follansbee SE, Gullett J, Mehalko SG, Gordon SM, Owen WF, Matthews TR, Buhles WC, DeArmond B (1991) Prevalence of resistance in patients receiving ganciclovir for serious cytomegalovirus infection. J Infect Dis 163: 716–719
65. Bozzette SA, Larsen RA, Chiu J, Leal MAE, Jacobsen J, Rothman P, Robinson P, Gilbert G, McCutchan JA, Tilles J, Leedom JM, Richman DD, California Collaborative Treatment Group (1991) A placebo-controlled trial of maintenance therapy with fluconazole after treatment of cryptococcal meningitis in the acquired immunodeficiency syndrome. N Engl J Med 324: 580–584
66. Masur H (1990) Problems in the management of opportunistic infections in patients infected with human immunodeficiency virus. J Infect Dis 161: 858–864
67. Berzofsky JA (1991) Approaches and issues in the development of vaccines against HIV. J Acquir Immune Defic Syndr 4: 451–459
68. Brundage JF, McNeil JG, Miller RN, Gardner LI, Harrison SM, Hawks C, Craig DB, Redfield R, Burke DS, U.S. Army Retrovirus Research Group (1990) The current distribution of CD4+ T-lymphocyte counts among adults in the United States with human immunodeficiency virus infections: Estimates based on the experience of the U.S. Army. J Acquir Immune Defic Syndr 3: 92–94
69. Gwinn M, Pappaioanou M, George JR, Hannon WH, Wasser SC, Redus MA, Hoff R, Grady GF, Willoughby A, Novello AC, Petersen LR, Dondero TJ, Curran JW (1991) Prevalence of HIV infection in childbearing women in the United States. JAMA 265: 1704–1708
70. Verghese A, Berk SL, Sarubbi F (1989) Urbs in rure: Human immunodeficiency virus infection in rural Tennessee. J Infect Dis 160: 1051–1055
71. U.S. Public Health Service (1991) Healthy People 2000. National Health Promotion and Disease Prevention Objectives. Washington, D.C., DHHS Publication No (PHS) 91-50213
72. Hingson R, Strunin L, Berlin B (1990) Acquired immunodeficiency syndrome transmission: Changes in knowledge and behaviors among teenagers, Massachusetts statewide surveys, 1986 to 1988. Pediatr 85: 24–29
73. Turner CF, Miller HG, Moses LE (eds) (1989) Facilitating change in health behaviors. In: AIDS. Sexual Behavior and Intravenous Drug Use. Washington, National Academy Press, pp 259–315
74. Osborn JE (1990) AIDS: Challenges to our health care systems. Cleve Clin J Med 57: 709–714
75. Van de Perre P, Jacobs D, Sprecher-Goldberger S (1987) The latex condom, an efficient barrier against sexual transmission of AIDS-related viruses. AIDS 1: 49–52
76. Des Jarlais DC, Friedman SR (1989) AIDS and IV drug use. Science 245: 578
77. Stryker J (1989) IV drug use and AIDS: Public policy and dirty needles. J Health Polit Policy Law 14: 719–740

Strategies for Control of Viral Hepatitis in the Age of Molecular Biology

Stanley M. Lemon and **Daniel S. Shapiro**

Department of Medicine, The University of North Carolina at Chapel Hill, Chapel Hill, North Carolina

Abstract

Five distinct human viruses are commonly associated with viral hepatitis in man. Two agents, hepatitis A virus (HAV) and hepatitis E virus (HEV) cause only acute hepatitis and are predominantly transmitted by the fecal-oral route. The others, hepatitis B virus (HBV), hepatitis D virus (HDV), and hepatitis C virus (HCV), are transmitted by parenteral and sexual exposure, and in the case of HBV and HCV are also transmitted to infants born of infected mothers. All have a worldwide distribution, although the prevalence of each varies significantly among different populations. The viruses belong to very different virus families and have in common only a tropism for the liver. Each has a distinctive structure and replication strategy. Infection with three of these agents (HBV, HCV and HDV) often leads to chronic hepatitis and possibly cirrhosis, while two of these viruses (HBV and HCV) have been associated with development of liver cancer. Effective vaccines offer hope for control of HAV, HBV, and HDV (through immunization against HBV), while recent advances in our understanding of HCV and HEV suggest that vaccines may soon be available for these agents as well.

Viral Agents of Hepatitis in Man

An Introduction: Hepatitis Virology and Modern Molecular Biology

Although reports of epidemic jaundice extend back into antiquity, the era of modern hepatitis virology opened in 1965 with the identification of "Australia antigen", an antigen found circulating in the blood of multiply transfused individuals (1). Shortly thereafter, it was discovered that this antigen was in fact a marker of infection with the agent of "homologous serum hepatitis", or "type B" viral hepatitis. Since those early days, when it appeared that all viral hepatitis might be due to one of two viruses, we have come to realize that the human hepatitis viruses comprise at least five distinct agents, each with unique antigenic and biologic attributes. In 1973, the second agent, that of infectious hepatitis ("type A viral hepatitis") was identified in human feces by immune electron microscopy (2). Shortly thereafter, it was recognized that most cases of posttransfusion hepatitis in the United States could not be attributed to infection with either hepatitis A virus (HAV) or hepatitis B virus (HBV), initiating a long and frustrating search by many virologists for the elusive agent(s) of "non-A, non-B hepatitis" (3). In 1977 came the identification of the "delta agent", now called hepatitis delta virus (HDV) and known to be a unique defective satellite virus of HBV (4), and in 1983 came the discovery of a new type of enterically transmitted hepatitis virus, the agent responsible for "enterically transmitted non-A, non-B hepatitis" or more simply hepatitis E virus (HEV) (5).

Throughout this period of time, the field of hepatitis virology advanced in parallel with developments in modern molecular biology. A new vaccine for hepatitis B, containing a component of the HBV envelope expressed from recombinant DNA in the yeast *Saccharomyces cerevisiae*, became the first triumph of the new molecular biology in the prevention of human disease (6). HBV was shown to be a novel type of DNA virus, replicating via reverse transcription of an RNA intermediate and thus with distant phylogenetic ties to the retroviruses (7). The genome of HAV was molecularly cloned. This fecally transmitted agent of viral hepatitis ultimately was shown to represent a new and unique genus of the family Picornaviridae, only very distantly related to the polioviruses and other enteroviruses (8). HDV was found to be distinct from all other animal viruses, with an exceptionally small RNA genome that is catalytically active (9) and has features bearing a striking resemblance to the viroids, replicating RNAs found in plants (10). Indeed, HDV may represent an echo of the ages when all life on earth was based on the chemistry of RNA, before DNA and proteins made biology the complex process it is today.

Perhaps there is no greater contribution of molecular biology to our understanding of the hepatitis viruses, however, than the recent identification of hepatitis C virus (HCV), the dominant agent of non-A, non-B hepatitis in the United States and probably many other regions as well (11). After numerous false starts, it was the combination of a carefully monitored series of experimental infections in chimpanzees, resulting in the generation of a high titered plasma pool, coupled with a determined effort to apply to this problem the tools of modern molecular biology which led to the recognition of the first HCV-specified antigen. Thus HCV, which we now recognize to be a new RNA virus type having distant relatedness to the flaviviruses and pestiviruses, was the first human pathogen to be initially identified using a planned molecular strategy.

New developments continue at a dizzying pace, but much remains to be done. First, we may not be at the end of the list of human hepatitis viruses – there is already talk of a "hepatitis F" agent. More important, however, is the distance we have yet to go in learning how best to control those viruses that we have already identified. Vaccines for hepatitis B are becoming increasingly inexpensive, raising hopes that immunization against HBV will become an increasingly more common practice worldwide. New formalin-inactivated vaccines for HAV are now in phase III trials, but there is a need for less expensive hepatitis A vaccines that can be used in developing regions of the world (12) and an urgent need to better understand the antigenic nature of HCV and to develop candidate HCV vaccines. Although we know a great deal about the molecular events that accompany HBV and HDV replication, we have yet to design specific and effective antiviral agents capable of modifying the course of chronic infections with these agents. With HCV there may be an even greater need for effective antiviral therapy, but knowledge of the replication strategy of this virus must be considered in its infancy. Lastly, there is the issue of hepatocellular carcinoma (HCC), on a worldwide basis one of the most frequent and deadly of all human cancers (13). Epidemiologic evidence clearly links chronic HBV infection with HCC and increasingly suggests that chronic hepatitis C may also lead to HCC, although the mechanisms of hepatocarcinogenesis remain obscure. In this brief review, we will attempt to highlight current frontiers in the control of these virus infections, making special reference to recent advances in understanding the molecular biology of the viruses and the general strategies by which we may ultimately limit the disease burden they continue to inflict.

Biological Unity and Diversity among the Human Hepatitis Viruses

We now know that acute viral hepatitis may follow infection with any of at least five distinct human viruses. In the individual patient, it is usually not possible to differentiate between these infections on the basis of clinical manifestations alone. Generally speaking, hepatitis A is more abrupt in its onset than hepatitis B, and acute hepatitis C is usually a less impressive illness than either hepatitis A or B. On the other hand, infection with each of these viruses (with the possible exception of HCV) may result in fulminant hepatitis, massive hepatic necrosis and death. HDV infection is particularly associated with severe acute episodes of hepatitis (14), while infection of pregnant women with HEV results in death in over 10% of cases (15). Nonetheless, the clinical and pathological manifestations of acute infection with each of these five viruses are sufficiently similar to render a diagnosis impossible in the individual case without serological testing and to suggest that each virus may be causing acute disease through similar pathogenetic mechanisms.

Immunopathologically-mediated Disease

All of these viruses appear to share a tropism for the hepatocyte, but our understanding of the way in which they cause disease remains incomplete. We suspect that acute hepatitis B is an immunopathologically mediated disease, less likely to develop in the immunosuppressed patient who becomes acutely infected with HBV, and there is growing evidence that acute hepatitis A may have a similar pathogenetic mechanism. Although some have speculated that hepatitis D may be due to a direct viral cytopathic effect of HDV, there are no strong data to support this view. Whether or not hepatitis C and hepatitis E also result from immune attack on infected hepatocytes is not known, but the striking portal mononuclear cell infiltrates found with each of these infections suggests that this might be the case.

What types of lymphocytes are these, and to what target molecules are they responding? Again, our knowledge is limited. In acute hepatitis B, these cells appear to be cytotoxic, CD8+ T lymphocytes responding to hepatitis B core antigen (HBcAg) and possibly HBsAg determinants (16, 17). Human leukocyte antigen (HLA)-restricted, cytotoxic T lymphocytes with specificity for virus-infected cells have also been identified in acute hepatitis A (18), but very little is known of the cellular immunology of these or other hepatitis virus infections. T cells may contribute to the disease process in several ways, including the release of interferons which may upregulate the normally low level display of HLA markers by hepatocytes, thereby rendering virus-infected hepatocytes better targets for cytotoxic T cells.

Viral Persistence

Although these infections cannot be distinguished from each other clinically, human hepatitis viruses may be cleanly separated into two groups on the basis of their potential to cause persistent infection and chronic liver disease (Fig. 1). HAV and HEV apparently never do this. Individuals who survive the acute infection go on to complete resolution of the disease and apparent lasting immunity. On the other hand, HBV, HCV, and HDV infections have the potential to become persistent. In the case of hepatitis B, only a small proportion of infected persons develop persistent infection (19). These persons are usually relatively immunocompromised, such as neonates (of whom 90% or more develop persistent infection) or individuals infected with human immunodeficiency virus (about 50%). Persistent HBV infection may be clinically silent, or it may lead to chronic liver disease of varying severity. Superinfection of otherwise healthy HBV carriers with

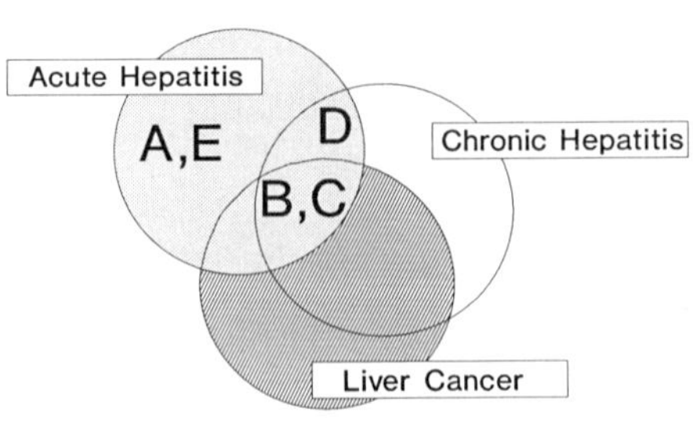

Fig. 1. Human hepatitis viruses and their disease associations

HDV not only leads to severe (often fulminant) acute hepatitis, but in those patients who survive the acute superinfection episode it often results in chronic HDV infection with a much increased risk of both chronic active hepatitis and progression to cirrhosis.

The problem of HCV persistence may be much greater. Current evidence suggests as many as half of all HCV-infected persons fail to clear the virus and become persistently infected (20, 21). (Somewhat arbitrarily, hepatitis virus infections are considered "chronic" once evidence of infection exceeds 6 months in duration). While early studies suggested that persistent infection with transfusion-transmitted, non-A, non-B viruses did not lead to serious liver disease, we now know that this is not the case. Persistent HCV infection is associated with chronic liver disease of variable severity, including cirrhosis and chronic liver failure (20,21). However, there remains much to be learned of the natural history of this infection including the frequency with which serious liver disease can be expected to develop in the HCV carrier and the latent period before such disease becomes manifest. We have no understanding of the mechanisms underlying the very high rate of persistence of HCV, or why persistence should be so common with HCV and apparently nonexistent with HAV. Both are positive-strand RNA viruses, sharing substantial similarities in their genomic organization.

Viral Carcinogenesis

Finally, two of these viruses, HBV and HCV may be singled out as potentially important factors in the development of primary liver cancer. HCC is one of the most common tumors in the world and is a major cause of mortality among middle aged adult males in regions of the world (such as China) where HBV infection is endemic. In a landmark study in Taiwan, Beasley and his coworkers demonstrated that the risk of developing HCC was over 200-fold greater in persons who were carriers of HBsAg, the envelope antigen of HBV and a serum marker of viral persistence (22). The mechanism(s) by which HBV, a virus with a DNA genome which frequently becomes integrated into the host cell DNA, promotes tumor development remain uncertain. This is an area of intensive investigation. Recently, it has become evident that persistent HCV infection may also be associated with the development of HCC (23). This is a particularly intriguing observation, because HCV is an RNA virus which is not likely to replicate through a DNA intermediate nor even involve the cell nucleus in its replication scheme. The association of HCV with HCC appears to have been quite clearly demonstrated in Japan, but it remains to be shown whether this association will be found in all other HCV-infected populations.

Epidemiologic Diversity among the Hepatitis Viruses

The human hepatitis viruses exhibit a diversity of transmission mechanisms, but these two groups of viruses (HAV and HEV on the one hand, and HBV, HDV and HCV on the other), may also be separated from each other based on common patterns of transmission (Fig. 2). HAV and HEV are shed in feces, and the predominant means by which these two viruses are transmitted is the fecal-oral route (5, 24). In the case of HAV and possibly also HEV, most if not all fecally shed virus originates in the liver, from which it reaches the intestinal contents via the bile. In contrast HBV, HDV and probably HCV as well are not shed in feces and are thus not transmitted by the fecal-oral route. The most likely reason for this difference is that the lipid-containing envelopes of HBV, HCV and HDV would render these viruses subject to rapid inactivation in bile. Thus, the transmission of these latter three viruses appears to be more dependent upon the level and probably also the duration of the attendant viremia. There is as yet no evidence for replication of any of these viruses at peripheral sites which might facilitate their shedding into secretions.

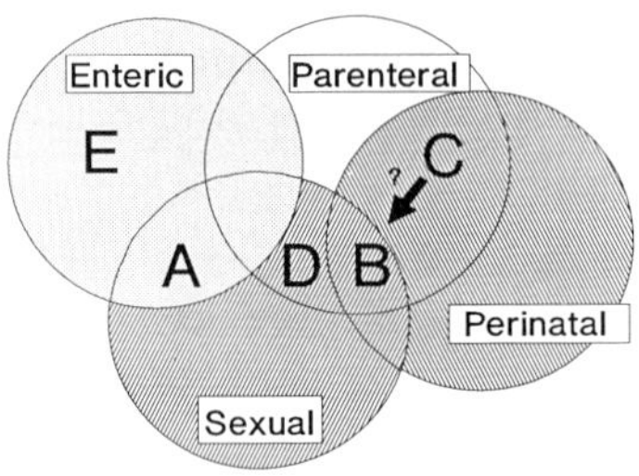

Fig. 2. Transmission patterns of hepatitis viruses

HBV, HCV, and HDV are hazards of blood transfusions and each is a common infection among needle-sharing drug addicts. Perinatal infection with HBV, very common in hepatitis B endemic regions, most likely results from maternal microtransfusion of the neonate prior to or much more often at the time of birth. However, direct percutaneous spread of HBV (including perinatal transmission) accounts for only a relatively small proportion of all HBV infections. In well developed, non-endemic countries like the United States, sexual transmission is probably the major means by which HBV is transmitted (25). Large quantities of virus may be present in the semen of HBV carriers. Worldwide, however, most HBV infections are acquired after the neonatal period but prior to adolescence (19). The mechanisms responsible for this "horizontal" transmission of HBV among relatively young children remain obscure, but may relate to the significant quantities of virus found in saliva. The quantity of HBV present in saliva appears to be related to the magnitude of viremia, which suggests that the virus is not replicated in the oropharynx (26). It is more likely that salivary shedding of HBV represents leakage of virus circulating in the blood, but this is not known for certain. The important point is that the magnitude of salivary shedding in some patients exceeds the levels of viremia in many others, and saliva has probably been underestimated as a source of virus for transmission. In several countries, however, improved economic conditions appear to have diminished the risk of horizontal transmission of HBV, raising questions as to whether western medicine (through the use of contaminated needles) may have contributed previously to horizontal spread of the virus. The precise mechanisms by which HBV is transmitted between people in the absence of sexual contact or direct percutaneous injection remain surprisingly vague.

The same may also be said for HCV. HCV infection is commonly seen in patients who have no history of blood transfusion or drug abuse, and it is fair to say that we have a great deal to learn about the epidemiology and modes of transmission of this virus. Recent evidence supports the possible sexual transmission of HCV (27) as well as HDV (28), but on a much lower scale than HBV. The relative importance of sexual transmission in the spread of these viruses has yet to be determined.

Finally, it should be mentioned that HAV has been increasingly noted to be a problem among intravenous drug users (29). There are multiple possible explanations for this, but it is likely that needle-borne transmission of HAV is at least partially responsible. We know that the viremia associated with acute HAV infection may be 3–4 weeks in duration, and that the magnitude of the viremia may be greater than that which is typically found in HCV infection (up to 10^5 infectious HAV particles per ml of serum). In addition, as with many other enterically transmitted pathogens, sexual activity may contribute to the spread of HAV by promoting fecal-oral transmission of the virus (25). Thus HAV shares at least some of the transmission mechanisms observed with HBV and the other chronic, blood-borne agents of hepatitis.

Approaches to the Control of Hepatitis Viruses

Hepatitis A – Progress and Problems in Vaccine Development

The need for control of HAV infections. Since HAV causes only acute disease and is rarely fatal, one could question the need for sophisticated approaches to the control of this virus. Indeed, within the United States and other well developed countries, HAV is generally considered to be of relatively limited public health importance. However, this somewhat narrow view overlooks the fact that the annual HAV disease burden within the United States costs in excess of US $ 200,000,000 (30). Moreover, hepatitis A is recognized to be an emerging problem in countries that are in transition from an underdeveloped to a more highly developed status (24). As public health sanitation improves in these transitional regions, the overall prevalence of HAV declines and the mean age at infection increases. However, since the severity of illness associated with HAV infection is directly related to the age of the individual, such improvements in public health sanitation may lead to paradoxical increases in the disease burden. This is probably the key factor underlying the massive outbreak of hepatitis A which occurred in Shanghai during 1988, involving over 350,000 mostly young men and women. Although an epidemic of this size represents a thankfully rare event, it underscores the importance HAV can assume in transitional regions due to its potential to cause epidemic disease, not to mention the relatively protracted nature of the resulting illness.

The molecular virology of HAV. The HAV virion is a small, spherical, nonenveloped particle containing a single-stranded, positive-sense RNA genome of approximately 7500 bases (8). By analogy with other picornaviruses, the HAV capsid consists of 60 copies of each of four (possibly three) structural proteins. The antigenic structure of the virus has been quite well characterized by the partial genomic sequencing of neutralization escape variants that have been generated by the growth of virus in the presence of monoclonal antibodies. Those antibodies recognize a series of overlapping, conformationally defined epitopes involving amino acid residues located within several surface loops of the capsid proteins VP3 and VP1 (31). Unfortunately, the highly conformational nature of these epitopes has thus far precluded most attempts to generate antigenic materials by expression from recombinant cDNA.

Genomic RNA from several HAV strains has been molecularly cloned as cDNA, and the partial or complete nucleotide sequences of a number of HAV strains have been available for several years (32). Epidemiologically diverse strains of HAV have been characterized by reverse transcription/polymerase chain reaction (RT/PCR) amplification of virus RNA present in fecal samples, followed by dideoxy sequencing of PCR amplimers. This work has led to the identification of several distinct HAV genotypes which differ at over 15% of base positions within the genome and has provided a novel view of the way in which this virus circulates within populations (33). In China, Greece and the United States, virus isolates are genetically quite closely related to each other, indicating the presence of a predominant circulating virus. In Northern Europe, however, a variety of HAV genotypes have been identified, suggesting that virus responsible for most cases may be imported from other regions.

HAV RNA shares many organizational features in common with RNA of other picornaviruses (Fig. 3). Indeed, much of what we know about the molecular biology of HAV has been extrapolated from or otherwise built upon the considerable understanding of the molecular structure and replication strategy of other picornaviruses that is enjoyed by virologists today. The first 735 bases (from the 5' end) of the viral RNA are not translated, but contain important control elements involved in replication of viral RNA and translation of viral proteins. Recent work in our laboratory suggests that this 5' nontranslated region (5'NTR) possesses a secondary structure resembling that of the 5'NTR of the murine cardioviruses (34). Additional studies suggest that the 3' half of the HAV 5'NTR contains a complex RNA structure which may function as a "ribosomal landing pad", directing the internal binding of the 40S ribosomal subunit along with putative cellular translation initiation factor(s) to a region in the viral RNA which is over 700 bases downstream of the 5' terminus.

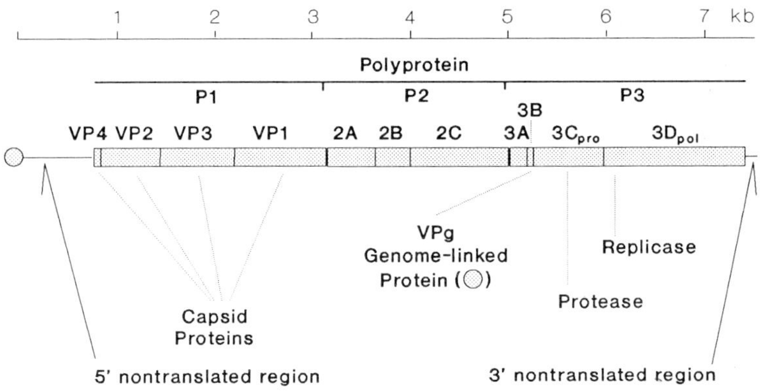

Fig. 3. Genomic organization of HAV. VPg is a small protein which is covalently linked to the 5' end of virion RNA

Translation of the RNA results in a large viral polyprotein which is encoded by a single open reading frame extending over 6500 bases (Fig. 3). This polyprotein is thought to be processed into a number of smaller proteins which are both structural (become part of the virus particle) and nonstructural (involved only in replication of the virus). For convenience, and in keeping with the nomenclature adopted for other picornaviruses, the polyprotein has been divided into three major domains: P1 (the structural proteins found in the virus capsid), P2 and P3 (both of which include nonstructural proteins essential for replication of the viral RNA). At least one protease involved in processing of the polyprotein has been identified within the P3 region ($3C^{pro}$), but most of the details of the processing of the HAV polyprotein remain to be determined. Moreover, the functions of most of the nonstructural proteins remain very obscure.

HAV is unique among all the human hepatitis viruses in that it can be propagated in conventional cell cultures (35). A variety of primate cell lines are permissive for the virus. Wild virus replicates very slowly, however, requiring several weeks to reach appreciable virus yields. There are no cytopathic effects, and the infection uniformly becomes persistent in cell culture. However, with serial passage, the virus becomes progressively adapted to growth in cell cultures. Virus which is well adapted replicates more rapidly and may induce specific cytopathic effects, but replication remains slow (requiring about 24 hrs. to reach maximum yields) and inefficient compared to the growth of poliovirus in monkey kidney cells (36). Unlike poliovirus, HAV does not induce shut-off of host cell macromolecular synthesis. The initial demonstration that HAV could be propagated in cell cultures has had an enormous impact on our ability to study this virus and has opened the way to development of conventional inactivated and attenuated vaccines.

An equally important advance came with the construction of the first infectious cDNA clone of HAV by Cohen and coworkers (37). As HAV is a positive-strand RNA virus, isolated virion RNA is infectious when transfected into permissive cells and results in virus production. Similarly, transfection of monkey kidney cells with synthetic HAV RNA transcribed in vitro from genomic-length cDNA constructs (or even transfection of the plasmid DNA itself) results in an infection from which virus may be rescued. Thus, we now have the ability to manipulate the viral genome as DNA and to determine the effect of specific mutations on virus functions. This ability to do "reverse genetics" has wide-reaching implications for our ability to characterize the attenuating mutations of HAV vaccine candidates, or even to generate new vaccine candidates by genetic engineering.

HAV vaccine development. Symptomatic hepatitis A may be prevented by passive administration of pooled immune serum globulins, but this is not practical as a general approach to control of this infection. Active immunization is the best strategy for control, and several candidate vaccines are now under development. As with hepatitis B, it is likely that a program of universal immunization will be required for ultimate control of hepatitis A.

The development of conventional formalin-inactivated vaccines for HAV has been pursued aggressively by industry following the initial practical demonstration that such a vaccine could be produced from virus propagated in cell culture (38). These inactivated vaccines are now in advanced stages of clinical testing and show promise of being both safe and very immunogenic (39). It is likely that doses of as little as 100 to 200 ng of virus antigen will suffice; a single dose of 400 ng may even provide sufficient protection for the short-term traveller who plans a trip to HAV endemic regions. The production and safety testing of these inactivated vaccines will be costly, however, and it is likely that their use will be restricted to high risk individuals in affluent societies. The present generation of inactivated HAV vaccines thus show little promise of contributing to the control of type A hepatitis in developing and transitional regions, where the need is unquestionably greatest but where only meager resources can be devoted to disease control efforts. One possible solution to this problem may be the use of HAV empty capsids which assemble in cell cultures infected with recombinant vaccinia virus expressing the Pl region of the HAV genome in addition to the $3C^{pro}$ protease. Such an approach will be economically feasible, however, only if it is shown that such capsids have antigenicity and stability comparable to virus produced in HAV infected cultures and that greater production efficiencies can be achieved during scale-up to industrial level production.

In addition to cost, a major concern is the duration of protective immunity that may be achieved by administration of inactivated vaccines. While this is not yet known, anything less than very long-term immunity may not benefit developing nations. The risk and severity of associated disease is directly related to age at acquisition of HAV infection (24). Use of a vaccine which provides even 10–20 years of protection against HAV infection in a developing region may lead only to an increase in the mean age at infection and possibly a paradoxical worsening of the HAV disease burden. Moreover, the duration of immunity achieved by an inactivated vaccine is likely to be related to the magnitude of the initial antibody response, which in turn is related to the amount of antigen per dose and number of doses administered. Thus, those inactivated vaccines providing the longest lasting immunity will be the most expensive to produce and administer, and thus the least available to developing nations. However, it should be emphasized that the length of protection afforded by immunization with inactivated HAV antigen is yet to be determined. It is possible that the lengthy incubation period associated with HAV infection may allow anamnestic antibody responses to be protective. If this is the case, immunologic memory (even in the absence of detectable levels of antibodies to the virus) may result in continuing protection against symptomatic infection, making the major barriers to use of inactivated vaccines cost and the need for multiple doses. Both of these variables might be favorably influenced by the use of novel vaccine formulations allowing for delayed release of antigen or the use of new adjuvants.

Since the future of inactivated vaccines for prevention of hepatitis A in the developing world remains uncertain, the development of a safe and immunogenic attenuated HAV vaccine is an attractive goal. In theory, an attenuated HAV vaccine could be less expensive to produce, could be effective with single dose administration, and could provide long-lasting, perhaps life-long, immunity such as that which follows infection with wild-type virus. Efforts to develop attenuated HAV vaccines have focused on the use of virus variants that have been adapted to growth in either continuous monkey kidney cells or human lung fibroblasts (12). Such virus variants have been shown to be attenuated in susceptible primates as well as in limited human clinical trials. However, these variants have relatively poor immunogenicity, inducing only low levels of antibody which in some cases may not be evident until several months after parenteral injection (40, 41). Less highly passaged virus may be more immunogenic, but likely to be significantly hepatovirulent. Thus, cell culture adaptation appears to have led to reduced viral replication within the hepatocyte and less disease, but there are as yet no candidate vaccine strains which have been shown clearly to have an acceptable balance between infectivity (that is, immunogenicity) and attenuation. Although an attenuated vaccine has had extensive clinical testing in China within the past few years (42), this virus is shed in the feces of some immunized persons. Its overall safety is not well documented as the capacity for reversion to virulence is not known.

At the molecular level, the genetic changes associated with attenuation and adaptation and passage of HAV in cell culture have been studied in several laboratories. Although we have shown that certain mutations within the 5'NTR of the genome are frequently present in cell culture adapted variants and contribute to the ability of these variants to replicate in monkey kidney cell cultures (43, 44), the limited data that are currently available suggest that it is the 2B/2C region of the genome that is most directly involved in determining the attenuation phenotype of the HM175 strain HAV vaccine candidate (45). The apparent lack of involvement of the HAV 5'NTR in determining the attenuation phenotype contrasts sharply with evidence that the 5'NTR sequences of poliovirus, mengovirus and foot-and-mouth virus play important roles in defining attenuation phenotypes of these other picornaviruses. We suspect that greater attention will focus on the 5'NTR of HAV in the characterization and possibly even genetic engineering of attenuated HAV vaccine candidates in the future.

Hepatitis B Virus – a Need for Less Expensive Vaccines

Worldwide status of hepatitis B. The prevalence of HBV infections varies widely among different regions of the world, with the highest rates of past and current infection found in East Asia and Sub-Saharan Africa. In addition to the morbidity and occasional mortality associated with acute hepatitis B, chronic infection may lead to cirrhosis and hepatocarcinogenesis. In regions where HBV carrier rates are high (in some regions up to 15–20% of adults), HCC is one of the most common malignant tumors. In less endemic regions, HBV remains a major cause of morbidity and an occasional cause of mortality. Within the United States, where less than 1% of the general population tests positive for HBsAg and where less than 10% has serologic evidence of previous HBV infection, HBV is common in certain high risk groups such as promiscuous male homosexuals and needle-sharing drug users (46). In addition, the relatively high carrier rate found in certain ethnic groups overseas remains present in at least the first generation of immigrants to the U.S., thereby adding to the overall burden of HBV infections. In 1985, it was estimated that the overall annual cost of hepatitis B infections in the U.S. approximated $ 300,000,000, half of which was considered to be vaccine preventable (30).

Hepatitis B virus. The application of modern molecular techniques has contributed dramatically to our understanding of the pathobiology of HBV, including the replication strategy of this virus. This level of knowledge is all the more remarkable because of the continuing absence of widely available, conventional cell culture systems allowing the propagation of this virus.

HBV is an hepadnavirus (47). The virion is a double-shelled structure with a lipid-containing surface envelope surrounding a well-defined core particle. This envelope contains the three glycosylated surface antigens of the virus: the major determinant (the S protein, or HBsAg) and two other C-terminally identical proteins, pre-S1 and pre-S2. The core contains multiple copies of an antigenically distinct core protein (HBcAg), a partially double-stranded, circular DNA genome, held together by overlapping 5' termini and a DNA polymerase activity necessary for viral replication. This DNA is converted to a covalently closed, approximately 3200 base pair, fully double-stranded form (supercoiled DNA) following penetration and uncoating of the virus. Within this DNA genome are four large open reading frames, present in all three potential reading frames and overlaping with each other extensively: these encode the surface proteins (pre-S1, pre-S2, and S), the core protein, the polymerase, and a small protein known as "X". Thus most bases in the genome encode two proteins, in two different reading frames, resulting in extraordinarily efficient use of the viral DNA.

Genomic replication proceeds with transcription of the supercoiled DNA to a greater than genomic length RNA species, the "pregenome", which becomes packaged in nascent core particles (7, 47). This RNA subsequently undergoes reverse transcription under direction of the polymerase to yield a negative-strand DNA, from which the positive strand is subsequently copied. In the process, all of the RNA pregenome is degraded with the exception of a small oligoribonucleotide found at the 5' terminus of the positive DNA strand, and which apparently serves as primer for this strand. From this brief outline of the replication strategy of HBV, it can be appreciated that this DNA virus shares several features in common with the retroviruses. Many further details of the replication cycle are known, some of which are relevant to mechanisms of disease production but are beyond the scope of this discussion. These may be found elsewhere (47).

Antiviral therapy for HBV. Despite a considerable number of clinical trials involving a variety of potential antiviral agents, only interferon has shown promise as a therpy for chronic HBV infection. The response to interferon is limited, however, and its use in HBV carriers with chronic hepatitis has not achieved general acceptance. Considerable industry interest now focuses on the use of nucleoside analogs as potential anti-hepadnaviral agents, and it is likely that progress will be made in this area in the next several years. This research in this field has been accelerated by the development of screening assays involving HBV DNA-transfected cell cultures, and continuing progress in elucidating the replication cycle of HBV.

Immunization against HBV. The first effective immunization against HBV was provided to at-risk children by Krugman and co-workers in the 1960s (48). Serum from children known to be infected with HBV was briefly boiled to inactivate the virus and used as a crude vaccine. The protective immunity which followed administration of this vaccine firmly established the principle that circulating viral antigens may serve as useful immunogens. This initial observation was followed by the development of very effective and safe plasma-derived vaccines containing the envelope antigen, HBsAg, in more or less pure forms (49, 50). Although discovery of the human immunodeficiency virus (HIV) raised fears concerning the possibility that these plasma-derived HBV vaccines might be contaminated with HIV, undoubtedly slowing the distribution of HBV vaccine, these fears proved unfounded. Moreover, any residual concerns were laid to rest by the subsequent development of HBsAg vaccines produced from recombinant DNA in yeast (51, 52). Although the HBsAg contained in the recombinant vaccines is not glycosylated and consists of the 22,000 dalton S protein only, the plasma-derived and recombinant immunogens are indistinguishable from each other in practice. Both vaccines are safe and highly immunogenic, particularly in very young children. A recent study has suggested that an extensive immunization program in The Gambia has reduced the carrier prevalence among young children (53). However, the development of effective vaccines for hepatitis B has done relatively little to change the burden of HBV-related disease in most countries. Why is this?

In the United States, the introduction of HBV vaccine in 1982 was followed over several years by a slight *increase* in the reported incidence of hepatitis B. By 1990 it became apparent that the chosen strategy of targeting immunization to high risk individuals (that is health care workers, homosexual men, infants born to HBsAg-positive mothers, etc.) would not be effective in reducing the overall disease burden. Most individuals at risk for the infection were not being identified or immunized, even with the recommended screening of pregnant women thought to be likely carriers of HBsAg. This realization has prompted a recent reorientation of the vaccine program towards a strategy of universal immunization. While it is too early to see if this will result in improved control of hepatitis B infection in the U.S., it is very likely to do so over time. The major limitations to achievement of universal immunization remain the relatively high cost of the vaccine and the perceptions of the medical profession and public concerning the cost vs. benefit of immunization.

The immunization strategy in more endemic regions of the world is much the same and is jeopardized by similar constraints. In HBV endemic regions, a relatively small proportion of children are infected at birth (usually less than 20%, consistent with the HBsAg carrier rate among pregnant women) while the remainder of the population is generally infected during childhood and early adolescence (19). Nonetheless, infants born to HBV infected mothers should be the prime targets for immunization in such regions, as these infants almost always become long-term carriers of the virus and thus represent the major reservoir for maintenance of the virus in the population. Given with hyperimmune globulin at birth, HBV vaccine is very effective at preventing neonatal infection (52). The ideal strategy would be to immunize all newborns regardless of the serologic status of the mother. Such an approach not only obviates the need for serological screening of pregnant women but also protects the vast majority of children from infection later in childhood. It may still be necessary to screen mothers, however, if newborns are to benefit from administration of hyperimmune globulin.

The possibility of successfully implementing a universal vaccine policy is dependent upon the cost of vaccine and the resources available to a society for this purpose. In well-to-do countries that have high HBV infection rates (e.g., Singapore and Japan), a strategy of multiple doses of vaccine given to all children beginning at birth may be reasonably achieved. However, given the relatively high cost of vaccine, this strategy is not yet possible in most highly endemic regions. Hope may be on the horizon, however, as the cost of vaccine has fallen substantially in recent years and may be expected to continue to drop with larger scales of production and the introduction to the market place of multiple competing manufacturers. In fact, the cost has recently reached the point where inclusion of this vaccine in multiple national programs may soon become a reality. Much more work is needed, however, on the development of

HBV vaccines formulated for delayed-release and capable of single dose immunization. Such vaccines would greatly reduce the costs of immunization. Better adjuvants that are safe for humans would also benefit hepatitis B immunization programs enormously. However, the development of safe and effective, replicating vector vaccines for hepatitis B, based possibly on recombinant poxviruses, adenovirus, or even picornaviruses such as poliovirus, may be needed to achieve a vaccine sufficiently inexpensive to permit its use in the poorest of endemic countries.

Will it ever be possible to eradicate hepatitis B? Effective immunization of all newborns will dramatically diminish the carrier prevalence in the next generation. With continuing immunization programs carried out over a period of multiple generations HBV would eventually become a very rare infection indeed. It remains to be seen, however, whether such a strategy could ever lead to elimination of the virus. We should not be too complacent about the future of HBV control, however, as there has been a recent report of breakthrough infection in immunized children born to HBV carrier mothers. Virus recovered from the infants has been shown to have an apparent amino acid substitution within the S antigen molecule. It remains to be seen, however, whether this virus is a true neutralization escape mutant, and whether this problem represents a significant threat to immunization programs.

HCC associated with HBV. Several mechanisms have been proposed as possible explanations for hepatocarcinogenesis associated with HBV infection (54). One general theory is that immunologically mediated liver damage, caused by cytotoxic lymphocytes or antibodies reacting to virus-specified proteins expressed by infected hepatocytes, results in a secondary regeneration of hepatocytes that leads to or otherwise promotes tumor development. According to this theory, the development of HCC reflects the inflammation accompanying HBV infection, rather than a direct tumor promoting effect of any virus gene product. There are good data to support such a model, including the development of carcinoma in transgenic mice that develop hepatocellular cytopathology due to overexpression of an HBV pre-S1 transgene (55). However, there is also support for a direct role played by one HBV gene product, the HBV X protein. This protein appears to be involved in the regulation of HBV replication, as it has the ability to transactivate a variety of heterologous promoters (56) and could possibly be involved in tumor production through the transactivation of a cellular proto-oncogene. These two very different mechanisms of hepatocarcinogenesis are not mutually exclusive, however, and it is possible that both play a role in causing liver cancer in HBV infected persons. In addition, HBV DNA frequently integrates into cellular DNA during chronic infection, and it is conceivable that HBV DNA integrations could lead to loss of normal control of hepatocyte growth and differentiation. However, insertional mutagenesis does not seem likely to play a major role because the location of HBV insertions within the host genome varies widely among those tumors which contain HBV DNA (about 70% of all tumors), arguing against a specific integration associated with tumor development. Finally, it should be noted that mutations are frequently present in the p53 tumor supressor gene in HCC tissue.

In some countries with high prevalences of HBV infection, considerable efforts have been expended on developing sensitive screening methods for early detection of liver cancer. These methods have included the measurement of serum levels of alpha fetoprotein as a tumor marker. Early partial hepatectomy may be curative in a fraction of cases, and thus such screening programs may be useful among known HBV carriers. However, prevention of the primary infection by immunization, as described above, offers a much more attractive and cost-effective strategy to the control of this malignancy. It is likely that HCC will be shown to be the first vaccine-preventable malignancy.

Hepatitis D Virus – Multiple Functions of the Delta Antigen

Hepatitis delta virus and delta hepatitis. HDV is an unclassified satellite virus of HBV. The viral particle, which is 35 nm in diameter, contains a unique RNA and a single virus-specified protein, hepatitis delta antigen (HDAg) (57–59). HDV RNA and HDAg are packaged within a lipid envelope containing HBsAg, the envelope antigen of HBV. Significant replication of HDV occurs only in persons who are also infected with HBV and is often associated with an aggressive chronic hepatitis which may lead to cirrhosis and death (14, 60). HDV also replicates in woodchuck carriers of woodchuck hepatitis virus (WHV), thus providing a useful animal model of delta infection. Recombinant interferon-α has shown promise in the treatment of chronic delta hepatitis, but side effects are common and relapses are frequent (61). There is a need for alternative treatment approaches.

In recent years, a considerable body of knowledge has accumulated concerning the unusual life cycle of HDV. The HDV genome, among the smallest of all animal virus genomes, has been molecularly cloned, and the complete nucleotide sequence of several HDV strains has been determined. The viral RNA is a single-stranded, circular molecule approximately 1700 bases in length and with a G+C content of 60%. Under native conditions, it assumes a rod-like, double-stranded structure due to extensive (up to 67%) intramolecular base pairing (62). Although both genomic and antigenomic RNA contain multiple open reading frames, the available evidence suggests that only one of these is actually expressed during delta infection (63). This open reading frame is present in antigenomic RNA and potentially encodes HDAg species of 195 or 214 amino acids, depending on the variable presence of an amber stop codon at position 196. Two antigenically similar forms of HDAg which differ in their migration characteristics in SDS-PAGE electrophoresis ($p24^d$ and $p27^d$) are found within the virus particle. We have recently confirmed that the large form of HDAg ($p27^d$) possesses a unique carboxy-terminal amino acid sequence, as predicted by nucleotide sequence microheterogeneity present in the open reading frame. HDAg forms dimers in vivo and appears to have RNA-binding activity that is specific for HDV RNA.

Replication of HDV RNA occurs within the nucleus of infected hepatocytes and has been shown to initiate within cells transfected with HDV cDNA (or RNA) in the absence of HBV gene products (64). Thus we know that the essential helper functions of HBV do not extend to replication of RNA and are probably limited to the provision of the HBsAg-containing envelope.

One of the most striking features of HDV is that both genomic and antigenomic RNAs are catalytically active and capable of self-cleavage and ligation under appropriate conditions (9). This activity resembles the ribozyme activity of the replicating RNA viroids of plants, but appears to be dependent upon an alternative RNA secondary structure. The ribozyme cleavage sites of HDV RNA are near one end of the double-stranded rod-like structure, within a region of the genome (the "viroid-like" domain) which is distinct from that encoding HDAg. HDV RNA probably replicates via a rolling-circle mechanism, with ribozyme directed cleavage and ligation playing important roles in the process. However, Taylor and his colleagues have elegantly demonstrated that efficient replication of HDV RNA is dependent upon expression of the small component of HDAg ($p24^d$) (64). While the polymerase directing RNA replication is not known, $p24^d$ is a relatively small protein and lacks homology with any known RNA polymerase. Thus, the current thinking is that a cellular polymerase (perhaps RNA polymerase II) directs replication of the viral RNA. It may be that p24d interacts with the cellular RNA polymerase complex to alter its template specificity from DNA to RNA. Unlike $p24^d$, however, $p27^d$ is a dominant negative regulator of HDV RNA replication (65). Its expression may play an important role in control of virus replication and assembly.

Towards the control of delta hepatitis. Is it possible that some of this recent knowledge may be put to use in designing new strategies for the control of HDV? We can already immunize against HDV by administering HBV vaccine to susceptible individuals, as in the absence of HBV infection there will be no HDV disease. However, what about the HBV carrier who is already at risk for delta infection? Unfortunately, attempts to immunize hepadnavirus susceptible animals with recombinant HDAg have not succeeded in producing the kind of protective immunity one might have hoped for against HDV. Indeed, the immunized animals appear to have had an exaggerated disease course following challenge with HDV (suggesting, parenthetically, an immunopathologic basis for delta hepatitis). It might be that protective immunity could eventually be generated by specific HDAg segments, but this has yet to be studied.

What, then, about the potential for antiviral therapy? As described above, recombinant interferon-α may have some benefits but also has its problems. Long-term treatment is required, side-effects are significant, and relapses appear common. Specific antiviral therapy directed against HBV replication (were it available) might not have much of an effect on HDV disease, as HBsAg expression may be directed by HBV DNA integrated into cellular chromosomes and this may be the only HBV gene product required for HDV replication. Little or no effort has been spent thus far in attempts to develop effective antiviral strategies for delta hepatitis, but several possibilities are suggested by our increasing understanding of HDV. As described above, HDAg expression is a prerequisite to efficient viral RNA replication, and to function properly HDAg must interact with a number of macromolecules: other HDAg molecules, nuclear transport proteins, HDV RNA, and possibly cellular RNA polymerase complexes. Interference with any of these virus-specific macromolecular interactions could be expected to greatly attenuate viral replication. The RNA replication down-regulating activity of $p27^d$ may itself be a clue to a novel antiviral strategy. In addition, transfection systems which mimic the molecular events in HDV RNA replication are available and could be used for in vitro screening of candidate antivirals. Delta hepatitis is an orphan disease, however, and it is unlikely that any major pharmaceutical manufacturer will invest the resources that would be required for such an effort.

Hepatitis C Virus – a New Agent Revealed by Molecular Biology

During the 1970s, cases of post-transfusion hepatitis were recognized which serologically were not due to infection with either HAV or HBV (3). These cases of "non-A, non-B" (NANB) hepatitis were thought to be due to infection with an as yet unidentified hepatotropic virus. Chimpanzee studies of NANB hepatitis suggested that an etiologic agent of NANB hepatitis was inactivated by chloroform treatment and could pass through an 80-nm sharp cutoff membrane filter (66). This work suggested the possibility that the agent of NANB hepatitis was a small, enveloped virus.

This major agent of NANB hepatitis (HCV) was subsequently identified through the combined efforts of investigators who focused on a meticulous series of experimental chimpanzee infections carried out over a number of years and molecular biologists who persevered in their efforts to identify the nucleic acid associated with this virus despite many early setbacks (11). Ultimately, chimpanzee plasma containing a high infectious titer of virus was used as a source of viral RNA to construct a cDNA library in phage λ-gt11. Approximately one million recombinant phage were screened for the expression of viral antigen, using as a probe antibodies from a chronic NANB hepatitis patient. This work resulted in the identification of a single positive cDNA clone which was then used to identify other overlapping clones. The cDNA, encoding part of a viral antigen, was inserted into a plasmid containing the human superoxide dismutase (SOD) gene and expressed in yeast as a fusion polypeptide. An assay for detecting antibodies to this polypeptide was developed (67), paving the way for the licensed diagnostic tests for antibody to HCV that are currently available.

The complete nucleotide sequence of several different strains of HCV have since been published (68). The virus, a positive-strand RNA virus, possesses a genome of approximately 10 kilobases (Fig. 4). Analysis of this RNA indicates the presence of a 341 nucleotide 5' nontranslated region (5' NTR), a 9033 nucleotide open reading frame, and a 27 nucleotide 3' untranslated region (69). The 5' NTR is strongly conserved between differ-

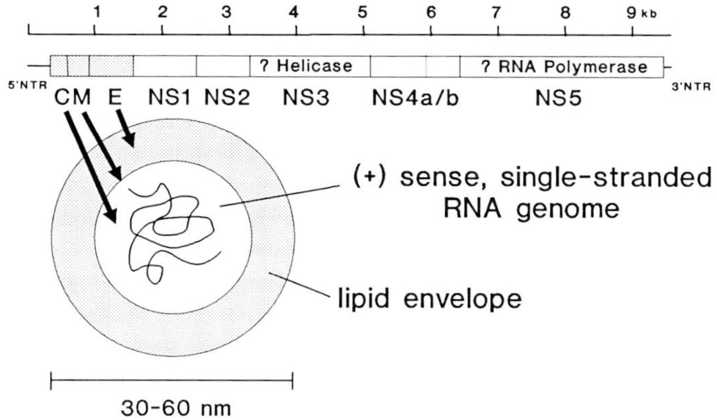

Fig. 4. Genomic organization of HCV. While NSl is a nonstructural protein in the flaviviruses (despite its ability to elicit protective immunity), it may be a structural component of the HCV particle

ent HCV isolates. The extreme 5' end is (G+C)-rich and is predicted to form a hairpin structure. This region of the genome is more similar to the 5' NTR of pestiviruses, as the 5' NTRs of flaviviruses are significantly shorter than that found in HCV. The large open reading frame encodes a 3011 amino acid polyprotein, with the coding regions for structural proteins (nucleocapsid, membrane protein, and major envelope protein) located 5' of a series of nonstructural proteins. One nonstructural protein (NS3) contains a domain that is consistent with a NTP-binding activity, while another protein appears to be a trypsin-like serine protease. Further downstream in the region that corresponds to NS5 is a region that may encode an RNA-dependent RNA polymerase (68). The genetic organization of HCV is most similar to that of the pestiviruses and the flaviviruses.

Sequence heterogeneity at the nucleotide level has been demonstrated among different strains of HCV. Strains collected from Japanese patients are more closely related to each other than they are to strains isolated from American patients, but there appear to be particular "hot spots" within the structural proteins where there is a great deal of sequence heterogeneity. These domains have been shown to change over time even among isolates from the same patient (70).

Clinically, HCV is responsible for the majority of cases of post-transfusion NANB hepatitis. It causes a chronic infection in approximately 50% of cases (20, 21). Chronic HCV infection can progress to hepatic cirrhosis, and recent evidence has associated HCV infection with the development of HCC. However, the frequency with which each of these events occurs is not clear and will require considerable study in different populations. Several studies have shown that longterm therapy with interferon-α results in chemical and histologic improvement in chronic hepatitis C, but the impact on life expectancy and the overall course of the disease remains unclear (71).

Most Japanese patients with HCC who are HBsAg-negative have serum markers of HCV infection; the HCV seroprevalence rate in this group is greater than among other Japanese of similar age (23). This association between HCV and liver cancer exists primarily in males. The pathogenesis of HCV-induced liver cancer remains very obscure, but it is possible that cancer development may reflect chronic inflammation and hepatocyte death and regeneration, as suggested for HBV-related liver cancer. Perinatal HCV infections have been described recently, in which the infant remains viremic for many months after birth, but fails to develop antibodies detectable by solid-phase immunoassay. The reasons underlying this phenonemon and its clinical significance remain to be determined. Much more work needs to be done to define the natural history of this infection.

Improved methods for serodiagnosis of HCV infections (so-called "second generation assays") are already being developed. These assays, which employ several different antigens from the HCV polyprotein (recombinant and synthetic peptides), have both improved sensitivity and specificity compared with the current, commercially available immunoassays. One difficulty in determining the sensitivity and specificity of an assay for HCV, however, is the lack of a "gold standard". The current gold standard is the demonstration of HCV nucleic acid in a serum sample by means of RT/PCR amplification. However, the use of PCR as a diagnostic assay is fraught with the possibility of false positive test results due to contamination of test samples or reaction mixes with viral RNA or plasmid DNA. In a setting where the risk of contamination is minimized, PCR can be used with DNA hybridization to demonstrate the presence of HCV nucleic acid. Alternatively, nested PCR, involving two rounds of PCR amplification with different sets of primers, can demonstrate amplified PCR products without the need for radionuclides (72). The use of primers derived from the 5' NTR region reduces the risk of false-negative PCR due to primer base mismatches, but does not totally exclude this possibility. The need for alternative, simpler diagnostic assays is obvious.

We have a long way to go before we will know the best strategies for control of HCV, or even how important such control might be. Further knowledge of conserved and non-conserved regions of the envelope protein may enable the design of a protective vaccine against this virus. The functions of the relatively lengthy 5' NTR, a highly conserved region, remain to be elucidated, but it is tempting to speculate that this region has functions similar to the HAV 5' NTR. If so, it may be a potential target for rational drug design or molecular approaches to vaccine development at some future date, although this is purely speculative. And finally, the association of chronic HCV infection with HCC may ultimately be a clue to a better understanding of the molecular basis of hepatocarcinogenesis. This virus, the first human pathogen to be discovered by a well thought out molecular cloning scheme, promises to be a fertile ground for further investigation.

Hepatitis E Virus

Hepatitis E virus (HEV) rounds out the alphabet soup of the hepatitis viruses. This agent was recognized in the 1970's as a cause of massive outbreaks of viral hepatitis in the Indian subcontinent that often appeared due to waterborne spread of virus – hence the term "epidemic NANB" or "waterborne NANB" hepatitis (73). The most striking of these outbreaks was that which occurred in Delhi in 1955, causing over 30,000 cases of jaundice (74). This outbreak was clearly associated with lapses in the quality of water supplies. The HEV particle was identified by immune electron microscopy in 1983 when it was also shown that cynomologus monkeys were susceptible to this virus and could be used as a model of the human infection (5). Since those early days, we have come to realize that HEV occurs in a worldwide distribution, with sporadic outbreaks identified in underdeveloped countries of both hemispheres. Isolates from Mexico and Burma appear to be antigenically closely related, if not identical.

In recent years, the genome of several HEV strains has been molecularly cloned and fully sequenced, opening the door to what will undoubtedly be a wealth of new and potentially very valuable information (75). The genome is positive-stranded RNA, about 7.5 kb in length, and thus similar in size and type to that of HAV. However, the genomic organization is remarkably different. The 5' end contains only a very short, nontranslated leader, followed by two open reading frames separated by only forty nucleotides. The most 5' of these reading frames appears to encode several nonstructural proteins, while the other encodes a single large protein of about 70,000 daltons. This is probably the major capsid protein, and recent evidence suggests that it may contain antigenic determinants that are useful in solid-phase immunoassays for HEV antibodies. There is a third, shorter reading frame which overlaps these other two reading frames centrally and which also appears to be expressed during infection. HEV is thus a novel RNA virus which has been suggested to be a member of the calicivirus family. Very recent evidence suggests that its genomic organization is similar to that of the Norwalk agent, a gastroenteritis virus originally described in North America.

Clinically, HEV causes only acute hepatitis and like HAV has not been associated with chronic liver disease. Unlike HAV, however, HEV tends to cause severe, often fatal, acute infections in pregnant women (15, 73). The reasons underlying this tendency remain completely unknown but are a focus of investigation. The epidemiology of HEV is also puzzling. Its potential for waterborne spread suggests that the virus may be relatively stable in the environment. However, the extent of the epidemics of HEV described in many developing regions suggests that population immunity may be relatively low. Whether this is due to the length of immunity following infection (which is brief in Norwalk virus infections) or simply to a low overall prevalence of HEV in these regions remains to be determined. It is difficult- to understand why infection with this virus, which has such a clearly documented potential for epidemic spread, would not be highly prevalent in regions of the world with poor sanitation and, for example, a high prevalence of HAV infection. Yet a third possibility which must be considered is that HEV is capable of undergoing significant antigenic variation. However, although our understanding of the virus is limited, there is as yet no evidence to support significant antigenic variability among HEV isolates.

The answers to these and many other questions will undoubtedly be forthcoming in the next few years. New antibody assays, based upon use of recombinant antigens or synthetic peptides may reveal unknown aspects of the epidemiology of the agent and may open avenues to vaccine development. Moreover, informal reports are already circulating concerning the propagation of this agent in cell culture. If true, this would represent a major step toward understanding the antigenic nature of the virus (as it has for hepatitis A) and developing an effective vaccine. Thus, scientific progress is likely to be excellent in the next few years. The major impediment to vaccine development may well be the fact that HEV is not present in well developed countries with the technological facilities for sophisticated vaccine development, and thus the development of an HEV vaccine has little commercial attractiveness.

References

1. Blumberg BS, Alter HJ, Visnich S (1965) A "new" antigen in leukemia sera. JAMA 191: 541–546
2. Feinstone SM, Kapikian AZ, Purcell RH (1973) Hepatitis A: detection by immune electron microscopy of a viruslike antigen associated with acute illness. Science 182: 1026–1028
3. Feinstone SM, Kapikian AZ, Purcell RH, Alter HJ, Holland PV (1975) Transfusion-associated hepatitis not due to viral hepatitis type A or B. N Engl J Med 292 :767–770
4. Rizzetto M, Canese MG, Arico S, et al (1977) Immunofluorescence detection of new antigen-antibodysystem (d/anti-d) associated to hepatitis B virus in liver and in serum of HBsAg carriers. Gut 18: 997–1003
5. Balayan MS, Andzhaparidze AG, Savinskaya SS, et al (1983) Evidence for a virus in non-A, non-B hepatitis transmitted via the fecal-oral route. Intervirology 20: 23–31
6. McAleer WJ, Buynak EB, Maigetter RZ, Wampler DE, Miller WJ, Hilleman MR (1984) Human hepatitis B vaccine from recombinant yeast. Nature 307: 178–180
7. Summers J, Mason WS (1982) Replication of the genome of a hepatitis B-like virus by reverse transcription of an RNA intermediate. Cell 29: 403–415
8. Cohen JI, Ticehurst JR, Furcell RH, Buckler-White A, Baroudy BM (1987) Complete nucleotide sequence of wild-type hepatitis A virus: comparison with different strains of hepatitis A virus and other picornaviruses. J Virol 61: 50–59
9. Sharmeen L, Kuo MYP, Dinter-Gottlieb G, Taylor J (1988) Antigenomic RNA of human hepatitis delta virus can undergo self-cleavage. J Virol 62: 2674–2679
10. Branch AD, Benenfeld BJ, Baroudy BM, Wells FV, Gerin JL, Robertson HD (1989) An ultraviolet-sensitive RNA structural element in a viroid-like domain of the hepatitis delta virus. Science 243: 649–652
11. Choo Q-L, Kuo G, Weiner AJ, Overby LR, Bradley DW, Houghton M (1989) Isolation of a cDNA clone derived from a blood-borne non-A, non-B viral hepatitis genome. Science 244: 359–362
12. Siegl G, Lemon SM (1990) Recent advances in hepatitis A vaccine development. Virus Res 17: 75–92

13. Di Bisceglie AM, Rustgi VK, Hoofnagle JH, Dusheiko GM, Lotze MT (1988) HCC. Ann Intern Med 108: 390–401
14. De Cock KM, Govindarajan S, Chin KP, Redeker AG (1986) Delta hepatitis in the Los Angeles area: a report of 126 cases. Ann Intern Med 105: 108–114
15. Khuroo MS, Teli MR, Skidmore S, Sofi MA, Khuroo MI (1981) Incidence and severity of viral hepatitis in pregnancy. Am J Med 70: 252–255
16. Mondelli M, Mieli Vergani G, Alberti A, et al (1982) Specificity of T lymphocyte cytotoxicity to autologous hepatocytes in chronic hepatitis B virus infection: evidence that T cells are directed against HBV core antigen expressed on hepatocytes. J Immunol 129: 2773–2778
17. Moriyama T, Guilhot S, Klopchin K, et al (1991) Immunobiology and pathogenesis of hepatocellular injury in hepatitis B virus transgenic mice. Science 252: 361–364
18. Vallbracht A, Maier K, Stierhof Y-D, Wiedmann KH, Flehmig B, Fleischer B (1989) Liver-derived cytotoxic T cells in hepatitis A virus infection. J Infect Dis 160: 209–217
19. Davis LG, Weber DJ, Lemon SM (1989) Horizontal transmission of hepatitis B virus. Lancet i: 889–893
20. Hopf U, Muller B, Kother D, et al (1990) Long-term follow-up of posttransfusion and sporadic chronic hepatitis non-A, non-B and frequency of circulating antibodies to hepatitis C virus (HCV). J Hepatol 10: 69–76
21. Alter HJ, Purcell RH, Shih JW, et al (1989) Detection of antibody to hepatitis C virus in prospectively followed transfusion recipients with acute and chronic non-A, non-B hepatitis. N Engl J Med 321: 1494–1500
22. Beasley RP, Hwang L-Y, Lin C-C, Chien C-S (1981) HCC and hepatitis B virus: a prospective study of 22 707 men in Taiwan. Lancet ii: 1129–1133
23. Saito I, Miyamura T, Ohbayashi A, et al (1991) Hepatitis C virus infection is associated with the development of HCC. Proc Natl Acad Sci USA 87: 6547–6549
24. Lemon SM (1985) Type A viral hepatitis: new developments in an old disease. N Engl J Med 313: 1059–1067
25. Lemon SM, Newbold JE (1990) Viral hepatitis. In: Holmes KK, Mardh PA, Sparling PF, et al (eds) Sexually Transmitted Diseases. New York, McGraw-Hill, 449–466
26. Jenison SA, Lemon SM, Baker LN, Newbold JE (1987) Quantitative analysis of hepatitis B virus DNA in saliva and semen of chronically infected homosexual men. J Infect Dis 156: 299–307
27. Tedder RS, Gilson RJC, Briggs M, et al (1991) Hepatitis C virus: Evidence for sexual transmission. Br Med J 302: 1299–1302
28. Solomon RE, Kaslow RA, Phair JP, et al (1988) Human immunodeficiency virus and hepatitis delta virus in homosexual men: a study of four cohorts. Ann Intern Med 108: 51–54
29. Centers for Disease Control (1988) Hepatitis A among drug abusers. MMWR 37: 297–305
30. Institute of Medicine (1985) New vaccine development: establishing priorities. Diseases of importance in the United States, Vol 1. Washington, D.C.
31. Ping L-H, Jansen RW, Stapleton JT, Cohen JI, Lemon SM (1988) Identification of an immunodominant antigenic site involving the capsid protein VP3 of hepatitis A virus. Proc Natl Acad Sci USA 85: 8281–8285
32. Ticehurst JR, Cohen JI, Feinstone SM, Purcell RH, Jansen RW, Lemon SM (1989) Replication of hepatitis A virus: new ideas from studies with cloned cDNA. In: Ehrenfeld E, Semler BL (eds) Molecular aspects of picornavirus infection and detection. Washington, D.C., ASM Press, 27–50
33. Jansen RW, Siegl G, Lemon SM (1990) Molecular epidemiology of human hepatitis A virus defined by an antigen-capture polymerase chain reaction method. Proc Natl Acad Sci USA 87: 2867–2871
34. Brown EA, Day SP, Jansen RW, Lemon SM (1992) The 5' nontranslated region of hepatitis A virus: secondary structure and elements required for translation in vitro. J Virol, in press
35. Provost PJ, Hilleman MR (1979) Propagation of human hepatitis A virus in cell culture in vitro. Proc Soc Exp Biol Med 160: 213–221

36. Cromeans T, Fields HA, Sobsey MD (1989) Replication kinetics and cytopathic effect of hepatitis A virus. J Gen Virol 70: 2051–2062
37. Cohen JI, Ticehurst JR, Feinstone SM, Rosenblum B, Purcell RH (1987) Hepatitis A virus cDNA and its RNA transcripts are infectious in cell culture. J Virol 1: 3035–3039
38. Binn LN, Bancroft WH, Lemon SM, et al (1986) Preparation of a prototype inactivated hepatitis A virus vaccine from infected cell cultures. J Infect Dis 153: 749–756
39. Andre FE, Hepburn A, D'Hondt E (1990) Inactivated candidate vaccines for hepatitis A. Prog Med Virol 37: 72–95
40. Provost PJ, Bishop RP, Gerety RJ, et al (1986) New findings in live, attenuated hepatitis A vaccine development. J Med Virol 20: 165–175
41. Midthun K, Ellerbeck E, Gershman K, et al (1991) Safety and immunogenicity of a live, attenuated hepatitis A vaccine in seronegative volunteers. J Infect Dis 163: 735–739
42. Mao JS, Dong DX, Zhang HY, et al (1989) Primary study of attenuated live hepatitis A vaccine (H2 strain) in humans. J Infect Dis 159: 621–624
43. Jansen RW, Newbold JE,Lemon SM (1988) Complete nucleotide sequence of a cell culture-adapted variant of hepatitis A virus: comparison with wild-type virus with restricted capacity for in vitro replication. Virology 163: 299–307
44. Day SP, Lemon SM (1990) A single base mutation in the 5' noncoding region of HAV enhances replication of virus in vitro. In: Brown F, Chanock RM, Ginsberg HS, Lerner RA (eds) Vaccines 90: Modern approaches to new vaccines including prevention of AIDS. Cold Spring Harbor: Cold Spring Harbor Laboratory Press, pp 175–178
45. Cohen JI, Rosenblum B, Feinstone SM, Ticehurst J, Purcell RH (1989) Attenuation and cell culture adaptation of hepatitis A virus (HAV): a genetic analysis with HAV cDNA. J Virol 63: 5364–5370
46. Francis DP, Hadler SC, Prendergast TJ, et al (1984) Occurrence of hepatitis A, B, and non-A/non-B in the United States: CDC sentinel county hepatitis study. Am J Med 76: 69–74
47. Ganem D, Varmus HE (1987) The molecular biology of the hepatitis B viruses. Ann Rev Biochem 56: 651–693
48. Krugman S, Overby LR, Mushahwar IK, Ling C-M, Frosner GG, Deinhardt F (1979) Viral hepatitis, type B: studies on natural history and prevention re-examined. N Engl J Med 300: 101–106
49. Hilleman MR, Buynak EB, Roehm RR, Tytell AA, Bertland AU, Lampson GP (1975) Purified and inactivated human hepatitis B vaccine: progress report. Am J Med Sci 270: 401–404
50. Szmuness W, Stevens CE, Harley EJ, et al (1980) Hepatitis B vaccine: demonstration of efficacy in a controlled clinical trial in a high-risk population in the United States. N Engl J Med 303: 833–841
51. Hilleman MR (1987) Yeast recombinant hepatitis B vaccine. Infection 15: 3–7
52. Stevens CE, Teylor PE, Tong MJ, et al (1987) Yeast-recombinant hepatitis B vaccine: efficacy with hepatitis B immune globulin in prevention of perinatal hepatitis B virus transmission. JAMA 1; 257: 2612–2616
53. Whittle HC, Inskip H, Hall AJ, Mendy M, Downes R, Hoare S (1991) Vaccination against hepatitis B and protection against chronic viral carriage in The Gambia. Lancet 337: 747–750
54. Rogler CE, Hino O, Shafritz DA (1989) Mechanisms of hepatic oncogenesis during persistent hepadnavirus infection. In: Notkins AL, Oldstone MBA (eds) Concepts in Viral Pathogenesis III. New York, Springer, pp 254–267
55. Chisari FV, Filippi P, Buras J, et al (1987) Structural and pathological effects of synthesis of hepatitis-B virus large envelope polypeptide in transgenic mice. Proc Natl Acad Sci USA 84: 6909–6913
56. Colgrove R, Simon G, Ganem D (1989) Transcriptional activation of homologous and heterologous genes by the hepatitis B virus X gene product in cells permissive for viral replication. J Virol 63: 4019–4026
57. Rizzetto M, Hoyer B, Canese MG, Shih JW-K, Purcell RH,Gerin JL (1980) d agent: association of d antigen with hepatitis B surface antigen and RNA in serum of d-infected chimpanzees. Proc Natl Acad Sci USA 77: 6124–6128

58. Wang K-S, Choo Q-L, Weiner AJ, et al (1986) Structure, sequence and expression of the hepatitis delta (d) viral genome. Nature 323: 508–514
59. Wang K-S, Choo Q-L, Weiner AJ, et al (1987) Corrigendum: structure, sequence and expression of the hepatitis delta (d) viral genome. Nature 328: 456
60. Rizzetto M, Verme G, Recchia S, et al (1983) Chronic hepatitis in carriers of hepatitis B surface antigen, with intrahepatic expression of the delta antigen. Ann Intern Med 98: 437–441
61. Di Bisceglie AM, Negro F, Smedile A, Bergmann K, Hoofnagle JH (1991) Alpha interferon therapy of chronic delta hepatitis: a pilot study. In: Gerin JL, Purcell RH, Rizzetto M (eds) The hepatitis delta virus. New York, Wiley-Liss, pp 393–397
62. Kos A, Dijkema R, Arnberg AC, van der Meide PH, Schellekens H (1986) The hepatitis delta (d) virus possesses a circular RNA. Nature 323: 558–560
63. Weiner AJ, Choo Q-L, Wang K-S, et al (1988) A single antigenomic open reading frame of the hepatitis delta virus encodes the epitope(s) of both hepatitis delta antigen polypeptides $p24^{d}$ and $p27^{d}$. J Virol 62: 594–599
64. Kuo MY-P, Chao M, Taylor J (1989) Initiation of replication of the human hepatitis delta virus genome from cloned DNA: role of delta antigen. J Virol 63: 1945–1950
65. Chao M, Hsieh S-Y, Taylor J (1990) Role of two forms of hepatitis delta virus antigen: evidence for a mechanism of self-limiting genome replication. J Virol 64: 5066–5069
66. Choo Q-L, Weiner AJ, Overby LR, Kuo G, Houghton M, Bradley DW (1990) Hepatitis C virus: the major causative agent of viral non-A, non-B hepatitis. Br Med Bull 46: 423–441
67. Kuo G, Choo Q-L Alter HJ, et al (1989) An assay for circulating antibodies to a major etiologic virus of human non-A, non-B hepatitis. Science 244: 362–364
68. Choo Q-L, Richman KH, Han JH, et al (1991) Genetic organization and diversity of the hepatitis C virus. Proc Natl Acad Sci USA 88: 2451–2455
69. Han JH, Shyamala V, Richman KH, et al (1991) Characterization of the terminal regions of hepatitis C viral RNA: Identification of conserved sequences in the 5' untranslated region and poly(A) tails at the 3' end. Proc Natl Acad Sci USA 88: 1711–1715
70. Ogata N, Alter HJ, Miller RH, Purcell RH (1991) Nucleotide sequence and mutation rate of the H strain of hepatitis C virus. Proc Natl Acad Sci USA 88: 3392–3396
71. Di Bisceglie AM, Martin P, Kassianides C, et al (1989) Recombinant interferon alfa therapy for chronic hepatitis C: A randomized, double-blind, placebo-controlled trial. N Engl J Med 321: 1506–1510
72. Garson JA, Tedder RS, Briggs M, et al (1990) Detection of hepatitis C viral sequences in blood donations by "nested" polymerase chain reaction and prediction of infectivity. Lancet 335: 1419–1422
73. Khuroo MS (1980) Study of an epidemic of non-A, non-B hepatitis: possibility of another human hepatitis virus distinct from post-transfusion non-A, non-B type. Am J Med 68: 818–824
74. Wong DC, Purcell RH, Sreenivasan MA, Prasad SR, Pavri KM(1980) Epidemic and endemic hepatitis A in India: evidence for a non-A, non-B hepatitis virus aetiology. Lancet ii: 876–879
75. Reyes GR, Purdy MA, Kim JP, et al (1990) Isolation of a cDNA from the virus responsible for enterically transmitted non-A, non-B hepatitis. Science 247: 1335–1339

Rickettsial Diseases: From Epidemiology to Molecular Biology, The Pathway Toward Disease Control

David H. Walker

Department of Pathology, The University of Texas Medical Branch, Galveston, Texas

Introduction

Definition and Catalogue of Rickettsiae

Rickettsial diseases comprise a heterogeneous group of illnesses that occur throughout the world (Table 1). They are remarkably underrecognized owing to the absence of clinical distinctiveness and unavailability of effective, specific laboratory diagnostic methods in many geographic areas (1).

Even the definition of rickettsiae as small gram negative, obligate intracellular bacteria that reside in arthropod hosts as their ecologic niche during at least a portion of their natural history suggests a great number and diversity of organisms (Table 2). Despite tenuous similarities of the ecology, clinical diseases, and laboratory techniques for their investigation, one's credulity is strained to maintain these agents as a cohesive taxonomic group. In fact, 16S ribosomal RNA sequencing reveals that the genera of *Rickettsia* (typhus and spotted fever groups), *Ehrlichia*, and *Rochalimaea* evolved from a relatively closely related common ancestor. In contrast, *Coxiella* is only distantly related to them and is much closer to *Legionella* (2). This chapter will focus primarily on the genetically and antigenically defined, more cohesive members of the typhus and spotted fever groups of the genus *Rickettsia*.

Epidemiology and Ecology of Spotted Fever Group and Typhus Group Rickettsioses

In the United States, the incidence of rickettsioses is often equated to that of Rocky Mountain spotted fever, which appears to fluctuate over long periods of time and in geographic distribution(3). The incidence of Rocky

Table 1. Rickettsial Diseases, Etiologic Agents, and Geographic Distribution

Disease	Etiologic Agent	Geographic Distribution
Spotted Fevers		
Rocky Mountain spotted fever	*Rickettsia rickettsii*	The Americas
Rickettsialpox	*Rickettsia akari*	USA, USSR
Boutonneuse fever	*Rickettsia conorii*	Europe, Africa, Asia
North Asian tick typhus	*Rickettsia sibirica*	Northern Asia
Queensland tick typhus	*Rickettsia australis*	Eastern Australia
Oriental spotted fever	*Rickettsia japonica*	Japan
Israeli spotted fever	*Rickettsia* sp. unnamed	Israel
Typhus Fevers		
Epidemic typhus	*Rickettsia prowazekii*	Africa, the Americas, Asia
Brill-Zinsser disease	*Rickettsia prowazekii*	Worldwide
Flying squirrel typhus	*Rickettsia prowazekii*	USA
Murine typhus	*Rickettsia typhi*	Worldwide
Scrub Typhus	*Rickettsia tsutsugamushi*	SE Asia, Japan, China, Sri Lanka, India, Asiatic USSR, Indonesia, Western Pacific, Northern Australia
Ehrlichioses		
Human ehrlichiosis	*Ehrlichia chaffeensis*	USA
Sennetsu rickettsiosis	*Ehrlichia sennetsu*	Japan
Q Fever	*Coxiella burnetii*	Worldwide
Trench Fever	*Rochalimaea quintana*	Europe & North America
Bacillary angiomatosis and peliosis	*Rochalimaea*-like organism, unnamed	USA

Mountain spotted fever was relatively high in the western U.S. in the years 1900–1945; however, it then declined dramatically in that region and has remained low until the 1990's. In contrast, the incidence in the southeastern U.S. rose steadily and remarkably during the 1970's and then declined during the 1980's. Passive surveillance reported 1126 patients in the U.S. in 1983 and approximately 600 patients annually in recent years. In contrast, in 1990 at Ft. Chaffee, Arkansas, 3.4% of the soldiers evaluated under prospective active surveillance had a four-fold or greater rise in titer to SFG rickettsiae (4). The incidence of spotted fever group (SFG) rickettsia-associated illness in this population was 300/100,000. The differences between data from active and passive surveillance, dramatic unexplained increases in incidence, and changes in geographic distribution should warn us that

Table 2. Properties of Rickettsiae Demonstrating Remarkable Dissimilarities

Genus	G+C content	LPS	Developmental Cycle	Axenic Cultivation	Major Target Cell	Intracellular Location
Rickettsia	29–33%	+	none	no	endothelium	cytosol
Orientia[a]	28.5–30.5%	none	none	no	presumably endothelium	cytosol
Ehrlichia	unknown	none	none	no	various leukocytes	phagosome
Coxiella	43%	+	proposed	no	macrophages	phagolysosome
Rochalimaea[b]	39%	+	none	yes	not applicable	extracellular attached to cell membrane

[a] Because of the major differences in cell wall composition and structure and in the genes studied to date, it has been proposed that *Rickettsia tsutsugamushi* belongs in a separate genus

[b] Although *Rochalimaea* does not meet the definition of a rickettsia owing to its cultivation on cell-free medium, it is substantially related to *Rickettsia prowazekii* with which it shares 30% DNA homology

these organisms, which are capable of killing the most vigorous, healthy person, are by no means under control.

SFG rickettsioses appear to have higher incidences in other parts of the world. Boutonneuse fever is highly endemic in Portugal, Spain, France, Italy, Yugoslavia, and areas in the southern USSR. A distinct *Rickettsia* species causes Israeli spotted fever, a prevalent endemic disease that has yet to be separated from other febrile diseases in the neighboring countries (5, 6). Queensland tick typhus has recently been recognized and diagnosed in a number of patients in Victoria and islands in the Bass Straits south of the Australian continent (7). A new SFG rickettsial species, *R. japonica*, has been identified in Japanese patients living on three of the four major islands (8). Antibodies to SFG rickettsiae are prevalent in many locations in southern Europe, northern Asia, Japan, Israel, and Africa where studies have been conducted. Seroprevalence of SFG rickettsioses is often reported as 10–20% of the population, but may reach as high as 75%. Possible explanations include previous missed diagnosis of the illness and asymptomatic seroconversion stimulated by nonpathogenic strains or species of SFG rickettsiae. My personal speculations are that mildly pathogenic SFG rickettsiae cause many undiagnosed infections and are successful parasites of ticks. Highly pathogenic SFG rickettsiae are somewhat deleterious for ticks, and therefore are less successful parasites of ticks. On the other hand, their mammalian pathogenicity including rickettsemia makes them more capable of horizontal transmission from tick-to-mammal-to-tick.

The least pathogenic SFG rickettsiae are the most prevalent and successful of these organisms in ticks (9). *Rickettsia montana,* the most prevalent SFG rickettsia in some places (e.g., North Carolina, Long Island, and Cape Cod), seems totally nonpathogenic. The East side agent, an intensely prevalent SFG rickettsia on the eastern portion of the Bitterroot Valley, interferes with the establishment of *R. rickettsii* in ticks. It is apparently nonpathogenic and seems to be maintained in nature solely by transovarian transmission(10).

Like many diseases of poor, developing countries, epidemic typhus occurs annually in remote, often mountainous, neglected regions (e.g., Latin America and Africa). Many governments have suppressed information about typhus epidemics. Epidemic typhus, which has exerted such a strong effect on human history, is one of the greatest threats that would be likely to follow societal disruption by natural disaster, war, or economic breakdown. Its prevention could be critical to the recovery of an effective socioeconomic condition. The ecology of *R. prowazekii* is important to recall. *Rickettsia prowazekii* is least adapted to its best known cycle: humans have a high case-fatality rate, and as Zinsser stated, "The louse shares with us the misfortune of being prey to the typhus virus ... In eight days he sickens, in ten days he is *in extremis,* on day 11 or 12 his tiny body turns red with blood extravasated from his bowel, and he gives up his little ghost." (11) *Rickettsia prowazekii* seems better adapted and perhaps has a longer relationship with the silent enzootic cycle of flying squirrels and their fleas and lice (12).

Murine typhus, perhaps the most prevalent and neglected of these rickettsioses, is usually not diagnosed correctly (13). *Rickettsia typhi* has adapted to fleas and some of their mammalian hosts with multiple means of transmission and maintenance in nature. Fleas transmit *R. typhi* in feces and less efficiently by bite or transovarian transmission (14). Murine typhus, although a frequent cause of morbidity as an incapacitating febrile disease of approximately two weeks duration, rarely kills except for patients who are elderly or have underlying disease (15).

Structural Composition and Adaptive Intracellular Physiology of Typhus Group and Spotted Fever Group Rickettsiae

Typhus group and spotted fever group rickettsiae have similar cell wall ultrastructure and composition (16–19). Both groups contain an abundant, S-layer protein of approximately 120 kDa, a 17 kDa lipoprotein, and a ladder of lipopolysaccharides. The S-layer protein contains heat labile epitopes that are unique for each species and serotype. Other epitopes exist that are more highly conserved within the genus. Antigenic differences between the lipopolysaccharides of the typhus group and of the SFG are distinctive and form the principal basis for the laboratory identification of each group. SFG rickettsiae have an additional major, immunodominant, heat-modifiable, high molecular weight, outer membrane protein that contains species-specific, surface-exposed epitopes and a large domain of multiple tandem repeat peptides (20, 21). There is also evidence for at least four other surface-exposed proteins and possibly a slime layer (22, 23). These rickettsiae are highly adapted to their niche in the cytosol which provides a high potassium ion concentration and an availability of different metabolic substrates and precursors for synthesis of proteins and nucleic acids than is available extracellularly (e.g., specific carrier-mediated membrane transport systems for potassium ions, uridine 5'-diphosphoglucose, nicotinamide adenine dinucleotide, AMP, ATP, ADP, lysine, proline, and other amino acids) (24).

Immunity to Typhus Group and Spotted Fever Group Rickettsiae

Currently, the only approaches to control rickettsial diseases are the development of vaccines and antibiotic treatment of acutely ill patients. Although immunity following typhus and spotted fevers is solid and longlasting, vaccines comprising whole killed organisms do not confer complete protective immunity (25). A live, attenuated *R. prowazekii* vaccine having protective properties has been reported to cause mild typhus fever in some patients, as well as to revert to a pathogenic state after *in vivo* passage. Even though this work shows great promise, vaccine development requires substantially more research. The rickettsial components which appear to be most important in protective immunity are the S-layer protein and the high molecular weight major outer membrane protein of the SFG rickettsiae. Vaccination with the purified S-layer protein of *R. typhi* provides partial protection to challenged guinea pigs (26). The S-layer protein contains epitopes recognized by human T-lymphocytes (27), and monoclonal antibodies to heat-labile epitopes of the S-layer protein of typhus group and SFG rickettsiae provide passive protection against illness in experimental animals (20, 28–30). Similarly, vaccination with a recombinant major outer membrane proteins of SFG rickettsiae confers measurable protection(31), and monoclonal antibodies against heat-labile, surface-exposed epitopes of these proteins provide passive protection to challenged experimental animals (18, 29–30).

The mechanisms of protective immunity against rickettsial diseases are incompletely understood. The preeminent importance of T-lymphocytes and cell mediated immunity has been demonstrated in studies involving lymphocyte depletion, genetic immunodeficiency states, and adoptive transfer. The available evidence suggests that the cytokines, interferon-γ and tumor necrosis factor, are important effectors (32–34). Cytotoxic T-lymphocytes and non-MHC-restricted cytotoxic cells can be harvested from infected hosts and assayed *in vitro* (35, 36). The significance of these effector mechanisms *in vivo* in clearing intracellular rickettsial infection from endothelial cells or in providing protective immunity to challenge with virulent rickettsiae is unknown. Once rickettsiae are released from host cells into the extracellular environment, antibodies opsonize rickettsiae for destruction by activated macrophages. It remains to be determined what essential steps of the concerted interaction of the various cell mediated and humoral elements of the immune system and phagocytes are required for the host to resist or recover from rickettsial infection. The optimal composition of a protective vaccine and formulation of an effective dosage and adjuvant regimen will depend upon future studies of the immunobiology of these organisms.

Pathogenesis of Typhus Group and Spotted Fever Group Rickettsioses

Understanding the pathogenetic steps of rickettsioses is essential for the design of effective preventive measures and innovative interventions to halt the progression of the disease process. Importantly vaccine and treatment research should be performed in animal models which parallel human disease in terms of portal of entry, route of spread, target cells, and immune and pathogenic mechanisms. Typhus and SFG rickettsiae enter the body via inoculation into the skin following the bite of infected ticks, mites, or fleas or by excoriation of infected louse or flea feces. Conceivably, infected louse and flea feces could be inhaled, and infected arthropod tissue, fluids or excreta could be inoculated via mucous membranes (e.g., conjunctiva). Subsequently, rickettsiae either proliferate locally causing an eschar (37) or spread immediately via the lymphatics and bloodstream throughout the body. Hematogenous dissemination brings rickettsiae into contact with endothelial cells throughout the body where attachment of the rickettsia to host cell membrane protein appears to occur by the rickettsial major outer membrane protein (38). This attachment process coupled with the rickettsial proton motive force induces the endothelial cells to engulf the organisms (39). The rickettsiae rapidly escape from the phagosome into the cytosol presumably by action of rickettsial phospholipase A. Rickettsiae propagate intracellularly by binary fission. *Rickettsia prowazekii* exits from the endothelium by burst lysis of the infected cell, which is the ostensible pathogenic event (40). *Rickettsia rickettsii* and *R. conorii* are released from the host cell by focal lysis of the host cell membrane at the end of filopodia, and cell injury occurs more insidiously in proportion to the quantity of intracellar rickettsiae (41). Only *R. rickettsii* is observed to spread to a substantial number of nonendothelial cells by invasion of adjacent vascular smooth muscle cells. Infection and injury to blood vessels lead to increased vascular permeability, edema, hypovolemia, and hypoperfusion, as well as signs and symptoms referable to the affected organ (e.g., brain lesions with seizures and coma, damage to the pulmonary microcirculation with noncardiogenic pulmonary edema and skin with rash) (42–46).

The pathogenic mechanisms that have been hypothesized include injury to the endothelial cell membrane by a contact-associated phospholipase A, protease, and/or lipid peroxidation by free radicals (47–49). Notably rickettsial lipopolysaccharide is nontoxic in the quantities that are present (50, 51), and no exotoxin or soluble destructive enzymes have been demonstrated.

Host-mediated events have also been proposed as hypothetical pathogenic mechanisms, based largely on *in vitro* data. These mechanisms include interferon-γ cytolysis of infected cells, cytokine-mediated acute phase response, prostacylin and thromboxane effects on platelet activity and vascular tone and permeability, leukotriene effects on vascular permeability, kallikrein-kinin effects on vascular tone and permeability, and killing of infected cells expressing antigens on their cell membranes by cytotoxic lymphocytes (35, 40, 52–55). The importance of most of these factors *in vivo* remains to be determined for humans and in appropriate animal models of infection. Although most host responses seem to produce effects that are in the overall balance beneficial to the host (e.g., fibrin-platelet thrombi located precisely in foci of severe rickettsial infection and vascular injury), it is probable that some of the effects of the disease involve host-mediated events (e.g., IL-1 and/or IL-6 roles in fever and the acute phase reaction).

Presently therapeutic intervention focuses on inhibition of rickettsial protein synthesis and growth by tetracyclines or chloramphenicol, or inhibition of rickettsial growth by fluoroquinolones. Supportive treatment emphasizes careful fluid replacement and management without precipitating or exacerbating noncardiogenic pulmonary edema (56). Patients still die of rickettsioses because of delayed diagnosis even when antirickettsial treatment was begun prior to death. Severe injury, inability to reverse all the pathogenic events quickly, and relative slowness of the host's clearance of rickettsiae under rickettsiostatic treatment illustrate why early diagnosis and a better understanding of the pathogenetic events could lead to a better outcome.

Directions for Control of Typhus Group and Spotted Fever Group Rickettsioses

Because the capabilities of clinicians and laboratorians to diagnose spotted fever rickettsioses, murine typhus, and epidemic typhus are inadequate, the true incidence of these illnesses is unknown (1, 57). Consequently, rickettsial diseases are seldom listed among the major causes of morbidity and mortality on a global basis. Where the data are known, it would appear that rickettsioses may indeed belong on such a list of important, potentially preventable, treatable infectious diseases (58, 59). The first step must be the demonstration of where rickettsial diseases are important and how severe the impact of the rickettsiae are on the public health. To evaluate these diseases, improved laboratory diagnosis will be required. It is essential to develop more sensitive, specific, timely, inexpensive assays that are simple to perform without sophisticated equipment (60). These tests and expertise in their use must then be distributed to the developing world. The improved diagnostic capability must be linked to improved epidemiologic surveillance. Just as passive surveillance underestimates the incidence of spotted fever rickettsiosis in the U.S., the WHO program for diagnosis and reporting of rickettsial diseases has failed to have a measurable impact on elucidation of the incidence of these infections around the globe.

Because these diseases are zoonoses with reservoirs in nature, eradication is not currently a possibility. The morbidity and mortality of rickettsioses could be reduced substantially by the development and delivery of vaccines against SFG and typhus group rickettsioses where epidemiologically indicated. It would be necessary to incorporate T-cell immunodominant epitope-stimulating antigens into a vaccine that provides long-term solid immunity: probably one set of cross-protective SFG antigens and one set of typhus group antigens would suffice to protect against all of these diseases. Determining the best approach depends on further investigation of the antigens and the protective immune response. The possibilities include a subunit vaccine (61) with appropriate adjuvant, a nonpathogenic live rickettsial vaccine, an engineered recombinant vaccinia-, BCG-, or other effective antigen expressing system. It would seem that a successful vaccine must stimulate T-memory lymphocytes.

The reduction of vector and reservoir populations also offers a possible approach to control the rickettsioses. Control of rat populations and their access to proximity with humans and insecticide control of rat fleas have been demonstrated to be effective in reducing murine typhus. Insecticides that effectively kill lice can help control epidemics of louse-borne typhus. Control of tick vectors of SFG rickettsioses is a wide-open challenge.

Critical Issues and Directions for Control of Scrub Typhus

The etiologic agent of scrub typhus, *R. tsutsugamushi,* differs remarkably from SFG and typhus group rickettsiae. Its cell wall comprises quite a different set of proteins and lacks lipopolysaccharide and peptidoglycan. These differences are reflected in ultrastructural and antigenic distinctiveness. *R. tsutsugamushi* is maintained in nature in an unusual ecologic niche, *Leptotrombidium* chiggers, which feed on mammals including humans only in the larval stage. Scrub typhus is highly prevalent in many of the most populous countries of Asia. It is usually misdiagnosed because of the infrequent occurrence of an eschar and rash. For example, a careful study at a rural hospital in Malaysia showed scrub typhus to be the most frequent cause of febrile admissions (62). Serologic investigations have demonstrated a very high prevalence of antibodies to *R. tsutsugamushi.* There are multiple, distinct strains of *R. tsutsugamushi* which stimulate poor, short-term cross-protection. Immunity is short-lived; people are fully susceptible to reinfection with even the homologous strain of *R. tsutsugamushi* after 2–3 years (63). Thus, reinfections are not uncommon. Because natural immunity is so evanescent, it would seem that a vaccine may never prove effective.

Human suffering from scrub typhus could be ameliorated by better diagnosis, acquisition of comprehensive epidemiologic data and its dissemination to health care workers in endemic areas, and the consequent more effective treatment of clinical cases. Although effective antimicrobial prophylaxis has been developed for persons with short-term exposure and resources to obtain antirickettsial drugs, it is difficult to conceive of a rational application of this approach to the vast, poor areas of the world where exposure to infected chiggers may extend through a large portion of the year (64). The prospects for control of scrub typhus are dim at present.

Directions for Understanding and Future Control of Human Ehrlichiosis

The emergence of a new tick-borne infectious disease in the U.S. emphasizes our continued lack of a complete inventory of human infections. Originally recognized as a life-threatening illness resembling Rocky Mountain spotted fever that often requires hospitalization, human ehrlichiosis is now known to range in severity from asymptomatic to fatal (65). Although only 260 cases have been reported in the U.S., active surveillance at Ft. Chaffee, Arkansas, demonstrated a high incidence of febrile illness associated with seroconversion to *Ehrlichia chaffeensis* (66). The latter is a newly identified species of intracellular bacterium recently isolated by workers at the CDC (67). It is likely that ehrlichiosis is a worldwide disease and that more than one species of *Ehrlichia* may cause human illness. Various species of *Ehrlichia* of veterinary importance have a tropism for either macrophages and lymphocytes or polymorphonuclear leukocytes. Ehrlichiae have been observed in the same types of human leukocytes. The only sensitive diagnostic test currently available is an indirect immunofluorescent antibody assay utilizing *E. chaffeensis,* an obligate intracellular bacterium that is difficult to propagate.

Present goals for the public health approach to ehrlichiosis should include development and distribution of effective diagnostic tools, determination of the vector(s), mammalian reservoir(s), geographic distribution and incidence, elucidation of the pathogenesis and immunity, and development of an effective regimen of antimicrobial prophylaxis and rational guidelines for its application.

References

1. Walker DH (1989) Rocky Mountain spotted fever: a disease in need of microbiological concern. Clin Microbiol Rev 2: 227–240
2. Weisburg WG, Dobson ME, Samuel JE, Dasch GA, Mallavia LP, Baca O, Mandelco, Sechrest JE, Weiss E, Woese CR (1989) Phylogenetic diversity of the rickettsiae. J Bacteriol 171: 4202–4206
3. Hattwick MAW, O'Brien RJ, Hanson BF (1976) Rocky Mountain spotted fever: epidemiology of an increasing problem. Ann Intern Med 84: 732–739
4. Fishbein DB, Yevich SJ, Sanchez JL, Dawson JE, Greene CR, Reid-Sanden F, Kardatzke JT (1991) Serologic studies of military personnel exposed to ticks during field exercises in Arkansas. Abstract from the American Society for Rickettsiology and Rickettsial Diseases Sesqui-Annual Meeting, May 1–5, 1991, abstract 19
5. Cwikel BJ, Ishbarieh J, Sarov I (1990) Antigenic polypeptides of Israeli spotted fever isolates compared with other spotted fever group rickettsiae. Ann NY Acad Sci 590: 381–388
6. Walker DH, Liu Q-H, Yu X-J, Li H, Taylor C (1991) Antigenic analysis of the major outer membrane proteins of *Rickettsia conorii, Rickettsia parkeri,* and the Israel spotted fever group rickettsia. Abstract of the American Society for Rickettsiology and Rickettsial Diseases Sesqui-Annual Meeting, May 1–5 1991, abstract 65

7. Sexton DJ, Dwyer B, Kemp R, Graves S (1991) Spotted fever group rickettsial infections in Australia. Rev Infect Dis 13: 876–886
8. Uchida T, Yu XJ, Uchiyama T, Walker DH (1989) Identification of a unique spotted fever group rickettsia from humans in Japan. J Infect Dis 159: 1122–1126
9. Phillip RN, Casper EA (1981) Serotypes of spotted fever group rickettsiae isolated from *Dermacentor andersoni* (Stiles) ticks in western Montana. Am J Trop Med Hyg 30: 230–238
10. Burgdorfer W, Hayes SF, Mavros AJ (1981) Nonpathogenic rickettsiae in *Dermacentor andersoni:* a limiting factor for the distribution of *Rickettsia rickettsii.* In: Burgdorfer W, Anacker RL (eds) Rickettsiae and Rickettsial Diseases. New York, Academic Press, pp 585–594
11. Zinsser H (1935) Rats, Lice, and History. New York, Little, Brown, and Co.
12. Sonenshine DE, Bozeman FM, Williams MS, Masiello SA, Chadwick DP, Stocks NI, Lauer DM, Elisberg L (1978) Epizootiology of epidemic typhus *(Rickettsia prowazekii)* in flying squirrels. Am J Trop Med Hyg 27: 339–349
13. Traub R, Wisseman CL, Farhang-Azad A (1978) The ecology of murine typhus – a critical review. Trop Dis Bull 75: 237–317
14. Farhang-Azad A, Traub R, Baqar S (1985) Transovarial transmission of murine typhus rickettsiae in *Xenopsylla cheopis* fleas. Science 227: 543–545
15. Walker DH, Parks FM, Betz TG, Taylor JP, Muehlberger JW (1989) Histopathology and immunohistologic demonstration of the distribution of *Rickettsia typhi* in fatal murine typhus. Am J Clin Pathol 91: 720–724
16. Silverman DJ, Wisseman CL Jr (1978) Comparative ultrastructural study on the cell envelopes of *Rickettsia prowazekii, Rickettsia rickettsii,* and *Rickettsia tsutsugamushi.* Infect Immun 21: 1020–1023
17. Ching W-M, Dasch GA, Carl M, Dobson ME (1990) Structural analysis of the 120 kDa serotype protein antigens of typhus group rickettsiae. Comparison with other S-layer proteins. Ann NY Acad Sci 590: 334–351
18. Anacker RL Mann RE, Gonzales C (1987) Reactivity of monoclonal antibodies to *Rickettsia ricketsii* with spotted fever and typhus group rickettsiae. J Clin Microbiol 25: 167–171
19. Anderson BE (1990) The 17-kilodalton protein antigens of spotted fever and typhus group rickettsiae. Ann NY Acad Sci 590: 326–333
20. Li H, Lenz B, Walker DH (1988) Protective monoclonal antibodies recognize heat labile epitopes on surface proteins of spotted fever group rickettsiae. Infect Immun 56: 2587–2593
21. Anderson BE, McDonald GA, Hones DC, Regnery RL (1990) A protective antigen of *Rickettsia rickettsii* has tandemly repeated, near-identical sequences. Infect Immun 58: 2760–2769
22. Williams JC, Walker DH, Peacock MG, Stewart ST (1986) Humoral immune response to Rocky Mountain spotted fever in experimentally infected guinea pigs: immunoprecipitation of lactoperoxidase ^{125}I-labeled proteins and detection of soluble antigens of *Rickettsia rickettsii.* Infect Immun 52: 120–127
23. Silverman DJ, Wisseman CL Waddell AD, Jones M (1978) External layers of *Rickettsia prowazekii* and *Rickettsia rickettsii*: occurrence of a slime layer. Infect Immun 22: 233–245
24. Winkler HH (1990) Rickettsia species (as organisms). Ann Rev Microbiol 44: 131–153
25. Weiss KL Walker DH (1990) New and improved vaccines against rickettsial infections. Rocky Mountain spotted fever, epidemic typhus, and scrub typhus. In: Woodrow GC, Levine MM (eds) New generation vaccines. New York, Marcel Dekker, pp 357–374
26. Bourgeois AL, Dasch GA (1981) The species-specific surface protein antigen of *Rickettsia typhi:* immunogenicity and protective efficacy in guinea pigs. In: Burgdorfer W, Anacker RL (eds) Rickettsiae and rickettsial diseases. New York, Academic Press, pp 71–80
27. Churilla A, Ching W-M, Dasch GA, Carl M (1990) Human T lymphocyte recognition of cyanogen bromide fragments of the surface protein of *Rickettsia typhi.* Ann NY Acad Sci 590: 215–220
28. Dasch GA, Burans JP, Dobson ME, Rollwagen FM, Misiti J (1984) Approaches to subunit vaccines against the typhus rickettsiae, *Rickettsia typhi* and *Rickettsia prowazekii.* In: Lieve L, Schlessinger D (eds) Microbiology 1984. Washington, Am Soc Microbiol, 251–256

29. Anacker RL, List RH, Mann RE, Hayes SF, Thomas LA (1985) Characterization of monoclonal antibodies protecting mice against *Rickettsia rickettsii.* J Infect Dis 151: 1052–1060
30. Feng HM, Walker DH, Wang JG (1987) Analysis of T-cell-dependent and -independent antigens of *Rickettsia conorii* with monoclonal antibodies. Infect Immun 55: 7–15
31. Vishwanath S, McDonald GA, Watkins NG (1990) A recombinant *Rickettsia conorii* vaccine protects guinea pigs from experimental boutonneuse fever and Rocky Mountain spotted fever. Infect Immun 58: 646–653
32. Turco J, Winkler HH (1983) Inhibition of the growth of *Rickettsia prowazekii* in cultured fibroblasts by lymphokines. J Exp Med 157: 974–986
33. Wisseman CL Jr, Waddell A (1983) Interferonlike factors from antigen- and mitogen-stimulated human leukocytes with antirickettsial and cytolytic actions on *Rickettsia prowazekii.* J Exp Med 157: 1780–1793
34. Manor E, Sarov I (1990) Inhibition of *Rickettsia conorii* growth by recombinant tumor necrosis factor alpha: enhancement of inhibition by gamma intereferon. Infect Immun 58: 1886–1889
35. Rollwagen FM, Dasch GA, Jerrells TR (1986) Mechanisms of immunity to rickettsial infection: characterization of a cytotoxic effector cell. J Immunol 136: 1418–1421
36. Carl M, Ching W-M, Dasch GA (1988) Recognition of typhus group rickettsia-infected targets by human lymphokine-activated killer cells. Infect Immun 56: 2526–2529
37. Walker DH, Occhino C, Tringali GR, DiRosa S, Mansueto S (1988) Pathogenesis of rickettsial eschars: the *tache noire* of boutonneuse fever. Human Pathol 19: 1449–1454
38. Li H, Jerrells TR, Walker DH (1991) Characterization of rickettsial attachment to target cells by flow cytometry. Abstract of the American Society for Rickettsiology and Rickettsial Diseases Sesqui-Annual Meeting, May 1–5, 1991, abstract 34
39. Walker TS (1984) Rickettsial interactions with human endothelial cells in vitro: adherence and entry. Infect Immun 44: 205–210
40. Wisseman CL Jr, Waddell AD (1975) In vitro studies on rickettsia-host cell interactions: intracellular growth cycle of virulent and attenuated *Rickettsia prowazekii* in chicken embryo cells in slide chamber cultures. Infect Immun 11: 1391–141
41. Walker DH, Cain BG (1980) The rickettsial plaque. Evidence for direct cytopathic effect of *Rickettsia rickettsii.* Lab Invest 43: 388–396
42. Harrell GT, Aikawa JK (1949) Pathogenesis of circulatory failure in Rocky Mountain spotted fever. Arch Intern Med 83: 331–347
43. Kaplowitz LG, Fischer JJ, Sparling PF (1981) Rocky Mountain spotted fever: a clinical dilemma. Curr Clin Top Infect Dis 2: 89–108
44. Horney LF, Walker DH (1988) Meningoencephalitis as a major manifestation of Rocky Mountain spotted fever. South Med J 81: 915–8
45. Walker DH, Crawford CG, Cain BG (1980) Rickettsial infection of the pulmonary microcirculation: the basis of interstitial pneumonitis of Rocky Mountain spotted fever. Human Pathol 11: 263–272
46. Wolbach SB, Todd JL, Palfrey FW (1922) Clinical observations, pp. 15–33, Pathology of typhus, pp 152–227. In: The Etiology and Pathology of Typhus. The League of Red Cross Societies, Cambridge, Harvard Press
47. Winkler HH, Daugherty RM (1989) Phospholipase A activity associated with the growth of *Rickettsia prowazekii* in L929 cells. Infect Immun 57: 36–40
48. Walker DH, Tidwell RR, Rector TM, Geratz JD (1984) Effect of synthetic protease inhibitors of the amidine type on cell injury by *Rickettsia rickettsii.* Antimicrob Agents Chemother 25: 582–585
49. Silverman DJ, Santucci LA (1990) A potential protective role for thiols against cell injury caused by *Rickettsia rickettsii.* Ann NY Acad Sci 590: 111–117
50. Schramek S, Brezina R, Kazar J (1977) Some biological properties of an endotoxic lipopolysaccharide from the typhus group rickettsiae. Acta Virol 21: 439–441
51. Kaplowitz LG, Lange JV, Fischer JJ, Walker DH (1983) Correlation of rickettsial titers, circulating endotoxin, and clinical features in Rocky Mountain spotted fever. Arch Intern Med 143: 1149–1151

52. Walker TS, Dersch MW, White WE (1991) Effects of typhus rickettsiae on peritoneal and alveolar macrophages: rickettsiae stimulate leukotriene and prostaglandin secretion. J Infect Dis 163: 568–573
53. Walker TS, Brown JS, Hoover CS, Morgan DA (1990) Endothelial prostaglandin secretion: effects of typhus rickettsiae. J Infect Dis 162: 1136–1144
54. Yamada T, Harber P, Pettit GW, Wing DA, Oster CN (1978) Activation of the kallikrein-kinin system in Rocky Mountain spotted fever. Ann Intern Med 88: 764–768
55. Rollwagen FM, Bakun AJ, Dorsey CH, Dasch GA (1985) Mechanisms of immunity to infection with typhus rickettsiae: infected fibroblasts bear rickettsial antigens on their surfaces. Infect Immun 50: 911–916
56. Walker DH, Mattern WD (1980) Rickettsial vasculitis. Am Heart J 100: 896–906
57. Fan MY, Walker DH, Yu SR, Liu QH (1987) Epidemiology and ecology of rickettsial diseases in the People's Republic of China. Rev Infect Dis 9: 823–840
58. Yagupsky P, Sarov B, Sarov I (1989) A cluster of cases of spotted fever in a kibbutz in southern Israel. Scand J Infect Dis 21: 155–160
59. Wilfert CM, MacCormack JN, Kleeman K, Philip RN, Austin E, Dickinson V, Turner L (1984) Epidemiology of Rocky Mountain spotted fever as determined by active surveillance. J Infect Dis 150: 469–479
60. Walker DH, Peacock MG (1988) Laboratory diagnosis of rickettsial diseases. In: Walker DH (ed) Biology of rickettsial diseases, Vol II. Boca Raton, CRC Press, pp 135–155
61. McDonald GA, Anacker RL, Garjian K (1987) Cloned gene of *Rickettsia rickettsii* surface antigen: candidate vaccine for Rocky Mountain spotted fever. Science 235: 83–85
62. Brown GW, Shirai A, Jegathesan M, Burke DS, Twartz JC, Saunders JP, Huxsoll DL (1984) Febrile illness in Malaysia- an analysis of 1,629 hospitalized patients. Am J Trop Med Hyg 33: 311–315
63. Smadel JE, Ley HL Diercks FH, Traub R (1950) Immunity in scrub typhus: resistance to induced reinfection. Arch Pathol 50: 847–861
64. Twartz JC, Shirai A, Selvaraju G, Saunders JP, Huxsoll DL, Groves MG (1982) Doxycycline prophylaxis for human scrub typhus. J Infect Dis 146: 811–818
65. Eng TR, Harkess JR, Fishbein DB, Dawson JE, Greene CN, Redus MA, Satalowich FT (1990) Epidemiologic, clinical, and laboratory findings of human ehrlichiosis in the United States. JAMA 264: 2251–258
66. Uhaa IJ, Sanchez JL Dawson JE, Greene CR, Kardatzke JT, Fishbein DB (1991) Epidemiologic, clinical, and serologic investigation of patients with suspected tick-borne illnesses. Abstract from the American Society for Rickettsiology and Rickettsial Diseases Sesqui-Annual Meeting, May 1–5, 1991, abstract 61
67. Dawson J, Anderson B, Fishbein D, Sanchez J, Goldsmith C, Wilson K, Duntley C (1991) Isolation and characterization of an *Ehrlichia* sp. from a patient diagnosed with human ehrlichiosis. J Clin Microbiol 29: 2741–2745

Diarrheal Diseases: New Challenges and Emerging Opportunities

Richard L. Guerrant

Division of Geographic Medicine, University of Virginia School of Medicine, Charlottesville, Virginia

Introduction

In keeping with the central theme, "Global Medicine: Current Status and Directions for the Twenty-First Century," a discussion of diarrheal diseases is particularly relevant, as diarrheal diseases constitute a leading global cause of morbidity and mortality and provide a useful "barometer" of health. Indeed, *health* is one of the most universal human values, transcending all cultural, political and geographic boundaries; everyone would rather be healthy than sick. In only this century has some measure of health, like education, become an attainable goal for most, with existing societal resources. Despite this potential, growing disparity threatens global health and perhaps civilization itself. Diarrheal diseases provide a useful barometer of health or neglect of a people, as well as a poignant example of the tremendous potential that public health and recent scientific advances have for alleviating human suffering. We must dare to consider the possibility of a world with a certain minimum level of health for all, with food and energy potentially freely available by molecular biologic or other methods, such as engineered *E. coli* or cyanobacteria to produce carbohydrates for food and hydrocarbons for energy.

After initial examination of diarrheal diseases in places that tend to be forgotten, the incredible advances in understanding of the etiologies and pathogenesis of diarrhea (recalling that the leading bacterial, viral and parasitic causes have only been recognized in the last 25 years) will be addressed. Finally, an overview of the unique opportunities for control that lie immediately before us will be considered.

Recognizing the Problem

The first challenge is recognition of the full magnitude of the problem presented by diarrheal diseases. Describing the blindness to the sufferings of others, Solzhenitsyn in his 1972 Nobel prize acceptance speech has stated, "What seems to us more important, more painful and more unendurable is not really what is more important, more painful and more unendurable, but merely that which is closer to home. Everything distant which for all its moans and muffled cries, its ruined lives and millions of victims, and does not threaten to come rolling up to our threshold today, we consider endurable and of tolerable dimensions."

In just the first four months of 1991, three events have brought diarrheal diseases "to our threshold." First, the seventh pandemic of cholera has now reached the western hemisphere for the first time in nearly a century. Between January and May of 1991, over 170,000 cases of cholera with more than 1,200 deaths have been reported from Peru. Genetic studies show that these Inaba, El Tor isolates are clonal, related to the Seventh Pandemic isolates from Asia and Africa, and are genetically and biochemically different from the endemic U.S. Gulf Coast isolates seen in recent years. Cholera has already affected 0.8% of Peru's 21 million population, with a remarkably low 0.7% case fatality rate, the latter being attributable to Peru's attention to control of diarrheal diseases and widely available oral rehydration therapy.

Secondly, early in the Persian Gulf deployment, as many as 10% of U.S. troops suffered diarrheal illnesses per week, a rate that exceeded by more than ten-fold the heat-related illnesses reported. The vast majority of these were due to enterotoxigenic *E. coli*, the same organisms that constitute the leading causes of endemic diarrhea among children in developing areas throughout Asia, Africa and Latin America.

Thirdly, diarrhea has again emerged as a major killer in Kurdish refugees and Bengali cyclone survivors, again demonstrating how diarrheal illnesses constitute a major barometer or indicator of disadvantaged people or disrupted public health measures at the present time.

In contrast, however, to the epidemics and crises that reach the headlines, I would like to emphasize three places where we tend to overlook diarrheal diseases, and where they are even more important.

Global Mortality and Morbidity from Endemic Diarrhea

First and by far most important is the tremendous mortality and perhaps even greater morbidity due to endemic diarrheal diseases among children throughout tropical, developing areas. As shown in Table 1, the annual mortality is estimated between 4.6 and 6 million children per year in Asia, Africa and Latin America; that is, each *day* more than 12,600 children die with diarrheal illnesses. Of perhaps even greater societal impact is the inestimable morbidity associated with 8 to 15 or more dehydrating, malnourishing diarrheal illnesses per child each year in their most critical developmental years of life in many impoverished areas (1–3). This contrasts with an estimated 10,000 deaths in the United States due to diarrhea (4), with 500 reported childhood deaths due to diarrhea in the United

Table 1. Mortality and Morbidity of Diarrheal Diseases

	Annual Mortality	Annual Morbidity
Global (predominantly Asia, Africa and Latin America)	4.6–6 million (>12,600 children/day)	2–11 illnesses/person (15–19 illnesses/child in some impoverished areas)
U.S.	est. 10,000 (500 children/yr)	1.9–2.1 illnesses/person (5 illnesses/child in day-care centers)

States (5). Like children in more affluent homes in tropical countries (6), illness rates in prospective community-based studies among children in the U.S. average 1.9 to 2.1 illnesses per person per year, with rates reaching as high as 5 illnesses per child per year among those who attend day-care centers (1, 7, 8). Furthermore, in areas where attack rates due to diarrheal illnesses are high and malnutrition is common, recurring diarrheal illnesses clearly have a profound effect on blunting or eradicating critical "catch-up" growth that is normally seen in malnourished children without diarrhea as well as that normally seen following diarrheal illnesses (9) (Fig. 1). In addition, malnutrition predisposes to increased frequency as well as duration of diarrheal illnesses, thus completing a vicious cycle (Fig. 1) (10).

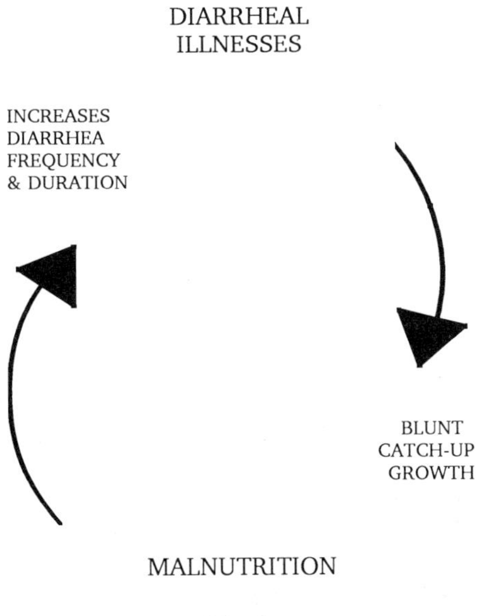

Fig. 1

With the increasing use of lifesaving oral rehydration therapy for acute diarrheal illnesses, persistent diarrhea is now emerging as a leading cause of diarrhea morbidity and mortality in many areas (2, 11). We are just beginning to appreciate the roles of enteroaggregative *E. coli* and *Cryptosporidium* in this setting (12–14). Despite the attention it attracted as a cause of intractable diarrhea in AIDS patients, cryptosporidiosis is even more common as a cause of endemic diarrhea throughout the world (Table 2) (15–18) and is increasingly associated with persistent diarrhea and malnutrition (19–21).

Table 2. Frequencies (and ranges) of *Cryptosporidium* in Sporadic Diarrhea and Controls in Developed and Developing Countries (15–18)

	Cases (%)	Controls (%)
Developed countries	2.1	0.2
(from 16 reports from Europe,	(0.1–9.1)	(0–1)
N. America, Austalia)	(n = 32,636)	(n = 589)
Developing countries	8.0	0.8
(from 14 reports from Asia,	(3.2–16.7)	(0–5.9)
Africa, Latin America)	(n = 4,301)	(n = 928)

Nosocomial Diarrhea

A second area where diarrheal illnesses pose increasingly recognized challenges is in institutions, particularly in day-care centers, hospitals and extended care facilities for the elderly. Diarrhea in day-care centers is often associated with organisms that require relatively low infectious doses and are easily spread such as *Shigella, Giardia lamblia, Cryptosporidium,* certain strains of *C. jejuni, C. diffcile* and *rotaviruses* (22, 23). Less widely appreciated are the impressive numbers of nosocomial diarrheal illnesses that may exceed the rates of any other nosocomial infection (1). Furthermore, nosocomial diarrhea may predispose to other nosocomial infections such as urinary tract infections, which have been found to be ten-fold more common following nosocomial diarrhea (24). Once again, as in developing countries, diarrheal illnesses and specific enteric pathogens such as *C. difficile* and *Cryptosporidium* infections acquired in our hospitals indicate the disturbing frequency with which fecal pathogens are spread from hospitalized patients to other patients or health care workers (25, 26) McFarland et al. (26) noted that an impressive 21% of patients acquired *C. difficile* on a general medical ward, with only 3.2 days until the organism was acquired if a roommate was infected. Despite the tremendous care we take with parenteral exposures to AIDS patients, acquisition of cryptosporidiosis from AIDS patients by health care personnel documents the ease with which this organism is acquired, presumably by the ingestion of fecal material from the AIDS patients being cared for (25).

Diarrhea in the Immunocompromised Host

The third setting in which challenges for control of diarrheal diseases lie before us is in the immunocompromised host. Now led by AIDS patients, in whom 50 to 98% either present with or develop diarrhea, immunocompromised patients often present with diarrhea that may be life threatening (27–29). In the United States, a remarkable two thirds of the AIDS patients eventually develop diarrhea that is often caused by recognizable pathogens such as cytomegalovirus, *Cryptosporidium*, microsporidia, mycobacteria, *Salmonella*, *Campylobacter* or other organisms (29, 30). In Zaire patients presenting to the hospital with diarrhea lasting 1 month or longer have an 84% chance of having AIDS (28). Clearly other patients immunocompromised by underlying disease, chemotherapy, or transplant-associated immunosuppression pose important challenges.

Pathogenesis: Etiologies, Host Defenses and Microbial Virulence Traits

As is apparent, the recognized etiologies of enteric infections are increasingly diverse. In just the last 25 years, the leading bacterial, viral, parasitic and now even fungal and possible algal causes of diarrhea have been discovered. These include the diverse types of *E. coli* ranging from enterotoxigenic to enterohemorrhagic, enteroinvasive, enteroadherent and enteropathogenic *E. coli*, as well as *Campylobacter jejuni* and other *Campylobacter* species, *Helicobacter pylori* (which may cause achlorhydria and thus predispose to other enteric infections), *Clostridium difficile*, rotaviruses and Norwalk-like viruses, *Cryptosporidium*, microsporidia, and now possibly *Candida albicans* and *Cyanobacterium*-like organisms. Yet common themes regarding host defenses and microbial virulence traits are emerging.

The host defenses critical to the gastrointestinal tract include personal hygiene (the number of organisms ingested characteristically determines the chance of acquiring an enteric infection), normal gastric acidity (when neutralized by antacids, surgery, or possibly *H. pylori* gastritis, patients are predisposed to increased susceptibility to many enteric infections), the gastrointestinal mucus barrier first encountered by an outside invader, normal motility and normal bowel flora. Impairment of any of these key enteric host defenses will increase the susceptibility of the host to a wide range of enteric infections. Preserving the integrity of these host defenses is an often overlooked goal in controlling enteric infections and diarrheal diseases.

An additional critical host defense is the intestinal mucosal immune system, often referred to as the gut associated lymphoid tissue (GALT). Important in both cellular and humoral immunity, the GALT is composed of

Peyer's patches, lamina propria lymphocytes and intraepithelial lymphocytes (31). Microfold (M) cells in Peyer's patches may provide access for certain invasive bacteria and constantly sample foreign antigen from the gut lumen for underlying macrophages which process this antigen for presentation to CD4, helper/inducer T lymphocytes. Via their cytokines such as IL-2 and gamma IFN, these T lymphocytes then stimulate follicular B lymphocytes to become IgA producing cells which migrate via lymph nodes, thoracic duct and bloodstream before returning for terminal differentiation into IgA producing plasma cells in the lamina propria . The secretory IgA is then transported to the gut lumen via epithelial cells, which add a stabilizing secretory component to the immunoglobulin dimer. In addition, one of six cells on the mucosal surface is an intraepithelial CD8 or gamma delta T lymphocyte that likely plays critical roles in cellular immune responses to both enteric pathogens and other foreign antigens. The complexity of the interplay between cytokines produced by macrophages and lymphocytes as well as the effect of these cytokines and neurohumoral transmitters on the secretory function of the epithelium itself is just beginning to be appreciated. We are increasingly recognizing the roles of these and other mediators such as gamma interferon, serotonin, prostaglandins, and other arachidonate metabolites in the diarrhea seen with enterotoxic and inflammatory processes (30, 32).

An improved understanding of microbial virulence traits not only enables better appreciation of the pathogenesis of secretory and inflammatory diarrheas, but also opens avenues of improved pharmacologic or immunologic control. These virulence traits include a growing range of recognized secretory enterotoxins, cytotoxins and neurotoxins, adherence traits, and invasiveness traits (Table 3). Perhaps the clearest demonstration of the importance of virulence traits in determining an enteric pathogen is the wide range of the types of *E. coli* that may cause secretory, cholera-like diarrhea via the production of heat labile (cholera-like) or heat stable enterotoxins or that may be invasive much like *Shigella*, depending on specific chromosomal and plasmid encoded virulence traits (Table 4). Other *E. coli* may produce a Shiga-like toxin, thereby causing enterohemorrhagic diarrhea and hemolytic uremic syndrome, and still other *E. coli* exhibit attaching and effacing localized adherence (including most classical "enteropathogenic" *E. coli*, EPEC) or aggregative or diffuse adherence patterns to cells such as HEp-2 cells in tissue culture. *E. coli* can produce one or more of three types of enterotoxins that induce intestinal secretion: (1) by acti-

Table 3. Enteric Microbial Virulence Traits

Secretory enterotoxins
Cytotoxins/neurotoxins
Adherence traits
Invasiveness

Table 4. Mechanisms of *E. Coli* Diarrhea

	Gene Code	Receptor	Mechanism
ETEC			
LT	plasmid	GM_1	ADPR-G_S → ac → Camp
ST_a	plasmid	? G.C.	direct pGC → cGMP
ST_b	plasmid	?	non-cA/G HCO_3-secretion
EHEC			
VT(SLT)	phage	Globotriaosyl ceramide (G-LC)	cleaves N-glycoside bond at position 4324 in target cells 28S $_r$RNA (like ricin)
EIEC	plasmid + chromosome	? inv	entry and dissolution of phagosome
EPEC	chromosome acf	–	actin condensation
EAEC	? plasmid	–	disruption of enzymes and absorption

vation of adenylate cyclase in a manner analogous to that of cholera toxin (heat labile toxins, LT-I and possibly LT-II) (33–36), (2) by activation of guanylate cyclase heat-stable toxin, STa, including STh or STp (37–39) or (3) through a guanylate- or adenylate cyclase-independent pathway (STb) (40, 41). In addition, *Klebsiella, Citrobacter, Salmonella,* and *Campylobacter* sp. produce cholera-like LTs that also activate adenylate cyclase, bind to ganglioside and display variable immunologic similarities to *E. coli* LTs (42–48). Furthermore, *Yersinia,* non-O1 *Vibrio cholerae,* and *Citrobacter freundii* produce antigenically cross-reacting and structurally homologous STs of 17–19 amino acids, with conservation of 6 cysteines (3 disulfide bonds) and a central asp-pro-ala region required for to ST-enterocyte binding and activation of guanylate cyclase (49–52). The exact roles of enterotoxins in the pathogenesis of many of these infections is not clear.

Other bacterial products that induce intestinal secretion include *C. difficile* toxin A (53), *C. perfringens* type A, *S. aureus* (and coagulase negative staphylococci) (54–55), *B. cereus,* and two recently described *E. coli* products that cause electrogenic secretion in Ussing chambers: (1) a chromosomally mediated 68–80 kDa secretory toxin produced in iron-deprived conditions by enteroinvasive *E. coli* (56); and (2) a 2–5 kDa heat stable, plasmid-encoded STa-like loop-negative toxin produced by enteroaggregative *E. coli* (57). *C. difficile* toxin A causes hemorrhagic secretion, possibly secondary to disruption of microfilaments and tight junctions (53, 58–61). Because of its different receptor specificity, toxin B is usually the cytotoxin detected in tissue culture. Enterotoxic and cytotoxic products of certain *Bacteroides fragilis* isolates from children and adults with diarrhea in Arizona and Montana have also been described (62–64).

Cytotoxic or neurotoxic products of enteric pathogens include Shiga toxin and the Shiga-like toxins (SLT, or Vero cytotoxins) that are produced by "enterohemorrhagic" *E. coli.* These toxins bind to globotriaosylceramide (Gb3) via their B subunit, and the enzymatically active A subunit (analogous to the plant toxin ricin) cleaves the N-glycoside bond of adenosine at position 4324 in the 28S rRNA of the 60S ribosomal subunit. This modification prevents elongation factor l-dependent aminoacyl tRNA binding to the ribosome and thereby halts protein synthesis (65–70). Subtle differences in the B subunit specificities for Gb4 or GbS as well as Gb3 may help explain differences in cell culture effects as well as in the disease manifestations of SLT-I and SLT-II, SLT-IIvh and SLT-IIvp (to cause bloody diarrhea or hemolytic uremic syndrome in patients, or edema disease in swine) (70–73). Shiga toxin causes limb paralysis and death in mice and rabbits, and axonal transport of toxin with vagal sensory neuron damage has been described (74–77). Examination of histopathologic sections, however, suggests that the neuronal damage may be indirect, via endothelial cell damage (74, 75). In addition, a 110 kDa heat- and trypsin-labile cytotoxin that is distinct from Shiga toxin has been recently implicated in patients with seizures or encephalopathy with shigellosis (78).

C. difficile toxin B, the cytotoxin typically detected in tissue culture assays for *C. difficile* toxin, is highly cytotoxic and lethal in mice (53), although its role in human disease is unclear. As with that of *C. difficile,* the cytotoxins of *C. perfringens, P. aeruginosa, S. aureus,* and coagulase-negative staphylococci have been implicated in necrotizing enterocolitis in neonates (55). The latter two organisms have been shown to produce a hemolytic, melittin-like delta toxin that activates phospholipase-A_2 to form platelet activating factor (PAF) and arachidonate metabolites that have been implicated in bowel damage or secretion (32, 54, 55, 60, 79).

In an elegant series of studies over the last 15 years, Lawrence and his colleagues have demonstrated the role of a trypsin-sensitive beta toxin of *C. perfringens* type C in causing the commonly fatal necrotizing enteritis (pigbel) following pig feasts in Papua New Guinea. Trypsin inhibitors in the sweet potatoes eaten at the feasts may play a role in the pathogenesis of "pigbel". Furthermore, active immunization against the beta toxin reduces mortality and hospital admissions for pigbel by 80% in vaccinated populations (80).

Additional cytotoxins have been described in *C. jejuni* and *H. pylori,* although the roles of these toxins in causing inflammatory enteritis and gastritis remain unclear (81–88). Finally, a 10–30 kDa "zonula occludens toxin" has recently been described with *Vibrio cholerae* that reversibly increases tissue conductance and tight junction permeability in stripped rabbit ileum in Ussing chambers, leaving glucose absorption intact. This toxin may help explain the diarrhea caused in volunteers given the live cholera vaccine strain CVD101, a ctxA deletion mutant of *V. cholerae* (89). Indeed, the microbial enterotoxins such as choleratoxin and ST have contributed significantly to our understanding of cyclic nucleotide regulation, while other enterotoxins such as STb, *C. difficile* toxin A and staphylococcal enterotoxins are elucidating new concepts about cyclic nucleotide-independent bicarbonate secretion, possible calcium-dependent chloride secretion and "superantigen" immune activation, respectively.

As important as toxin production to most enteric pathogens is the capacity to colonize in a relevant region of the bowel to cause disease. This fact is best defined with the plasmid-encoded (or plasmid-regulated) 2–7 nm surface fibrillae or fimbriae, CFA/I-V (colonization factor antigens) of enterotoxigenic *E. coli* (87–90). Analogous to K88, K99, 987P and F41 adhesins of animal enterotoxigenic *E. coli,* these immunologically distinct adhesins are critical to the pathogenicity of human enterotoxigenic *E. coli* (91–92). Analogous fimbriate or other adhesins may also aid in the initial colonization of enterohemorrhagic *E. coli* O157 and enteropathgenic *E. coli* (93–95). Classical "enteropathogenic" *E. coli* exhibit a qualitatively different attaching and effacing adherence in localized patterns to the brush border or to HEp-2 cells in culture (96–102). This attaching and effacing adherence is associated with polymerization of F-actin host cells (103), and with a specific chromosomal sequence identifiable by gene probe in enteropathogenic *E. coli* strains (104).

Distinct from the localized adherence of enteropathogenic *E. coli* to HEp-2 cells are "aggregative" and "diffuse" adherence patterns (102, 105). DNA probes have been developed that identify some, but not all, *E. coli* with the aggregative and diffuse patterns of HEp-2 cell adherence. To date, *E. coli* with the aggregate adherence phenotype, with or without being probe positive, have been associated with persistent diarrhea in studies in India and Brazil (12, 14, 106). Some investigators have suggested that the diffusely adhering *E. coli,* which produce a mannose-resistant hemagglutinin (107), may also be associated with diarrhea (108).

The expression of "invasiveness" is complex. In *Shigella* and enteroinvasive *E. coli,* invasiveness appears to involve a series of plasmid-encoded invasin and adhesin proteins that are regulated by key chromosomal codons (such as kcpA) (109, 110). A single *invasin* is encoded by *Yersinia pseudotuberculosis* that may enter via *integrin* receptors (111). In *Salmonella,* both adherence and invasion appear closely linked and may require bacterial proteins that are induced by trypsin- and neuraminidase-sensitive structures present on the epithelial cell surface (112). The capacity of *Entamoeba histolyica* to adhere and "invade" appears to relate at least in part to a GalNAc-inhibitable amebic lectin that leads to contact-dependent cytolysis of host cells, particularly attracted neutrophils (113–115). The distinctions between enterotoxigenic *E. coli* fimbriate adhesins to carbohydrates and glycolipids and the more intimate attachment of organisms such as *Yersinia, Salmonella, Shigella* and possibly enteropathogenic *E. coli* to transmembrane proteins such as integrins appear to provide critical determinants of surface colonization or cell invasion respectively (116).

Future considerations

Clearly the explosion of information regarding the etiologies and pathogenesis of enteric infections has tremendous implications for the improved control of these major causes of global morbidity and mortality. An orchestrated attack via epidemiologic, physiologic, pharmacologic, biochemical, immunologic and antimicrobial approaches is required. The epidemiologic control involves key issues of distribution and human behavior to provide acceptable minimum standards of improved water supplies and sanitation facilities that have been critical to the control of diarrheal diseases for the growing 75% of the world's population who reside in the tropical developing world. Improved physiologic control involves the application of existing and still improving oral rehydration therapy and continued key nutritional support with feeding at the community level to control and indeed prevent the major consequences of dehydration and malnutrition caused by diarrhea. At the pharmacologic and biochemical levels, antisecretory and antimicrobial agents require continued search and improvements for better understanding of secretory physiology and antimicrobial resistance patterns. Finally, an improved understanding of virulence traits has opened avenues for substantial advances in vaccine development for several enteric infections (117). Now available is the new Ty21a live gal-epimerase mutant typhoid fever vaccine that has 67–96% efficacy for 3 years with substantially fewer side effects than the killed whole cell parenteral typhoid vaccines previously available. There is additional promise with the Vi polysaccharide vaccine as well as aro-A and pur-A deletion auxotrophic mutants of *S. typhi.* Similarly, the oral whole cell/B subunit cholera vaccine provides protection not only against cholera but also significant protection against *E. coli* illnesses associated with heat labile toxin as well as a significant reduction in hospital visits overall (118), with some protection (best against classical cholera) lasting through the third year after oral immunization in adults (119). Additional promise lies ahead for both cholera and enterotoxigenic *E. coli* diarrheas with live, nontoxigenic colonizing toxin deletion or auxotrophic mutants. Live mutant and recombinant shigella vaccines that employ both chromosomal and plasmid virulence traits are also under study. Finally, initial encouraging results with rotavirus vaccines suggest that attenuated bovine and rhesus rotaviruses, particularly with reassortant genetic insertions from human rotaviruses, hold promise for effective polyvalent live rotavirus vaccines as well.

Conclusions

Never before have such capabilities to relieve human suffering been within our reach as they are with the control of diarrheal diseases today. In short, the challenge for our future is to awaken to diarrheal diseases as the barometer of health (or neglect) of a substantial majority of our global population. The measure of civilization itself may well be how we deal with the disparate health of the disadvantaged in our midst. We have the means at hand; only time will tell if we have the will or the insight to realize that how the poor fare will determine the destiny of us all.

References

1. Guerrant RL, Hughes JM, Lima NL, Crane JK (1990) Diarrhea in developed and developing countries: Magnitude, special settings, and etiologies. Rev Infect Dis [Suppl 1] 12: 41–S50
2. Schorling JB, Wanke CA, Schorling SK, McAuliffe JF, de Souza MA, Guerrant RL (1990) A prospective study of persistent diarrhea among children in an urban Brazilian slum: Patterns of occurrence and etiologic agents. Am J Epidemiol 132: 144–156
3. Bhatnagar S, Dosajh U (1986) Diarrhoeal disease morbidity in children below 5 years in urban slums of Delhi. Indian J Med Res 84: 53–58
4. Bennett JV, Holmberg SD, Rogers MF, Solomon SL (1987) Infectious and parasitic diseases. Am J Prev Med [Suppl] 3: 102
5. Ho M-S, Glass RI, Pinsky PR, et al (1988) Diarrheal deaths in American children are they preventable? JAMA 260: 3281–3285
6. Guerrant RL, Kirchhoff LV, Shields DS, et al (1983) Prospective study of diarrheal illnesses in northeastern Brazil: Patterns of disease, nutritional impact, etiologies, and risk factors. J Infect Dis 148: 986–997
7. Dingle JH, Badger DG, Jordan SW Jr (1964) Illness in the home: A study of 25,000 illnesses in a group of Cleveland families. Cleveland,OH, Case Western Reserve University Press
8. Bartlett AV, Moore M, Gary GW, Starko KM, Erben JJ, Meredith BA (1985) Diarrheal illness among infants and toddlers in daycare centers. II Comparison with daycare home and households. J Pediatr 107: 503–509
9. Schorling JB, Guerrant RL (1990) Diarrhea and catch-up growth. Lancet 1335: 599–600
10. Schorling JB, McAuliffe JF, de Souza MA, Guerrant RL (1990) Malnutrition predisposes to greater diarrhea incidence and duration among children in an urban Brazilian slum. Int J Epidemiol 19: 728–735
11. Lima AAM, Fang G, Schorling JB, et al (1992) Persistent diarrhea in Northeast Brazil: Etiologies and interactions with malnutrition. Acta Paediatr Scand (In Press)
12. Bhan MK, Raj P, Levine MM, et al (1989) Enteroaggregative *Escherichia coli* associated with persistent diarrhea in a cohort of rural children in India. J Infect Dis 159: 1061–1064
13. Bhan MK, Khoshoo V, Sommerfelt H, Pushker R, Sazawal S, Srivastava R (1989) Enteroaggregative *Escherichia coli* and *Salmonella* associated with nondysenteric persistent diarrhea. Pediatr Infect Dis J 8: 499–502
14. Fang GD, Lima AM, Wanke CA, Kaper JB, Levine MM, Guerrant RL (1991) HEp2 celladherent *E. coli:* Potential causes of persistent diarrhea of multiple genotypes and different adherence phenotypes. Clin Res 39: 223A, 39: 223A,
15. Soave R, Armstrong D (1986) Cryptosporidium and cryptosporidiosis. Rev Infect Dis 8: 1012–1023
16. Fayer R, Ungar BLP (1986) *Cryptosporidium* spp. and cryptosporidiosis. Microbiol Rev 50: 458–484
17. Janoff EN, Reller LB (1987) *Cryptosporidium* species, a protean protozoan. J Clin Microbiol; 25: 967–975
18. Guerrant RL, Petri WA, Weikel CS (1990) Parasitic causes of diarrhea. In: Lebenthal E, Duffey M (eds) Pathophysiology of secretory diarrhea. New York, Raven Press, Ltd., 273–280
19. Sallon S, Deckelbaum RJ, Schmid I, Harlap S, Baras M, Spira DT (1988) *Cryptosporidium,* malnutrition, and chronic diarrhea in children. Am J Dis Child 142: 312–316
20. MacFarlane DE, Horner-Bryce J (1987) Cryptosporidiosis in wellnourished and malnourished children. Acta Paediatr Scand 76: 474–477

21. Sarabia-Arce S, Salazar-Lindo E, Gilman RH, Naranjo J, Miranda E (1990) Case-control study of *Cryptosporidium parvum* infection in Peruvian children hospitalized for diarrhea: possible association with malnutrition and nosocomial infection. Pediatr Infect Dis J 9: 627–631
22. Pickering LK, Evans DG, DuPont HL, et al (1981) Diarrhea caused by *Shigella*, rotavirus and *Giardia* in daycare centers: Prospective study. J Pediatr 99: 51–56
23. Bartlett AV, Moore M, Gary GW, Starko KM, Erben JJ, Meredith BA (1985) Diarrheal illness among infants and toddlers in daycare centers. I. Epidemiology and pathogens. J Pediatr 107: 495–502
24. Lima NL, Guerrant RL, Kaiser DL, Germanson T, Farr BM (1990) A retrospective cohort study of nosocomial diarrhea as a risk factor for nosocomial infection. J Infect Dis 161: 948–952
25. Koch KL, Phillips DJ, Aber RC, Current WL (1985) Cryptosporidiosis in hospital personnel. Ann Intern Med 102: 593–596
26. McFarland LV, Mulligan ME, Kwok RYY, Starnm WE (1989) Nosocomial acquisition of *Clostridium difficile* infection. N Engl J Med 320: 204–210
27. Soave R, Johnson WD Jr (1988) Animal reservoirs of *Cryptosporidium* spp and *Isospora belli*. J Infect Dis 158: 910
28. Colebunders R, Francis H, Mann JM, et al (1987) Persistent diarrhea, strongly associated with HIV infeciton in Kinshasa, Zaire. Am J Gastroenterol 82: 859–864
29. Antony MA, Brandt LJ, Klein RS, Bernstein LH (1988) Infectious diarrhea in patients with AIDS. Dig Dis Sci 33: 1141–1146
30. Guerrant RL, Bobak DL (1991) Bacterial and protozoal gastroenteritis. N Engl J Med 325: 327–340
31. Brandtzaeg P, Halstensen TS, Kett K, et al (1989) Immunobiology and immunopathology of human gut mucosa: humoral immunity and intraepithelial lymphocytes. Gastroenterol 97: 1562–1584
32. Musch MW, Miller RJ, Field M (1982) Stimulation of colonic secretion by lipoxygenase metabolites of arachidonic acid. Science 217: 1255–1256
33. Kimberg DV, Field M, Johnson J, Henderson A, Gershon E (1971) Stimulation of intestinal mucosal adenyl cyclase by cholera enterotoxin and prostaglandins. J Clin Invest 50: 1218–1230
34. Chen LC, Rohde JE, Sharp GWG (1971) Intestinal adenyl-cyclase activity in human cholera. Lancet 1: 939–941
35. Guerrant RL, Chen LC, Sharp GWG (1975) Intestinal adenyl-cyclase activity in canine cholera: Correlation with fluid accumulation. J Infect Dis 125: 377–381
36. Guth BEC, Pickett CL, Twiddy EM, et al (1986) Production of Type II heat-labile enterotoxin (LT-II) by *Escherichia coli* isolated from food and human feces. Infect Immun 54: 587–589
37. Hughes JM, Murad F, Chang B, Guerrant RL (1978) Role of cyclic GMP in the action of heat-stable enterotoxins of *Escherichia coli*. Nature 271: 755–756
38. Field M, Graf Jr LH, Mata LJ (1978) Heat stable enterotoxin of *E. coli*. In vitro effects on guanylate cyclase activity, cyclic GMP concentration, and ion transport in small intestine. Proc Natl Acad Sci USA 75: 2800
39. Guerrant RL, Hughes JM, Chang B, Robertson DC, Murad F (1980)Activation of intestinal guanylate cyclase by heat-stable enterotoxin of *E. coli:* Studies of tissue specificity, potential receptors and intermediates. J Infect Dis 142: 220–228
40. Kennedy DJ, Greenberg RN, Dunn JA, Abernathy R, Ryerse JS, Guerrant RL (1984) Effects of *Escherichia coli* heat-stable enterotoxin STb on intestines of mice, rats, rabbits, and piglets. Infect Immun 46: 639–643
41. Weikel CS, Nellans HN, Guerrant RL (1986) The in vivo and in vitro effects of a novel enterotoxin, STb, produced by *Escherichia coli*. J Infect Dis 153: 893–901
42. Guerrant RL, Dickens MD, Wenzel RP, Kapikian AZ (1976) Toxigenic bacterial diarrhea: Nursery outbreak involving multiple bacterial strains. J Pediatr 89: 885–891
43. Wachsmuth K, Wells J, Shipley P (1979) Heat-labile enterotoxin production in isolates from a shipboard outbreak of human diarrheal illness. Infect Immun 24: 793–797

44. Honda T, Shimizu M, Takeda Y (1976) Isolation of a factor causing morphological changes of Chinese hamster ovary cells from the culture filtrates of *Vibrio parahemolyticus.* Infect Immun 14: 1028–1033
45. Sandefur PD, Peterson JW (1977) Neutralization of *Salmonella* toxin-induced elongation of Chinese hamster ovary cells by cholera antitoxin. Infect Immun 15: 988–992
46. Ruiz-Palacios GM, Torres J, Torres NI (1983) Cholera-like enterotoxin produced by *Campylobacter jejuni.* Characterization and clinical significance. Lancet 2: 250–252
47. Ruiz-Palacios GM, Lopez-Vidal Y, Torres J, Torres N (1985) Serum antibodies to heat-labile enterotoxin of *Campylobacter jejuni.* J Infect Dis 152: 413–416
48. Daikoku T, Kawagughi M, Takama K, Suzuki S (1990) Partial purification and characterization of the enterotoxin produced by *Campylobacter jejuni.* Infect Immun 58: 2414–2419
49. Aimoto S, Takao T, Shimonishi Y, et al (1982) Amino-acid sequence of a heat stable enterotoxin produced by human enterotoxigenic *Escherichia coli.* Eur J Biochem 129: 257–263
50. Takao T, Hitouji T, Aimoto S, et al (1983) Amino-acid sequence of a heat-stable enterotoxin isolated from enterotoxigenic *Escherichia coli* strain 18D. FEBS 152: 1–5
51. Guarino A, Giannella R, Thompson MR (1989) *Citrobacter freundii* produces an 18-amino-acid heat-stable enterotoxin identical to the 18-amino-acid *Escherichia coli* heat-stable enterotoxin (ST Ia). Infect Immun 57: 649–652
52. Takeda T, Balakrish Nair G, Suzuki K, Shimonishi Y (1990) Production of a monoclonal antibody to *Vibrio cholerae* Non-Ol heat-stable enterotoxin (ST) which is cross-reactive with *Yersinia enterocolitica* ST. Infect Immun 58: 2755–2759
53. Lyerly DM, Krivan HC, Wilkins TD (1988) *Clostridium difficile:* Its disease and toxins. J Clin Microbiol 1: 1–18
54. Kapral FA (1985) *Staphylococcus aureus* delta toxin as an enterotoxin. Ciba Found Symp 112: 215–229
55. Scheifele DW (1990) Role of bacterial toxins in neonatal necrotizing enterocolitis. J Pediatr 117 (No 1, Part 2): 45–S46
56. Fasano A, Kay BA, Russell RG, Maneval Jr DR, Levine MM (1990) Enterotoxin and cytotoxin production by enteroinvasive *Escherichia coli.* Infect Immun 58: 3717–3723
57. Savarino SJ, Fasano A, Robertson DC, Levine MM (1991) Enteroaggregative *Escherichia coli* elaborate a heat-stable enterotoxin demonstrable in an in vitro rabbit intestinal model. J Clin Invest 87: 1450–1455
58. Lima AAM, Lyerly DM, Wilkins TD, Innes DJ, Guerrant RL (1988) Effects of *Clostridium difficile* toxins A and B in rabbit small and large intestine in vivo and on cultured cells in vitro. Infect Immun 56: 582–588
59. Lima AAM, Innes DJ, Chadee K, Lyerly DM, Wilkins TD, Guerrant RL (1989) *Clostridium difficile* toxin A: Early sequential histopathologic effectts in rabbit small intestine. Lab lnvest 61: 419–425
60. Field M, Rao MC, Chang EB (1989) Intestinal electrolyte transport and diarrheal disease (Parts 1 & 2). N Engl J Med 32: 800–806 and 879–883
61. Moore R, Pothoulakis C, LaMont JT, Carlson S, Madara JL (1990) *C. difficile* toxin A increases intestinal permeability and induces Cl-secretion. Am Physiol Soc Gl 65–Gl 72
62. Myers LL, Shoop DS, Stackhouse LL, et al (1987) Isolation of enterotoxigenic *Bacteroides fragilis* from humans with diarrhea. J Clin Microbiol 25: 2330–2333
63. Myers LL, Shoop DS, Collins JE (1990) Rabbit model to evaluate enterovirulence of Bacteroides fragilis. J Clin Microbiol 28: 1658–1660
64. Weikel CS, Grieco FD, Reuben J, Myers LL, Sack RB (1990) HT29/C_1 cells treated with crude *Bacteroides fragilis* enterotoxin dramatically alter their morphology. Presented US Japan Cholera Conference, Kyoto (in press)
65. Keusch GT, Grady GF, Mata LJ (1972) The pathogenesis of *Shigella* diarrhea I. Enterotoxin production by *Shigella dysenteriae* 1. J Clin Invest 51: 1212–1218
66. O'Brien AD, Holmes RK (1987) Shiga and shiga-like toxins. Microbiol Rev 51 : 206–220
67. Karmali MA, Petric M, Lim C, Fleming PC, Arbus GS, Lior H (1985) The association between ideopathic hemolytic uremic syndrome and infection by verotoxin producing *E. coli.* J Infect Dis 151: 775–782

68. Obrig TG, Moran RP, Colinas RJ (1985) Ribonuclease activity associated with the 60-S ribosome inactivating proteins Ricin A, phytolaccin and shiga toxin. Biochem Biophys Res Commun 1300: 8790–8840
69. Reisbig R, Olsnes S, Eiklid K (1981) The cytotoxic activity of *Shigella* toxin: Evidence for catalytic inactivation of the 60-S ribosomal subunit. J Biol Chem 2560: 8739–8744
70. Jackson MP (1990) Structure-function analysis of Shiga toxin and the Shiga-like toxins. Microbial Pathogenesis 8: 235–242
71. Samuel JE, Perera LP, Ward S, O'Brien AD, Ginsburg V, Krivan HC (1990) Comparison of the glycolipid receptor specificities of Shiga-like toxin type II and Shiga-like toxin type II variants. Infect Immun 58: 611–618
72. Karmali MA(1989) Infection by verocytotoxin-producing *Escherichia coli.* Clin Microbiol Rev 2: 15–38
73. Riley LW, Remis RS, Helgerson SD, et al (1983) Outbreak of hemorrhagic colitis associated with a rare *E. coli* serotype. N Engl J Med 308: 681–685
74. Bridgewater FAJ, Morgan RS, Rowson KEK, Wright GP (1955) The neurotoxin of *Shigella shigae.* Morphological and functional lesions produced in the central nervous system of rabbits. Br J Exp Pathol 36: 447–453
75. Cavanagh JB, Howard JG, Whitby JL (1956) The neurotoxin of *Shigella shigae:* A comparative study of the effects produced in various laboratory animals. Br J Exp Med 370: 272–278
76. Howard JG (1955) Observations on the intoxication produced in mice and rabbits by the neurotoxin of *Shigella shigae.* Br J Exp Pathol 36: 439–446
77. Wiley RG, Donohue-Rolfe A, Keusch GT (1985) Axonally transported *Shigella* cytotoxin is neurotoxic? J Neuropathol Exp Neurol 440: 496–506
78. Ashkenazi A, Cleary KR, Pickering LK, Murray BE, Cleary TG (1990) The association of Shiga toxin and other cytotoxins with the neurologic manifestations of shigellosis. J Infect Dis 161: 961–965
79. Kasimir S, Schonfeld W, Alouf JE, Konig W (1990) Effect of *Staphylococcus aureus* delta-toxin on human granulocyte functions and platelet-activating-factor metabolism. Infect Immun 58: 1653–1659
80. Lawrence GW, Lehmann D, Anian G, et al (1990) Impact of active immunization against enteritis necroticans in Papua New Guinea. Lancet 336: 1165–1167
81. Johnson WM, Lior H (1984) Toxins produced by *Campylobacter jejuni* and *Campylobacter coli.* Lancet 1: 229–230
82. Yeen WP, Pothocheary SD, Pang T (1983) Demonstration of a cytotoxin from *Campylobacter jejuni.* J Clin Pathol 36: 1237–1240
83. Guerrant RL, Wanke CA, Pennie RA, Barrett LJ, Lima AAM, O'Brien AD (1987) Production of a unique cytotoxin by *Campylobacter jejuni.* Infect Immun 55: 2526–2530
84. Perez-Perez GL, Cohn DL, Guerrant RL, Patton CM, Reller LB, Blaser MJ (1989) Clinical and immunologic significance of cholera-like toxin and cytotoxin production by *Campylobacter* species in patients with acute inflammatory diarrhea in the USA. J Infect Dis 160: 460–467
85. Leunk RD, Johnson PT, David BC, Kraft WG, Morgan DR (1988) Cytotoxic activity in broth-culture filtrates of *Campylobacter pylori.* J Med Microbiol 26: 93–99
86. Leunk RD, Ferguson MA, Morgan DR, Low DE, Simor AE (1990) Antibody to cytotoxin in infection by *Helicobacter pylori.* J Clin Microbiol 28: 1181–1184
87. Guerrant RL, Lingwood CA (1991) Glycoconjugate receptors for adhesins and toxins. In: Marshall, McCallum and Guerrant (eds) Gastroduodenal Disease and Helicobacter pylori (in press)
88. Smoot DT, Mobley HLT, Chippendale GR, Lewison JF, Resau JH (1990) *Helicobacter pylori* urease activity is toxic to human gastric epithelial cells. Infect Immun 58: 1992–1994
89. Fasano A, Baudry B, Pumplin DW, et al (1991) *Vibrio cholerae* produces a second enterotoxin which affects intestinal tight junctions. PNAS (in press)
90. Evans DG, Silver RP, Evans DJ, Chase DG, Gorbach SL (1975) Plasmid-controlled colonization factor associated with virulence in *Escherichia coli* enterotoxigenic for humans. Infect Immun 12: 656–667

91. Satterwhite TK, Evans DG, DuPont HL, Evans DJ (1978) Role of *Escherichia coli* colonization factor antigen in acute diarrhea. Lancet 2: 181–183
92. Levine MM, Kaper JB, Black RE, Clements ML (1983) New knowledge on pathogenesis of bacterial enteric infections as applied to vaccine development. Microbiol Rev 47: 510–550
93. Karch H, Heesemann J, Laufs R, et al (1987) A plasmid of enterohemorrhagic Escherichia coli 0157:H7 is required for expression of a new fimbrial antigen and for adhesion to epithelial cells. Infect Immun 55: 455–461
94. Toth I, Cohen ML, Rumschlag HS, et al (1990) Influence of the 60-Megadalton plasmid on adherence of *Escherichia coli* 0157:H7 and genetic derivatives. Infect Immun 58: 1223–1231
95. Baldini MA, Kaper JB, Levine MM, Candy DCA, Moon HW (1983) Plasmid-mediated adhesin in enteropathogenic *Escherichia coli.* J Pediatr Gastroenterol Nutr 2: 534–538
96. Ulshen MH, Rollo JL (1980) Pathogenesis of *Escherichia coli* gastroenteritis in man, another mechanism. N Engl J Med 302: 99–101
97. Polotsky YE, Dragunskaya EM, Seliverstova GV, et al (1977) Pathogenic effect of enterotoxigenic *Escherichia coli* and *Escherichia coli* causing infantile diarrhoea. Acta Microbiol Acad Sci Hung 4: 221
98. Rothbaum R, McAdams AJ, Giannella R, Partin JC (1982) A clinicopathologic study of enterocyte-adherent *Escherichia coli:* A cause of protracted diarrhea in children. Gastroenterol 83: 441–454
99. Levine MM, Nalin DR, Hornick RB, et al (1978) *Escherichia coli* strains that cause diarrhea but do not produce heat-labile or heat-stable enterotoxins and are noninvasive. Lancet 1: 1119–1122
100. Guerrant RL (1980) Yet another pathogenic mechanism for *Escherichia coli* diarrhea. N Engl J Med 302: 113–114
101. Cravioto A, Gross RJ, Scotland S, et al (1979) An adhesive factor found in strains of *Escherichia coli* belonging to the traditional infantile enteropathogenic serotypes. Curr Microbiol 3: 95–99
102. Nataro JP, Kaper JB, Robins-Browne R, et al (1987) Patterns of adherence of diarrheagenic *Escherichia coli* to HEP-2 cells. Pediatr Infect Dis J 6: 829–831
103. Knutton S, Baldwin T, Williams PH, McNeish AS (1989) Actin accumulation at sites of bacterial adhesion to tissue culture cells: basis of a new diagnostic test for enteropathogenic and enterohemorrhagic *Escherichia coli.* Infect Immun 57: 1290–1298
104. Jerse AE, Martin WC, Galen JE, Kaper JB (1990) Oligonucleotide probe for detection of the enteropathogenic *Escherichia coli* (EPEC) adherence factor of localized adherent EPEC. J Clin Microbiol 28: 2842–2844
105. Mathewson JJ, Cravioto A (1989) HEp-2 cell adherence as an assay for virulence among diarrheagenic *Escherichia coli.* J Infect Dis 159: 1057–1060
106. Vial P, Robins-Browne R, Lior H, et al (1988) Characterization of enteroadherent-aggregative *Escherichia coli,* a putative agent of diarrheal disease. J Infect Dis 158: 70–79
107. Bilge SS, Clausen CR, Lau W, Moseley SL (1989) Molecular characterization of a fimbrial adhesin, F1845, mediating diffuse adherence of diarrhea-associated *Escherichia coli* to HEp-2 cells. J Bacteriol 171: 4281–4289
108. Giron JA, Fry J, Frankel G, et al (1991) Diffuse-adhering *Escherichia coli* (DAEC) as a putative cause of diarrhea in Mayan children in Mexico. J Infect Dis 163: 507–513
109. Sansonetti PJ, Hale TL, Oakes EV (1985) Genetics of virulence in enteroinvasive *Eschericia coli.* Microbiol 74–77
110. Maurelli AT, Sansonetti P (1988) Identification of a chromosomal gene controlling temperature-regulated expression of *Shigella* virulence. Proc Natl Acad Sci USA 85: 2820–2824
111. Isberg RL, Voorhis DL, Falkow S (1987) Identification of invasin: a protein that allows enteric bacteria to penetrate cultured mammalian cells. Cell 50: 769–778
112. Finlay BB, Heffron F, Falkow S (1989) Epithelial cell surfaces induce *Salmonella* proteins required for bacterial adherence and invasion. Science 243: 940–943

113. Ravdin JI, Guerrant RL (1981) Role of adherence in cytopathogenic mechanisms of *Entamoeba histolytica*. J Clin Invest 68: 1305–1313
114. Guerrant RL, Brush JE, Ravdin JI, et al (1981) Interaction between *Entamoeba histolytica* and human polymorphonuclear leukocytes. J Infect Dis 143: 83–93
115. Petri WA Jr, Chapman MD, Snodgrass T, Mann BJ, Broman J, Ravdin JI (1989) Subunit structure of the galactose and N-acetyl-D-galactosamine-inhibitable adherence lectin of *Entamoeba histolytica*. J Biol Chem 264: 3007–3012
116. Isberg R (1991) Discrimination between intracellular uptake and surface adhesion of bacterial pathogens. Science 252: 934–938
117. Guerrant RL (1988) Vaccines against enteric infections. Current Opinion in Infectious Diseases 1: 868–876
118. Clemens D, Sack DA, Harris JR, et al (1988) Impact of B subunit killed whole-cell and killed whole-cell-only oral vaccines against cholera upon treated diarrhoeal illness and mortality in an area endemic for cholera. Lancet 1: 1375–1378
119. Clemens JD, Sack DA, Harris JR, Van Loon F, Chakraborty J, Ahmen F (1990) Field trial of oral cholera vaccines in Bangladesh: results from three-year follow-up. Lancet 335(8684): 270–273

Prospects for Control of Malaria in the Twenty-First Century*

Carter L. Diggs

Atlantic Resources Corporation, Arlington, Virginia, U.S.A.

Abstract

After significant gains against malaria through control efforts earlier in the twentieth century, the malaria problem has increased for the last two decades. The thrust for global eradication of the disease was frustrated by the emergence of insecticide and drug resistance, concerns that vector control methods would damage the environment, and failure of the system to monitor for and correct deficiencies. The realignment of control strategy that resulted, although containing positive elements, has proven to be difficult to implement. In spite of the current situation, methods are available, and others can be developed through research and development, to mount a renewed attack on malaria. In order to mobilize an effective control program, careful central planning, coordination, and communication must be coupled with local area analysis and planning, tailored intervention programs, adequate surveillance systems, and appropriate operational research and evaluation. Above all, it will be necessary that decision makers have the will, and therefore provide the resources, for an effective malaria control effort.

Introduction

It is fashionable to promote programs against human problems by characterizing them as "wars". We are all cognizant of the "war on poverty", the "war on drugs", and Gordon Harrison's book on the struggle against malaria is subtitled "A history of the hostilities" (13). It is instructive to compare the expenditures in these "wars" with those of the more authen-

---

* Supported by Agency for International Development Contract DPE-5979-C-00-0039-00
The views expressed in this paper are those of the author and do not necessarily reflect those of Atlantic Resources Corporation or the Agency for International Development.

tic wars such as the 1990–1991 Persian Gulf War. The bill for that war is conservatively estimated at more than $30 billion (as of February 1991; U.S. Department of Defense Public Affairs Office). In contrast, expenditures for malaria control on a world wide basis is probably less than $100 million per year; The U.S. Agency for International Development, probably the major donor to malaria control, projected obligations for Fiscal Year 1991 of less than $28 million (Center for International Health Information). Far from a war being waged, malaria control has been all but ignored during the last two decades. A true war on malaria would have to be taken as seriously as was the Persian Gulf War and would cost more, perhaps much more, than is currently being expended. Can malaria be controlled in the twenty-first century? I believe so, if sufficient funds are allocated. Will it be controlled? Only if there is the will to make it happen.

In this presentation, I will highlight some of the major issues currently relevant to malaria control with emphasis on those areas impacting on the feasibility of a successful control effort. The outline of the presentation is as follows: first, I will review with you the magnitude of the current malaria problem, and how we arrived where we are. Second, I will discuss current methodologies for combatting malaria. Next, I will review recent research and development efforts aimed at malaria control. This will be followed by a speculative view of how an expanded malaria control effort might be approached. Finally, I will return to the somewhat philosophical mode of my opening remarks to see if we can glean any further insights or guesses as to what the future may hold.

The Current Status of the Malaria Problem

Malaria puts humans off guard. When you visit an area highly endemic for malaria, you are as likely as not to be impressed with the lack of pathogenicity of malaria. It is not at all unusual to visit a school with apparently healthy, active children, most of whom on thick film examination have parasites. This remarkable immunity to disease (malaria) but not infection (parasitemia) can persuade local health officials and the populace itself that malaria is not so bad. Indeed it might not be considered so bad if one considers the percentage of malaria cases that result in death. *Plasmodium vivax* and *P. ovale* almost never kill. *P. malariae* deaths are uncommon and usually associated with chronic infections that are inadequately treated, and even *P. falciparum*, the etiological agent of malignant tertian malaria, has an overall mortality of approximately 1% (11). It is when the absolute numbers of cases of malaria are considered that its true importance is appreciated. A recent estimate of the annual number of clinical cases of falciparum malaria is more than 200,000,000, (Fig. 1) so that the 1% case fatality rate translates into more than 2,000,000 deaths per year (32). This figure puts malaria among the top several causes of death, only exceeded by the generic categories of diarrheal diseases and respiratory infections. It is also important to be aware that the majority of these deaths are among young children who have not yet developed the

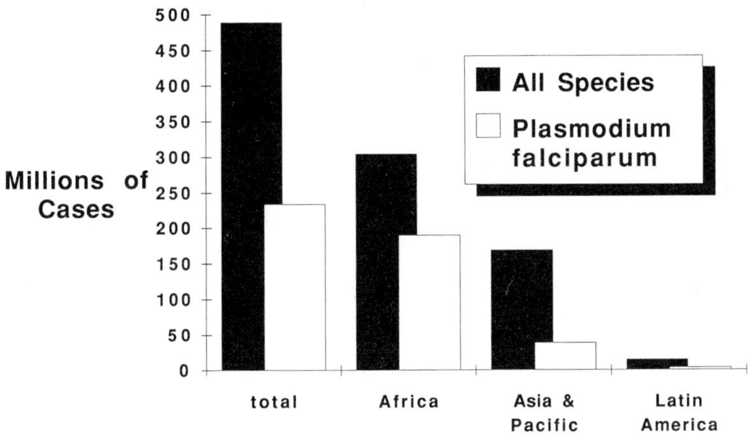

Fig. 1. Estimated annual malaria morbidity (from Sturchler, 1989)

immunity that can be observed in their older siblings. Whereas newborns appear to be protected by passive immunity derived from the mother, children of about one year of age are extremely vulnerable. Although accurate data are not available, the case fatality rate in this group may well be 25% in the absence of treatment.

This distinction between infection and disease has another complicating consequence; the identification of clinical malaria is difficult and somewhat arbitrary. The presence of parasites is not a very useful finding in this regard. A high parasitemia in a febrile patient suggests that the clinical illness may be due to malaria, but no other specific criteria are available. The diagnosis of severe malaria is primarily presumptive. CNS signs, parasitemia, and no obvious cause of some other CNS disease leads to the diagnosis of cerebral malaria. Because of the abundance of other etiologic agents causing acute diarrheal and respiratory diseases, it is impossible to determine what proportion of these syndromes are malaria related. However, it has been estimated that 25% of childhood deaths in Africa are due to malaria. [For detailed descriptions of malaria (2, 37).]

Twentieth Century Battles against Malaria

With the availability and remarkable insecticidal properties of DDT, the possibility of global eradication of malaria was entertained, and in 1955, WHO embarked on an eradication campaign with financial backing by a number of donor countries (10). Based primarily on the use of DDT as a residual insecticide, the objective was to decrease transmission in each geographical area (the attack phase) until it fell below a sustainable level, maintain surveillance for long enough to ensure that the parasite was in fact eradicated (consolidation phase), and finally to guard against reintroduction from other geographical areas (the maintenance phase). It was thus envisioned that, after a vigorous campaign, the problem would be solved and efforts would not have to be sustained indefinitely (26). The World Health Organization expended almost $230 million between 1955 and 1974 (10). The U.S. contribution to the effort between 1950 and 1972 was about $1 billion (31).

The attack was launched in those areas in which an infrastructure was already in place and where efforts were already underway. Italy, Greece, India, and Ceylon (Sri Lanka) were among the countries which already had programs in place. Significantly, no African country was on the list. It was recognized that sub-Saharan Africa would provide the greatest challenge, and attack of that area was deferred (13).

Successes in some areas were extremely impressive. Italy and Greece remain free of malaria today. Other areas lowered the incidence of malaria to a remarkable degree. One of the best known examples is Sri Lanka. Prior to the beginning of the effort, there had been a high incidence of malaria for many years. In 1934 and 1935, an epidemic killed 87,000 people in seven months (14). There were an estimated 1,000,000 cases per year in the early 1950s. In 1963, only 17 cases were recorded (31). A striking reduction in malaria incidence was achieved in many other areas as well. But then a series of reverses took place that culminated in the abandonment of the global eradication effort in 1968.

As is the case for most historical events, the causes which led to a reassessment of the global malaria eradication concept are multiple, and the contributions of each to the final outcome are debated. However, the easiest factor to incriminate is the emergence of resistance of mosquitoes to DDT. Demonstrated in only two species of *Anopheles* in 1946, resistance had been found in 46 species widely distributed throughout malaria endemic areas by 1976 (2). In addition to the emergence of mosquitoes which could function normally after exposure to DDT, some populations of anopheline mosquitoes developed "behavioral resistance" to the compound (15). This was expressed as a negative tropism or avoidance behavior of mosquitoes entering a house which had been sprayed. Although this repellent action was of immediate benefit to the residents of sprayed houses, it also enabled mosquitoes to survive and act as vectors in unprotected areas.

A second blow to the malaria eradication effort was the groundswell of concern that DDT, as well as other insecticides, might have an adverse effect on the health of animals, especially wildlife, and perhaps man. This development was a prime example of the power of the pen in the political process. Rachel Carson's book, *The Silent Spring*, which appeared in 1962, so aroused public opinion that support for the spraying activities which comprised the principal strategy of the eradication effort fell precipitously. Arguments that the benefits of vector control outweighed the risk to human health and the environment were made, but pragmatists soon accepted the fact that the public perception of the opposite, i. e., that insecticides wreak havoc while helping little, was a powerful reality with an independent existence quite apart from any evidence which might refute the conclusion. This reality made spraying activities infeasible on the scale required by the malaria eradication program.

Although the spearhead of the eradication effort was reduction of the vector population through the use of insecticide, an important secondary modality was the treatment of cases detected during the consolidation phase in any given area. Chloroquine was the almost perfect drug for this purpose. Highly effective and very well-tolerated, it could be depended upon to cure essentially all infections, when a standard regimen was administered. It is likely that this caveat, "in which a standard regimen was administered", is one of the keys to the catastrophic demise of chloroquine from its exalted status. The drug was widely available on the open market and self-administration was widespread. There is no doubt that subcurative regimens were used that alleviated symptoms but allowed the continued replication of the parasite with subsequent transmission and introduction of drug resistant mutants into the mosquito and human populations. The result was the progressive spread of chloroquine resistant malaria, from foci in South America (24) and Asia (12, 35), and finally in Africa, first appearing in a small area of East Africa (8) and spreading progressively until now, only small enclaves in a few countries on that continent have escaped (Fig. 2). Needless to say, these events were extremely discouraging to the eradication effort.

A problem not encountered, but one that would have had to have been met if the campaign had progressed to the point of attacking malaria on the continent of Africa, is the greater vectorial capacity of *Anopheles gambiae* compared with other species of anopheline mosquitoes. This characteristic, which is a function of the density of the vectors, the number of blood meals on humans per vector per day, the daily vector survival probability, and the incubation period of the parasite in the mosquito (9) probably includes the most important factors in the maintenance of the high level of malaria transmission on this continent. It has been estimated that even if the number of infected mosquito bites received from this mosquito was reduced ten fold, there would be no diminution in the incidence of malaria. In the face of such redundant transmission, a malaria eradication campaign based on vector control would have resulted in relatively little decrease in malaria incidence until the vector was eradicated.

Finally, the malaria eradication program suffered from system failure. Although the program never grew to its intended maximal size (efforts in Africa were never started), its complexity was already great and the management structure inadequate. What might have served well was a centralized organizational structure through which control of operations could be maintained through the management chain; i. e., a military-like command and control system. Lacking that, strong central coordination was an absolute necessity. But, as it was put by Gordon Harrison, "people ... were ... conditioned to thinking that the key to success was DDT, not organization" (13).

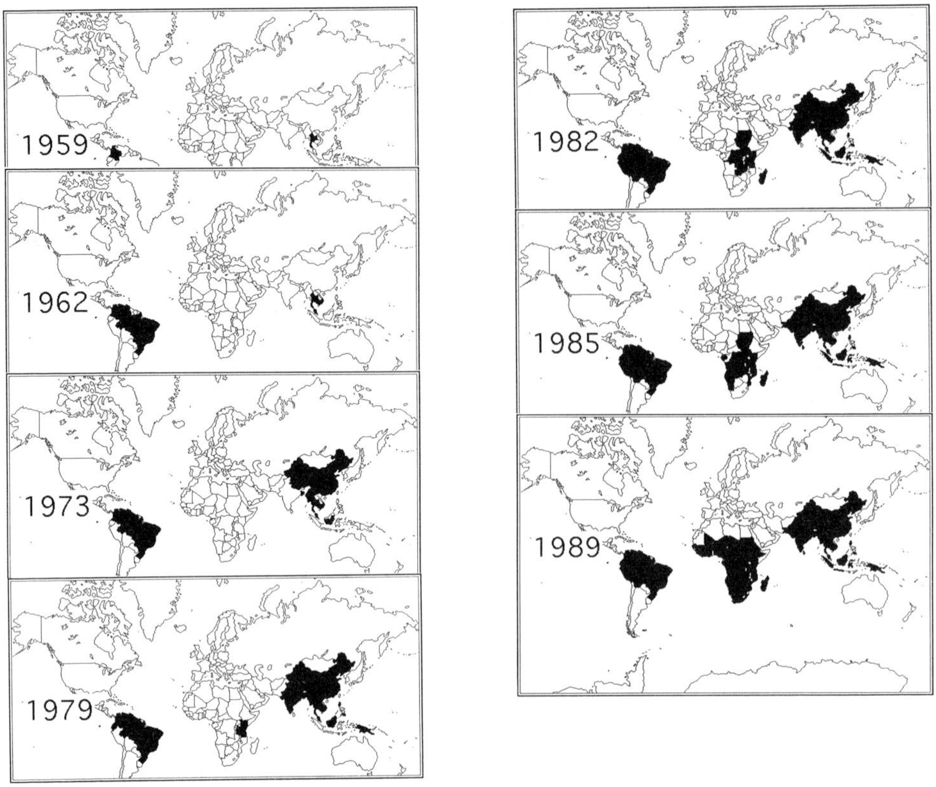

Fig. 2. Thirty years of chloroquine resistance. By 1959 Chloroquine resistance had been documented in both Thailand and Colombia, although the reports were published later. Other dates indicate years reports were published. (Data derived from Moore and Lanier, 1961; Harinasuta et al, 1962; Onori in Wernsdorfer and McGregor, 1988; and the 1989–1990 Annual Report of the Africa Child Survival Inititiative, U.S. Agency for International Development and Centers for Disease Control, U.S. Government Printing Office 1990-532-036/F4908.)

There was every reason to believe that centralized command and control was an appropriate plan; history had provided several rather amazing demonstrations of the efficacy of this approach. One especially compelling example bears relating. In 1930, *Anopheles gambiae* invaded Brazil. There was an immediate upsurge in the incidence of malaria. Less than a year after the presence of the mosquito was discovered, an epidemic occurred with 10,000 cases in a six-square mile area inhabited by 12,000 people. The Brazilian Yellow Fever Service undertook the problem and, in spite of heavy engagement in the effort against *Aedes aegypti,* successfully reduced the *Anopheles gambiae* population to very small numbers, after which no further measures could be taken. Only relatively small, sporadic outbreaks occurred over the next several years, but in 1938, major epidemics occurred and the vector was found to extend over a wide geographic area. In order to address the problem, the Antimalaria Service was organized in 1938, and in 1939 recruited the Rockefeller Foundation for assistance in controlling the problem. In an unusual move, the Brazilian government granted essentially total control over the effort to The Rockefeller Foundation, which delegated authority to Fred Soper. Within a few months, a highly regimented team was assembled and operated under strict command and control during 1939 and 1940. Paris Green was used to kill larvae and pyrethrum was used against adults. An extremely effective system of monitoring was instituted, and deviations from standard procedures were dealt with harshly. As a result, the last *Anopheles gambiae* mosquito was collected in late 1940 (7).

The global eradication program was not conducted with the same rigor as was "Soper's" campaign. Spraying was not always under adequate surveillance, and operations were sometimes incorrectly implemented or simply omitted. Perhaps of greatest importance was the lack of appreciation, at this point in history, of the vulnerability of complex systems designed by humans to fatal malfunctions, the redundancy of mechanisms in nature to evade detrimental forces, and the lack of operational research to uncover and correct these malfunctions and reactions in a systematic manner. Inevitably, the outcome of the eradication effort was degraded.

In 1968, with support waning, WHO acknowledged the necessity for a change in the antimalarial strategy. It was apparent that a time limited solution (i. e., global eradication) was not feasible at that time. It was concluded that, although eradication efforts should be undertaken where eradication was judged to be feasible, that strategy should be adapted to the epidemiological situation as well as to the administrative and economic resources available. The initiative for these efforts was largely left to national health departments (10). Already resurgent at that time, malaria has continued a gradual increase in incidence. In 1975, Sri Lanka had 600,000 cases of malaria, up from the 17 in 1963 at the pinnacle of the eradication era (31). Many of the old forces which have exacerbated the incidence of many infectious diseases throughout history are operative in causing a worsening of the malaria problem in many parts of the world today. Settlement of Irian Jaya by non-immune Javanese has resulted in a major malaria problem for Indonesia. Development and deforestation in the Amazon rain forest and the movements of nonimmune populations into and through this area have resulted in a striking increase in malaria in Brazil. In the meantime, Africa maintains its ancient status quo, with close to two million of its children dying from malaria each year.

The recommendations made by WHO in 1968 were difficult to implement for many reasons; the administrative and economic constraints recognized at that time were often too great to allow reasonable progress of control efforts. The tailoring of programs to the "epidemiological situation" has often proven to be too difficult a task, usually because little or no epidemiological assessment was possible with available resources. The declaration of Alma-Ata in 1978, which included the idea of the incorporation of malaria control activities into primary health care systems, provided some conceptual guidance but, except perhaps for isolated small instances, resulted in little or no actual impact on malaria control activities.

Certainly, the WHO analysis of 1968 was a pragmatic, if discouraging, starting point for further deliberations on how to approach control efforts. If "eradication", which is by definition a time-limited approach, is not possible, the alternative is "control", with a most optimistic endpoint of eliminating malaria as a major public health problem. Control, as opposed to eradication, recognizing the long-term, indeed indefinite, length of commitment, seeks to institutionalize antimalarial efforts into the permanent infrastructure of health systems, a "horizontal" as opposed to the "vertical" approach taken during the eradication era. Although the principles have been promulgated, many questions continue to be debated: What organizational structures should support control efforts? What interventions should be used? How and at what level should "adequate control" be defined? How will control efforts change as malaria incidence declines? How will resurgence be prevented? How much will all this cost? And most importantly, who will pay for it?

Methods Currently Available for Combatting Malaria

Most, if not all, who aspire to contribute to control of malaria agree that no single weapon is likely to be sufficient. On the contrary, an armamentarium which includes both currently available and new methodologies are urgently needed. Research and development to provide the latter will be discussed in the next section. What follows is an overview of what is currently available with some comments as to the usefulness of the various approaches in a control effort.

Antimalarial Drugs[1]

Although drugs have recently been the only method used against malaria in many endemic areas, they have only a limited impact on control of transmission. In the current social and economic climate in most malaria endemic areas, only a small proportion of cases reach a health facility where they can be adequately treated. Even if this were not the case, adequate treatment of the clinical disease does not necessarily influence transmission, since viable gametocytes capable of infecting mosquitoes continue to circulate in the blood of the convalescent patient treated with standard antimalaria drugs effective against blood stages of the parasite. Mass chemoprophylaxis is also problematic due to economic constraints, widespread drug resistance, and the hazards of long-term drug administration.

[1] This account is an overview only, and is not intended as a definitive guide to treatment or prophylaxis. Standard references, including the "Health Information for International Travel", published annually by the Centers for Disease Control, should be used for this purpose. CDC also has a 24-hour malaria hotline for current recommendations for the prevention of malaria. The number is (404) 332-4555

However, drugs have a major role in the health care system as a part of a more comprehensive approach to malaria control and in prevention of malaria in individuals transiently exposed.

Prior to the development of widespread drug resistance, a variety of drugs were available. Quinine, which has been in use for centuries, although effective against the blood stages of all of the malaria parasites, has the disadvantages of requiring a prolonged period of administration to achieve elimination of parasites and of having a number of unpleasant side effects; indeed the presence of tinnitus has been considered positive evidence that a therapeutic blood level of the drug has been achieved; vertigo and deafness are also common.

Chloroquine was an almost ideal agent for alleviation of the clinical manifestations of malaria due to all four species of human malaria parasites and for the radical cure of *P. falciparum* and *P. malariae*, which do not have persistent liver stages and therefore do not relapse. Neither chloroquine nor other 4-aminoquinolines are active against the liver stages of *P. vivax* and *P. ovale*. However, 8-aminoquinolines do have this activity, and the most useful member of this group of compounds, primaquine, is incorporated into *P. vivax* and *P. ovale* curative regimens. Unlike the essentially 100% efficacy of chloroquine on susceptible parasites, primaquine fails to cure relapsing malaria in about 10% of cases.

In addition to their use in therapy, chloroquine and primaquine in combination have also been used extensively for "true causal prophylaxis" of malaria. The combined chloroquine/primaquine formulation is taken weekly during and after exposure to risk of infection. However, due to chloroquine resistance and the potential for primiquine toxicity, this regimen is of limited usefulness in most areas.

In spite of the existence of chloroquine resistant strains of *P. falciparum* almost everywhere in the world, chloroquine continues to be used. Chloroquine resistance is categorized into four levels based on the clinical response to a standard treatment regimen. Only at the highest level (R IV) is there no diminution in parasitemia after treatment. Thus, in cases in which lower levels of resistance are exhibited (RI-RIII) clinical benefit is achieved, and undoubtedly, self-treatment continues to prevent morbidity and mortality from malaria. However, conversion of acute disease to a chronic state perpetuates rather than solves the problem, and some manifestations of disease may be observed with higher frequency. For example, clinicians in Kenya have observed an increased incidence of severe anemia in children in recent years, believed to be due to malaria made chronic by subcurative treatment (18). This is particularly disturbing since it results in more transfusions with blood that may itself be hazardous due to contamination with human immunodeficiency or hepatitis B virus in spite of state-of-the-art screening procedures. Thus malaria may accelerate the AIDS epidemic through a chain of events in which the health care system plays an unwitting role.

Other drugs which have been used for a number of years and are still useful against malaria include the antifolate group, which act at various biochemical levels to deprive the parasite of folic acid, which is essential to its viability. These include pyrimethamine, sulfadoxine, and proguanil. The first two drugs have been used extensively in combination under the proprietary name Fansidar®. This combination is highly effective in areas where the parasites are susceptible, but resistance has developed in areas where it has been widely used. Another disadvantage of Fansidar® is the relatively high incidence (1/15,000) of Stevens-Johnson syndrome in recipients. Fansidar® is recommended as a self-treatment drug in individuals on chloroquine prophylaxis who experience symptoms suggestive of malaria and who do not have readily available medical assistance. This is most appropriate in Africa where Fansidar® resistance is not yet pervasive. Resistance to proguanil has become widespread as well, but it is still recommended as an adjunct to chloroquine prophylaxis for travelers to Africa. It is not licensed in the United States.

Another class of compounds with antimalarial activity consists of the tetracyclines. Although their activity was discovered several decades ago, their slow action and the short half life in the circulation have prevented their widespread use. Recently, the efficacy of daily deoxytetracycline as a prophylactic agent has been demonstrated, and the drug is now recommended for this purpose in certain circumstances (27).

Mefloquine, which was developed in response to the rapid spread of resistance to the older antimalarials, has recently been licensed in the United States. A quinoline methanol, this compound is structurally similar to quinine, but does not have the disadvantages of quinine. It has few side effects in most recipients and a long half life. Unfortunately, resistance was described even before it was licensed. In addition, with widespread use, relatively low incidence side effects, some serious, have been discovered. However, mefloquine is currently the best single drug for the treatment and prophylaxis of chloroquine resistant malaria.

Personal Protective Measures

Like drugs, personal protective measures have a limited but important role in the overall approach to malaria control. In areas where malaria incidence is highest, socioeconomic barriers severely limit access to the resident population. Nevertheless, these methods are important in the overall antimalarial effort. Currently, all such methods are directed towards prevention of mosquito bites. General protective measures include avoidance of high-risk exposure such as outdoor activities during peak mosquito feeding periods, the wearing of protective clothing, the use of repellents, the use of screens to discourage entrance of mosquitoes into houses, and the use of bed nets to help prevent bites during sleep. The best known repellent, N,N diethlymetatoluamide (DEET) is highly effective. A few cases of encephalopathy apparently due to high level exposure in workers have been reported (25); the agent can probably still be used without harm under most circumstances, but these reports signal the need for caution (23).

As can be inferred from previous comments in this paper, insecticide also has a direct role in personal protection aside from its general reduction in the size of mosquito populations. Insecticides are useful in the clearance of mosquitoes from living quarters, in the repellent action of some insecticides against mosquitoes as they enter the vicinity of the treated areas, and in the killing of mosquitoes before they have a chance to bite. A development of the last few years which is particularly promising is the use of permethrin as a residual agent which is rapidly lethal to mosquitoes that land on a treated surface. The compound has been most often used to impregnate bednets which are used during the sleeping hours. It can also be used to treat clothing. Unlike most personal protection measures, impregnated bednets can decrease the mosquito population in some locales.

Vector Control

Reducing the population of anopheline mosquitoes would appear to be the only approach that currently can result in diminishing the incidence of malaria infection to a significant degree, although future approaches might be capable of controlling the disease without controlling the vector (see Research, below). What are the alternatives since the demise of much of the usefulness of the agent which has had the greatest impact on malaria incidence in history, DDT? Other insecticides as effective as DDT have been developed, and some of these have not (yet) been shown to be as dangerous to human health and the environment as DDT is alleged to be. Application of newer residual insecticides has, in fact, been shown to be effective in decreasing the transmission rate in areas of high endemicity. However, each generation of insecticide that has been developed has been more expensive to produce than the one before it. As a result, the use of most insecticides in large-scale applications is beyond the reach of most current or contemplated budgets. Nevertheless, the use of insecticides to reduce populations of adult mosquitoes remains as one important component in the mounting of control efforts.

Arguably of greater potential in reducing mosquito numbers than interventions against the adult insects is a variety of measures which can be taken against larvae, either directly or by depriving them of their habitat. Direct measures include the use of larvicidal chemical agents. Although some of these are apparently quite safe, the perception of environmental pollution is often an effective deterrent to use, as is the case for adulticidal methods. More acceptable from this point of view are mechanical methods such as the use of polystryrene beads which interfere with the emergence of the adult mosquitoes from pupae at the time of maturation. An approach which may be even more acceptable is the use of larvivorous fish which can not only limit the numbers of insects which survive to adulthood but, depending on the species of fish, can serve as a source of food. This approach is particularly attractive as a part of the use of submerged rice growing areas. The resulting fertilization of the rice and the additional crop (i. e., the fish) obtained from the land motivates the farmer to exercise the necessary husbandry and the entire community benefits from the decreased vector numbers (30).

It is likely that the most powerful (and perhaps also the most expensive) method for controlling mosquito breeding is the modification of the breeding sites. Drainage of swamps can often effectively deprive the larvae of an environment which allows their survival. However, the ecological consequences of large-scale destruction of wetlands are profound, and any effort of this type can only be undertaken in conjunction with a careful environmental impact assessment and with measures to prevent adverse effects of the intervention.

Less profound modifications of breeding sites require a greater knowledge of the local ecosystem, since different species of anopheline mosquitoes have different preferences with respect to the amount of sunlight available, the amount and type of current in the body of water, the salinity of the water, the types of other organisms present, and other variables. These preferences allow for a wide range of choices in planning for intervention (29). In some instances, it is impossible to gain access to the larvae. An often cited example is the habit of some populations of *Anopheles gambiae* to oviposit in the hoofprints of large animals; in this case, it is essentially impossible to devise a practical method to interfere with the development and subsequent emergence of the mosquitoes.

Current Status of Control Efforts

Although many countries have nominal control programs, most suffer from lack of personnel with an adequate understanding of all of the factors required to initiate and maintain such an effort and all suffer from a lack of sufficient funds for the purpose. Although the objectives and strategies of malaria control are quite different from those of malaria eradication, many countries adhere to the methods and sometimes even the terminology of the eradication era. Thus, "Departments of Malaria Eradication" still exist, and there are still residual insecticide administration efforts which were originally instituted as a measure which was to be applied only during a short time period during which the area would be rid of the mosquitoes. While in some cases these efforts are helpful, a more thoughtful approach to the nature of the problem in each area would almost certainly improve the effectiveness of the effort. More will be said later about improvements that might be made in the approach to control efforts.

Research Efforts to Improve Malaria Control Methods

Drug Development

Following the emergence of resistance to chloroquine, the United States Army mounted a program to identify new antimalarial agents at the Walter Reed Army Institute of Research (WRAIR), which was to span more than two and one-half decades and cost more than $100 million. The approach was empirical, and more than 400,000 compounds were screened. One of the main products of this program was mefloquine. Although the ability of the Army to deal with malaria in a military context was markedly enhanced by the availability of this drug, the rapid emergence of resistant parasites makes it clear that the utility of the remedy is limited in time.

With increasingly numerous demands on its resources, it is unlikely that the Army will soon mount another effort of the type and magnitude as the one that led to mefloquine. Although there are obviously more compounds which could be obtained or synthesized, those easiest and cheapest to obtain have already been tested. In addition, the strategy of maintaining the screening program to keep one step ahead of the parasite, while perhaps necessary and rational, is less appealing to decision makers than a similar expenditure for a definitive solution. For these reasons, the WRAIR program continues with a shift in recent years to a more diverse multidisciplinary approach. In particular, computer modeling of drugs is expected to accelerate rational drug development progress. There are a number of promising developments, both from the WRAIR effort and from elsewhere.

- **New drugs in the pipeline**

The search for new drugs to replace those to which the parasites have become resistant and those that are for other reasons less than optimally effective continues in the WRAIR program. Halofantrine is currently in clinical trials.

Qinghaosu, a traditional Chinese herbal medicine, has been shown to have remarkable efficacy against falciparum malaria. Although the traditional formulations are not ideal for parenteral use, extensive investigations of the medicinal chemistry of the material has led to several derivatives including arteether which holds great promise for the treatment of severe malaria.

- **Reversal of drug resistance**

One of the most intriguing recent developments in antimalarial drug research is the discovery of agents which reverse the resistance of parasites to chloroquine. As so often happens in science, this discovery was made as a result of a cross disciplinary insight. Dr. Samuel Martin had for some time noted the reversal of resistance of neoplasms to cancer chemotherapeutic agents and speculated that a similar phenomenon might apply in malaria. He subsequently demonstrated that one of the same drugs that reverses resistance to antineoplastic agents, verapamil, also reverses chloroquine resistance (19). In addition to its obvious implications for enhancing the usefulness of chloroquine, the discovery has led to better insight into the mechanism of resistance. Chloroquine concentrates in sensitive but not resistant parasites, and verapamil and a number of other drugs reverse both the efflux of the drugs and the resistance of the parasites. Chloroquine has moderate activity against many microorganisms, and it appears that the exquisite sensitivity of malaria parasites is due to the accumulation of the drug by the parasites; resistant parasites have acquired the ability to reverse this process (17).

The phenomenon of reversal of resistance to tumors that inspired Dr. Martin's hypothesis also has another intriguing aspect: tumors which develop resistance to one drug are often resistant to a variety of other drugs of different chemical classes. Cross resistance among antimalarial drugs of different classes has also been noted, and recently it has been shown that certain drugs, including chlorpromazine, can both reverse chloroquine resistance and enhance the activity of quinine and quinidine. Similarly, a piperidine analog has been shown experimentally to reverse resistance to mefloquine, halofantrine, and artemisinin, compounds of three different chemical classes (20). These developments suggest that not only may older drugs be resurrected but that life for new drugs may be prolonged.

- **Molecular biology of antimalarial drug action**

As is the case for all of biology, the techniques of molecular biology have allowed major inroads to be made in the understanding of drug action and resistance. The gene for *P. falciparum* dihydrofolate reductases, from both sensitive and antifolate-resistant parasites, has been cloned and sequenced (16). Multiple mutations are responsible for antifolate resistance, and mutations in different parts of the gene result in resistance to pyrimethamine and cycloguanil, respectively (28). These insights provide a basis for the design of new antifolate drugs which may be able to circumvent parasite resistance.

The genetic locus of chloroquine resistance has also been defined. This achievement not only will allow the development of gene probes to enable the rapid identification of resistant parasites, but may also lead to new approaches to drug design. Interestingly, chloroquine resistance does not appear to be linked genetically with a gene which exhibits homology with a mammalian gene involved in multidrug resistance of tumors (36).

Vector Control

In addition to operational research, which will be further discussed later, entirely new approaches to vector control are being explored. It has been proposed that it might be possible to genetically select and/or modify anopheline mosquitoes to produce insects that are both refractory to malaria and possessive of survival characteristics which would allow them to replace a wild population, thus depriving the parasite of a means of transmission (5). Studies directed towards this long-term goal have been initiated at the National Institute of Allergy and Infectious Diseases (NIAID). Obviously, much work is needed to define the desired genetic characteristics, but if such engineered mosquitoes could be realized, a major malaria control tool would be available.

Vaccine Development

The initiation of the drug development effort was not the only response of the US Army to the twofold threat of resistance of parasites to drugs and of mosquitoes to insecticides. At about this same time, both WRAIR and the Agency for International Development (A.I.D.) initiated programs to explore the feasibility of the development of vaccines against malaria. The A.I.D. program was relatively well-funded even at this early stage, and support has continued until the present time. WRAIR's program was quite small initially, but has been increased over the years as evidence mounted that the approach would eventually yield practical results. Insights gleaned from the NIAID basic research program have also played a key role in the vaccine development effort. At the same time, outside the US, the Special Programme for Research and Training in Tropical Diseases (TDR) has played a seminal role in these efforts, and efforts by an Australian consortium have moved the field forward in a major way.

During much of this modern era of malaria immunology (1962 to the present), there has been considerable controversy over which stages of the parasite, merozoites or sporozoites, were the best targets for vaccine development. During the 1970s, which could be called "the decade of the cell", a great deal of information was obtained supporting both sides of the argument. Immunization of monkeys with purified merozoites produced impressive protection. The *in vitro* culture of *P. falciparum* led to speculations that blood stage vaccines would be produced in culture, but although this technology revolutionized the field, it did not prove to be a practical means of large-scale production of parasite material. Also during this period, there was rapid accumulation of knowledge regarding the induction of immunity using living sporozoites that had been irradiated to prevent proliferation as the immunogen. Most of this work was done using rodent models, but it was also demonstrated that the method worked in man, albeit through methods that fell short of offering a feasible way to mount a practical vaccine development effort. By the end of the decade workers were left excited by the new insights but frustrated by the lack of any way to obtain enough antigen for either a blood stage or a sporozoite vaccine development effort.

The 1980s completely reversed this pessimism. The advent of monoclonal antibody and molecular cloning technology resulted in completely new approaches for malaria vaccine development and ushered in what could be called "the decade of the molecule". A monoclonal antibody to a rodent malaria parasite which neutralized the infectivity of sporozoites allowed the visualization of the major circumsporozoite surface protein (CSP) in western blots. With the publication of this work, the agenda for the decade in sporozoite vaccine development was set. Similar CSPs were demonstrated in other parasites and, in due course, the genes for a number of these antigens were cloned and sequenced. The molecules have in their central portions long stretches in which a relatively short sequence of amino acids is repeated many times. Absorption experiments demonstrated that all the detectable antibody resulting from immunization with irradiated parasites reacted with these central repeat regions. This and other results led to the construction and testing of a number of vaccines based on the repeat region of the *P. falciparum* CSP. The antigen used in one of the first two vaccines was the twelve-mer $(NANP)_3$ conjugated to tetanus toxoid; the other was a recombinant fusion protein consisting of thirty-two *P. falciparum* repeats plus 32 amino acids from the tetracycline resistance gene adjacent to the malaria antigen gene in the construct $R_{32}tet_{32}$. Both $(NANP)_3$-TT and $R_{32}tet_{32}$ were administered with the adjuvant alum. Although highly immunogenic in preclinical studies, these vaccines proved to be of limited immunogenicity in humans, failing to stimulate a secondary serologic response to second and third doses of the vaccines. However, two of the volunteers with the highest antibody titers, one of whom received $(NANP)_3$-TT and one who received $R_{32}tet_{32}$, did not develop malaria after challenge. In spite of the small numbers, this was a very significant result, since failure to infect unprotected individuals under the conditions used is very unlikely.

The reasons for the difference in immunogenicity between, for example, mice and humans is only partially understood. Studies in inbred mice have shown that the immune response to CSP is genetically restricted and that CSP central repeat epitopes are not recognized by helper T cells in some mouse strains. However, it has been shown that human helper T cell clones reactive with *P. falciparum* central repeat epitopes can be isolated from individuals immunized with irradiated parasites. Continued clinical investigation has demonstrated that much higher levels of antibody can be obtained when adjuvants containing monophosphoryl lipid A and mycobacterial cell wall antigen or monophosphoryl lipid A and liposomes are used. The efficacy of such advanced vaccines is currently being evaluated.

Many blood stage antigens have been described, and a number tested in monkeys, but with one exception, they have been very slow to reach the clinic. Among the most studied antigens of *P. falciparum* is the major merozoite surface antigen (MMSA), in a sense analogous to CSP, and has been shown to be capable of protecting monkeys from challenge. Another is the major erythrocyte binding antigen (EBA), to which antibodies have been shown to block development of the parasite in culture with erythrocytes, as have antibodies to MMSA. These antigens and others show promise of being capable of giving rise to antibodies that can interfere, in one way or another, with the growth and development of the parasite.

Another category of blood stage antigen is the molecule or molecules responsible for the adherence of parasites to endothelial cells, a phenomenon which probably is involved in the pathogenesis of cerebral malaria and, perhaps, other forms of severe malaria. It is likely that this is a mechanism whereby mature parasites are protected from circulation through the splenic circulation where they would, because of their altered surface properties, be cleared and destroyed. Antibodies against a cytoadherence molecule have been shown to enhance clearance of parasites. Molecules of this type offer another avenue towards vaccine development [(21) and associated papers].

Large-scale field trials of one synthetic blood stage vaccine are already taking place in South America. Unpublished reports indicate success. Although controversial, these developments are of great interest, and, if confirmed, signal a great leap forward (22).

Many obstacles stand in the way of the development of practical vaccines. There is much that is unknown regarding the effector mechanisms that mediate protection against malaria. It is clear that both antibodies and cytotoxic T cells are operative in the immunity induced by irradiated sporozoites; antibodies work against the sporozoite and T cells (or cytokines produced by T cells) work against infected hepatocytes; but the antigenic specificity of these interactions is likely to involve more than the CSP; there is now evidence for both additional sporozoite antigens and for antigens specific for the liver stages of the parasite (34). In rodent models, at least, there is also evidence for both antibody and non-antibody mediated effector mechanisms. This situation has obvious implications for the usefulness of *in vitro* correlates of immunity in the evaluation of immune status of, for example, recipients of experimental vaccines.

Another obstacle to vaccine development is the polymorphism of the antigens (6). If vaccines with limited numbers of epitopes are to be used, those epitopes should be highly conserved in order for the vaccine to be effective against a large proportion of the parasites in nature. Many epitopes are polymorphic and it is too early to know if the hope can be realized that some will be both highly conserved and capable of giving rise to protective immunity.

Finally, in the presence of considerable perceived uncertainty regarding the feasibility of malaria vaccine development, or at least regarding when it will be feasible, willingness of commercial enterprises to invest in vaccine research and development efforts is either lacking or agreed to with reluctance on the part of the elements of the company that allocate research and development dollars. [See (4, 33) for current reviews of vaccine development efforts.]

What Can Be Done?

The Institute of Medicine of the National Academy of Science has recently performed a study of the U.S. effort towards solution of the malaria problem. Also being developed is a study by the American Association for the Advancement of Science for the Africa Bureau of the Agency for International Development with the purpose of recommending a new strategy for the control of malaria in Africa. Finally, WHO is planning a malaria "summit" with the intent of bringing together Ministers of Health from the countries endemic for malaria. The expected outcome of the summit meeting is as follows (38):

"1. Recognition of malaria as a major public health problem and detrimental factor to socioeconomic development in many countries; that commitments and investments are insufficient to address it; that routine control operations need reassessment and reorientation;

2. Strengthening the commitment to malaria control among political and health leaders, both of the countries where the disease is endemic and of the international community in its entirety;

3. A formal declaration of approval of and sustained support for a global strategy for malaria control."

The Summit, which is to be held in 1992, will be preceded by three technical meetings in countries endemic for malaria, one each on the continents of Africa, Asia, and South America.

These developments would appear to indicate a renewed determination to attack the global malaria problem. It will be very interesting to see the results of these efforts. Considerable thought has been put into the theory of malaria control, although it has not been possible to implement many of the proposals on a sufficiently large scale because of fiscal constraints. It is useful, however, to conceptualize what needs to be done, even if projected funding patterns will not allow it, in order to retreat to pragmatism in a more reasoned way. Further, a "straw man" proposal is a reasonable starting point in the development of a realistic plan. Towards this end, I will share with you some of my thinking along these lines.

Framework for an Idealized Malaria Control Plan

In devising any strategic plan, it is necessary to enunciate its goals and objectives. Goals for tropical diseases for the next century, eradication, control, and containment, are useful to think about in the context of the malaria problem. Eradication is the obvious first choice, but we have tried that and it did not work. Shall we try again with our modern insights and technology, even in the face of widespread resistance to antimalarial drugs and insecticides? Among the many factors on which the feasibility of eradication depends, the potential of epidemic disease from a single or a few cases ranks high. Each case of smallpox, in modern times, had the potential of infecting a relatively few other individuals. Each case of malaria, with most of the credit going to the vector, can serve as a source of infection for hundreds of individuals. However, the title of this talk allows more than 109 years to accomplish such a goal. We should not discard it. Certainly, as indicated in 1968 by WHO, eradication in locales where it is feasible should be accomplished, even though continued monitoring would be necessary to prevent reintroduction. In the final analysis, however, the issue may not be whether eradication is possible, but whether the cost of final eradication to prevent a few cases per year is worth the benefit obtained as compared to benefits which could be obtained in other areas. Under these circumstances, it would be fair to say that the malaria problem will have been solved, i. e., control in the best sense of the word achieved, even though the parasite would not have been eradicated. The precise definition of problem solution needs not concern us at this point in time. On the way to reaching the goal of eradication/problem solution, first containment and then an intermediate level of control short of the ideal, are certainly laudable interim measures. With these goals in mind, then, we can go on to the elements of a strategic plan. These could be listed as follows:

- Research and development
- Education and training
- Surveillance
- Local area analysis and planning
- Central coordination and communication
- Intervention, operational research, and evaluation

Each of these deserves comment:

Research and Development

The horrible morbidity and mortality of malaria tempts an attitude that we should expend any available resources on any interventions available rather than on the acquisition of knowledge in the hopes of having better interventions in the future. The end result is obvious; no better interventions would ever become available. It is absolutely imperative that research continue, not only as applied research toward all possibilities of improved intervention methods, but also as basic research to obtain a better understanding of the biology of the parasite and the host's response to it, as well as of the larger ecosystem in which malaria operates. Further, a distinction needs to be made between research and development. The first has to do with the acquisition of knowledge; the second with using that knowledge to devise intervention methods. Development efforts must not be discouraged either because they do not provide new knowledge or because they would be more successful if more knowledge were available. Development efforts often ask the critical questions which are then answered through research efforts. Choosing which research efforts and which developmental efforts to support is, of course, a difficult task and is beyond the scope of this discussion.

Education and Training

It is true that "the only thing eradicated by the malaria eradication campaign was the malariologists", as has been often said. New generations of both specialists and generalists will be necessary if malaria is to be attacked successfully. The most obvious disciplines on the list include epidemiologists, parasitologists, entomologists, and clinicians, but the skills of civil engineers, managers, educators, and experts in operations research will be no less critical. Another dimension of the problem is the absolute necessity for experts to be on site to deal with local issues. This condition will most likely require that local governments take the initiative to ensure that experts are available to their areas.

Training in the rituals of a discipline are not enough. Malaria is a "smart" enemy. Those who participate in fighting this enemy must learn to learn in order to be able to ask the right questions and get the right answers to devise the most effective tactics and to modify those tactics, in response to changing conditions. Thus, the insistence on education and not only training.

Surveillance

Just as important as defining the goals of a strategy is defining the problem, both qualitatively and quantitatively. Although approximate figures are quoted, we do not know either the incidence of malaria or the mortality due to malaria. Information acquisition and quality is compromised first by the fact that malaria means different things to different people, as discussed above. Aside from this, few systems are in place to determine incidence outside of hospitals and other health care centers. As has been often said, what is seen therefore is the "tip of the iceberg". The sampling and diagnostic methods, as well as data management and analytic techniques are available to address this problem.

Local Area Analysis and Planning

Much has been said recently about the paradigm approach to defining malaria endemicity and the stratified approach to planning of control measures. This reflects the increasing appreciation of the fact that the epidemiological parameters of malaria differ drastically in different ecological situations, resulting in different problems to be faced in attacking the disease. Local area analysis is, therefore, essential to define which of the recognized paradigms obtain, or if in fact the local situation does not conform well to any of the recognized paradigms. Outside expert consultants will be invaluable at this stage, but responsibility for the effort must rest with the local workers. After analysis, definite measurable objectives, with the goals of containment or control, with discrete milestones, should be formulated for the chosen ecologic area(s). In certain instances (e.g., small islands), objectives could be set within the framework of the eradication goal in the near future. For most, this would be a distant goal to be undertaken after the success of less ambitious efforts. The geographic area within which the ecological unit is to be located also needs to be defined in coordination with workers in adjacent areas. It would likely be local governments that would have the responsibility of making the administrative units responsible for intervention congruent with ecological units. It is also at the local level that the continued surveillance, implementation, operational research, evaluation, and replanning cycle need to be completed. Thus the system would decentralize most of the decision making for implementation in the endemic areas.

Central Coordination and Communication

In spite of the decentralized character of the effort, for a variety of reasons, central coordination of an attack on malaria is necessary. A hierarchical structure involving governments and WHO would seem most feasible. Oversight, review, and approval of plans at each level would provide a venue for communication and discussion and encourage the discipline needed to optimize the effectiveness of the operation. Ideally, teams that review tactical plans would consist of

a) a permanent group of experts who would participate in such reviews at all levels,

b) a group of peers to the unit whose plan was being reviewed, and

c) health officials at the administrative level immediately above the one being reviewed, who would have the authority for approval/disapproval of plans.

Although most important at the unit level, this review process would take place at all levels. The hierarchical structure would also serve to provide a mechanism for compilation and analysis of surveillance data and for dissemination of this information. It would also be responsible for the extensive communication system necessary for the management of oversight and review and would play an active role in education and training.

Intervention, Operational Research, and Evaluation

Depending on the paradigm and on other local factors, intervention would take many different forms and would involve diverse groups and individuals. As indicated above, the failure of the eradication effort has resulted in much analysis and contrasting of eradication versus control efforts. Eradication has been characterized as a "vertical" effort, directed towards malaria without reference to other health problems or to sectors outside of the health area which it might have influenced or which might have influenced it. "Horizontal" efforts are now recommended in which efforts against malaria are a part of an integrated health system and which involve intersectoral collaboration, for example with agronomists to plan in a coordinated fashion to prevent the creation of anopheline breeding sites by agricultural projects. Thus far, it might appear that the framework presented here espouses a vertical approach. This is not the case. First, coordination with general preventive medicine planners and the health care system is essential to ensure meshing of efforts. How malaria units are integrated administratively into these systems is less important than functional integration through coordination and collaboration. No doubt, the former expedites the latter, but where separate malaria control units are working smoothly, it might not be wise to change the structure simply to satisfy a formula. Second, active collaboration with government agencies and private organizations concerned with agriculture, forestry, water utilization, and other areas will be essential in implementing certain intervention tactics. Similarly, enlistment of support, both in fiscal and in human resources, from local offices of donor organizations such as A.I.D. missions and private voluntary organizations will be essential. Nevertheless, it is critically important that the complex issues involved in an attack on malaria not be glossed over or neglected in an attempt at an "integrated" program. In a recent meeting on the malaria problem at the London School of Tropical Medicine and Hygiene, Dr. Awash Teklehaimanot, in speaking on the organization of malaria control efforts, provided an excellent analysis of the issues. At the end of his presentation, it was concluded that what is needed is a "diagonal" approach, taking what is needed from both of the extreme points of view.

As mentioned above, surveillance must be a part of a coherent attack on malaria and needs to be built into local plans at the outset. The overall design should include as much opportunity as possible for evaluation of the effectiveness of measures taken. Local plans for antimalarial efforts should include not only direct interventions against the parasite and/or the vector, but should also incorporate operational research on the implementation, effectiveness, and cost of the interventions themselves. For example the failure to actually deliver insecticide was cited as one of the deficiencies of the global eradication campaign. The recognition of the importance of the interdependencies within the overall system, and the institution of appropriate mechanisms for detecting malfunctions and naturally occurring alternative pathways which evade control efforts is essential.

The data from surveillance and operational research are the fundamental bases for evaluation and replanning. This can be done continuously on an informal basis, but it is important not to change tactics so often as to not allow adequate comprehension of outcomes. More formal evaluation must be done at appropriate intervals; this can best be done by the implementing unit but should also be reviewed as a part of the review process for the plan for the next period.

Reality Testing

How much would all of this cost? Is it likely that we will be able to pay for it between now and the end of the twenty first century? The first question is answerable, to a first approximation, by budget building on the plan proposed, although this in itself would be a substantial undertaking. The second question cannot be answered at this time. However, within the framework outlined above is the possibility of working with less than optimal resources and still gaining significant benefits, in some if not all, local areas. Certainly more funds than are currently being expended need to be applied to result in improvement in the situation, and indications that they are coming are not evident. We are left, then, with the clear indication that, although the problem is enormously complex and available technology less than optimal, progress could be made in this area, and, that in the long run, the malaria problem could be solved, *if* resources were available. What is left to be said?

A Mobilizing Idea

Russell L. Ackoff in his book, *Redesigning the Future*, comes to the crux of the resource problem in a series of quotations that fit our topic well. He quotes C. P. Snow as saying:

"Since the gap between the rich and the poor can be removed, it will be. If we are shortsighted, inept, incapable of good will or enlightened self interest, then it may be removed to the accompaniment of war and starvation; but removed, it will be. The questions are how, and by whom."

Ackoff continues with a quotation from the British author C. F. Powell, whose figures are old (1964), but whose point is nevertheless timely:

"At present, the total amount given for aid and development amounts to $6 B per annum. A number of estimates have been made of the material resources required for the radical transformation of the present situation [the disparity in health and living conditions between the "developed" and the "developing" world]. They vary considerably, but most of them fall in the range from $10–15 B per annum for a period of about twenty years. These estimates, while representing great expenditures are well within the resources of the advanced countries. They could be provided, for example, by even a modest measure of disarmament."

Ackoffs quotation from the then Secretary General of the United Nations continues the argument:

"The truth, the central stupendous truth, about developed countries today is that they have – in anything but the shortest run – the kind and scale of resources they decide to have ... It is no longer resources that limit decisions. It is the decision that makes the resources."

If we accept these arguments, then a solution to the malaria problem and to other problems being discussed in this book depends on the right decisions being made by those in power. To do this they (and we) need to be educated in the possibilities for change. What then can we do? Ackoff even offers an answer to this question by a quotation from the Spanish philosopher Jose Ortega y Gasset. The answer, in brief, is to produce a mobilizing idea. The quotation is as follows:

"...man has been able to grow enthusiastic over his vision of ...unconvincing enterprises. He has put himself to work for the sake of an idea, seeking by magnificent exertions to arrive at the incredible. And in the end, he has arrived there. Beyond all doubt it is one of the vital sources of man's power, to be thus able to kindle enthusiasm from the mere glimmer of something improbable, difficult, remote."

Surely the goal of solving the malaria problem fits this description. In addition to continuing to exert efforts to implement the tools we have against malaria and to devise new tools, we must take every opportunity to foster an increased awareness of the impact of the problem on human welfare and of the mobilizing idea of the feasibility of its solution in the consciousness of all who will listen, including ourselves.

Acknowledgements

The helpful suggestions of Richard Andre, Andrew Arata, Nancy de Moraes, Steven Landry, Kirk Miller, Will Milhous, and Catherine Savino are gratefully acknowledged.

References

1. Ackoff RL (1974) Redesigning the future. New York, John Wiley & Sons
2. Bruce-Chwatt LJ (1980) Essential malariology. London, William Heinemann
3. Center for International Health Information Standard Report (1990) No 9–90. Arlington, Va
4. Certa, U (1991) Malaria vaccine. Experientia 47: 158–163
5. Collins FH, Sakai RK, Vernick KD, Paskewitz P, Seeley DC, Miller LH, Collins WE, Campbell CC, Gwadz RW (1986) Genetic selection of a *Plasmodium*-refractory strain of the malaria vector *Anopheles gambiae*. Science 234: 607–610
6. Cox FEG (1991) Variation and vaccination. Nature 349: 193
7. Davis JR, Garcia R (1989) Malaria mosquito in Brazil. In: Dahlsten DL, Garcia R (eds) Eradication of exotic pests. New Haven London, Yale University Press
8. Fough S, Jepsen S, Effersoe P (1972) Chloroquine resistant *Plasmodium falciparum* in Kenya. Trans R Soc Trop Med Hyg 73: 228–229
9. Garrett-Jones (1964) The human blood index of malaria vectors in relation to epidemiological assessment. Bull WHO 30: 241–261
10. Gramiccia G, Beales PF (1988) The recent history of malaria control and eradication. In: Wernsdorfer WH, McGregor I (eds) Malaria. Principles and practice of malariology. Edinburgh London Melbourne New York, Churchill Livingstone
11. Greenwood BM, Bradley AK, Greenwood AM, Byass P, et al (1987) Mortality and morbidity from malaria among children in a rural area of The Gambia, West Africa. Trans R Soc Trop Med Hyg 81: 478–486
12. Harinasuta T, Migascos D, Bunnag D (1962) Chloroquine resistance in *Plasmodium falciparum* in Thailand, UNESCO First Regional Symposium on Scientific Knowledge of Tropical Parasites, Singapore. Rome, UNESCO
13. Harrison G (1978) Mosquitoes, malaria, and man. New York, Dutton
14. Hayworth J (1988) The global distribution of malaria and the present control effort. In: Wernsdorfer WH, McGregor I (eds) Malaria. Principles and practice of malariology. Edinburgh London Melbourne New York, Churchill Livingstone
15. Hayes J, Charlwood DC (1977) *Anopheles darlingi* avoids DDT in an area where malaria is resistant to drug. Acta Amazonica 7: 289
16. Hyde JE (1990) The dihydrofolate reductasethymidylate synthetase gene in the drug resistance of malaria parasites. Pharmacol Ther 48: 45–59
17. Krogstad DJ, Gluzman IY, Kyle DE, Oduola AMJ, Martin SK, Milhous WK, Schlesinger PH (1987) Efflux of chloroquine from *Plasmodium falciparum*: mechanism of chloroquine resistance. Science 238: 1283–1285
18. Lackritz EM, Campbell CC, Hightower AW, Ruebush TK, Were JB (1990) The epidemiology of anemia and malaria parasitemia in Western Kenya: Implications for the prevention of blood transfusion. American Society for Tropical Medicine & Hygiene Annual Meeting

19. Martin SK, Oduola AMJ, Milhous WK (1987) Reversal of chloroquine resistance in *Plasmodium falciparum* by verapamil. Science 235: 899–901
20. Milhous W, Schuster B (1990) Malaria studies aim at drug resistance. US Med 26: 27–28
21. Miller LH (1990) Introduction to the Symposium on Cytoadherence and Cerebral Malaria. Am J Trop Med Hyg 43 [Suppl]
22. Mitchell GH (1991) Malaria research in Colombia: has a useful malaria vaccine arrived? Vaccine 2: 219–220
23. Moody RP (1989) The safety of diethyltoluamide insect repellents (letter). JAMA 262: 28–29
24. Moore DV, Lanier JE (1961) Observations on two *Plasmodium falciparum* infections with an abnormal response to chloroquine. Am J Trop Med Hyg 10: 5–9
25. Centers of Disease Control (1989) Seizures temporally associated with use of DEET insect repellant; New York and Connecticut Morbidity and Mortality Weekly Report 38: 678–680
26. Pampana EA (1969) Textbook of malaria eradication. London, Oxford University Press
27. Pang L, Limsomwong N, Singharaj P (1987) Doxycycline prophylaxis for *falciparum* malaria. Lancet i: 1161–1164
28. Peterson DS, Milhous WK, Wellems TE (1987) Molecular basis of differential resistance to cycloguanil and pyrimethamine in *Plasmodium falciparum* malaria. Proc Natl Acad Sci USA 87: 3018–3022
29. Rafatjah HA (1988) Malaria vector control: environmental management. In: Wernsdorfer WH, McGregor I (eds) Malaria. Principles and practice of malariology. Edinburgh London Melbourne New York, Churchill Livingstone
30. Service MW (1989) Rice, a challenge to health. Parasit Today 5: 162–165
31. Shuler AV (1985) Malaria; Meeting the global challenge (AID Science and Technology Series). Boston, Oelgeschlager, Gunn & Hain
32. Stürchler D (1989) How much malaria is there worldwide? Parasitol Today 5: 39–40
33. Siddiqui WA (1991) Where are we in the quest for vaccine for malaria? Drugs 41: 1–10
34. Stevenson MM, Nowotarski M, Yap G (1990) Review: cytokines and malaria. Clin Invest Med 13: 353–359
35. Young MD, Contaos PG, Stitcher JE, Miller JW (1963) Drug resistance in *Plasmodium falciparum* from Thailand. Am J Trop Med Hyg 12: 305
36. Wellems TE, Walker-Jonah AW, Panton LJ (1991) Genetic mapping of the chloroquine-resistance locus on *Plasmodium falciparum* chromosome 7. Proc Natl Acad Sci USA 88: 3382–3386
37. Wernsdorfer WH, McGregor I (1988) Malaria. Principles and practice of malariology. Edinburgh London Melbourne New York, Churchill Livingstone
38. WHO (1990) Report of the First Meeting of the Malaria Summit Consultative Group. Geneva, 31 October–2 November, 1990

Black Fungi: A Model for Understanding Tropical Mycosis

Michael R. McGinnis

Department of Pathology, University of Texas Medical Branch, Galveston, Texas, U.S.A.

Introduction

Regardless of specific etiology, fungal infections can be clinically classified as either superficial, cutaneous and corneal, subcutaneous, systemic, or allergic. Such a classification scheme is based upon the fact that fungal infections are the result of dynamic host-pathogen interactions. These interactions can be monitored by observing and measuring clinical, pathological, and mycological changes. Each observation that is made represents a single instance in an evolving continuum of host-pathogen interactions and subsequent host-pathogen responses to each other.

In tropical regions, the spectrum of fungi capable of causing mycoses is enormous. Factors such as temperature, humidity, photoperiods, solar radiation, indigenous flora and fauna, soil types, and host related factors like population genetics, customs, socio-economic considerations, and health care delivery systems have a profound impact upon the incidence, types of mycotic infections, and their management. The black fungi, which are characterized by having melanin in their cell walls, can serve as an excellent example for understanding mycoses occurring in tropical regions.

Role of Melanin in Fungal Protection and Pathenogensis

Melanins are high molecular weight pigments formed by the oxidative polymerization of phenolic compounds. These pigments are characterized by their chemical and physical properties. Fungal melanins may occur as electron-dense granules located in the fungal cell wall, polymers in the cytoplasm, as extracellular polymers in the medium surrounding the fungus, or in any combination. Melanin pigments are important for the survival of fungi because they function as protectants against environmental stresses like UV radiation (26, 72, 76), desiccation and high temperatures (82), and for the survival of fungi in soil ecosystems (36, 37, 61, 66). For example, Geis and Szaniszlo (25) have shown that the carotenoid and melanin pigments formed by *Wangiella dermatitidis* help provide resistance to photo-induced damage.

Medically important dematiaceous fungi typically form melanin via the pentaketide pathway using the natural precursor 1,8-dihydroxynaphthalene (DHN) (Table 1). Even though 3, 4-dihydroxyphenylalanine (DOPA) has been reported to serve as the melanin precursor in fungi like *Aureobasidium pullulans*, Wheeler and Bell (76) believe that the melanins in this and other dematiaceous opportunistic pathogens are derived from DHN rather than DOPA. Their conclusion is based upon the observations that the amino acid tyrosine occurs universally in fungi and that tyrosinase, which is a polyphenoloxidase necessary for the oxidation of L-tyrosine to DOPA and then DOPA to dopaquinone, has not been conclusively demonstrated in the fungal outer cell wall where melanin is synthesized. Other polyphenoloxidases, such as catecholases (*o*-diphenoloxidases) and laccases (*p*-diphenoloxidases) which do not oxidize tyrosine, can be confused with tyrosinase.

Table 1. Some Medically Important Fungi Having Melanin Produced from 1, 8-dihydroxynaphthalene (DHN)

Alternaria alternata	*Nattrassia mangiferae*
Aspergillus nidulans	*Phaeoannellomyces werneckii*
A. niger	*Phaeococcomyces spp.*
Aureobasidium pullulans	*Phialophora richardsiae*
Bipolaris spp.	*P. verrucosa*
Cladosporium carrionii	*Piedraia hortae*[a]
Curvularia spp.	*Pseudallescheria boydii*[a]
Exophiala jeanselmei	*Sporothrix schenckii*[a]
Exserohilum spp.	*Stenella araguata*[a]
Fonsecaea compacta	*Wangiella dermatitidis*
F. pedrosoi	*Xylohypha bantiana*
Madurella grisea[a]	
M. mycetomatis[a]	

[a] Suspected DHN melanin

Although fungi like *Aspergillus niger* form cytoplasmic melanins such as aspergillin, most melanins are either formed in the outer cell wall or extracellularly near the hyphae. Wheeler and Bell (76) have suggested two possible mechanisms for extracellular melanin formation. First, the fungus may secrete phenoloxidases such as tyrosinase, laccase, or peroxidase into the external environment. These enzymes then oxidize phenolic compounds already present in the external environment. Secondly, the fungi may secrete phenolic compounds into the external environment. At a later time, the phenolic compounds undergo autoxidization or are oxidized by phenoloxidases that the fungi subsequently release into the external environment. The brown to black coloration of culture media inoculated with fungi like *Madurella mycetomatis* and *Nattrassia mangifera* can be accounted for by the presence of extracellular melanins.

Extracellular melanin combining with host tissue debris and proteins that are associated with the hyphae composing the sclerotia (syn. granules, grains) of *M. mycetomatis* appears to protect the fungus from host antibodies and damage caused by antifungal agents. In addition, the melanized sclerotia probably protect the fungus against hydrolytic enzymes that could digest the fungal cell walls. Low molecular weight extracellular melanins apparently function as cement that helps to hold the fungal cells composing the sclerotia together (20). It has been suggested that the natural precursor for the extracellular melanins may be proteins originating from the host. The amorphous material found between the hyphal cells of sclerotia is derived from both the host and fungus (50). In *Exophiala jeanselmei,* the extracellular and cell wall melanins are similar, but not identical (23, 69).

Microfibrils, or fimbriae, have been found to be associated with the outer cell wall in a number of medically important fungi such as *A. pullulans, Candida albicans,* and *Sporothrix schenckii* (12). Microfibrils associated with the cell walls of the hyphal elements composing sclerotia of *M. mycetomatis* have been described as being polysaccharides (75). In other fungi, they are often conserved surface proteins that extrude in varying lengths and have a great deal of variation in their antigenicity (12). In dematiaceous fungi, the microfibrils may also contain melanin pigments which are difficult to characterize. In bacteria, fimbriae assist with adhesion to living and inert substances, pellicle formation, nucleic acid transfer, and motility, and serve as virulence factors. Microfibrils formed by fungi may have similar roles. Sclerotia formed by *M. mycetomatis* having microfibrils, which may contain melanin in addition to polysaccharides, typically have polymorphonuclear leukocytes and host cell debris attached in tissue. These components appear to create an inert protective buffer for the fungus.

The sclerotic bodies (syn. muriform cells) characteristic of the tissue form of the agents of chromoblastomycosis are frequently described as being darkly pigmented with a golden brown crusty material on their cell walls. *In vitro,* the sclerotic synanomorph of *W. dermatitidis* has five times more melanin in its cell wall than the cell walls of the yeast synanamorph (67). In natural infections, the heavily melanized cell wall and material on the cell walls of the sclerotic bodies may be important protective mechanisms against humoral and cell-mediated host defense mechanisms for fungi like *Fonsecaea pedrosoi.* For example, based upon studies in animal models, a melanin-deficient isolate of *W. dermatitidis* was less virulent than the parent isolate (13, 14). The melanin-deficient isolate was associated with decreased mortality, although the chronic neurological signs still occurred. *In vitro* susceptibility studies using melanin-deficient isolates of *W. dermatitidis* have shown that melanin does not appear to protect the fungus against contemporary antifungal agents (57). Mutants of *C. neoformans* that do not form the polyphenoloxidases needed to produce melanin from *o*-diphenolic compounds (catecholamines) exhibit decreased virulence in animal models (35, 58, 59).

In vivo Fungal Morphology

When dematiaceous fungi cause disease, they frequently exhibit a great deal of morphological variation in size, shape, and structure. Fungal elements in tissue vary from hyaline to black, depending upon how much melanin is present in their cell walls. In tissue, these fungi exist as sclerotia, hyphae of varying shapes and sizes, pseudohyphae, yeast cells, muriform cells, or a combination of several of these different forms. The current clinical nomenclature used to describe infections caused by the black fungi is based upon, in part, the fungal morphology of the etiologic agent in tissue. Diseases caused by the dematiaceous fungi include mycetoma, phaeohyphomycosis, and chromoblastomycosis (Fig. 1). Hyphae are the fundamental form that gives rise to sclerotia (syn. granules, grains) on one side of the scale and yeast cells on the other end. Muriform cells are unique structures that are arrested between a hyphal and yeast morphology.

Sclerotia, which are nearly without exception referred to as either granules or grains in the medical literature, are macroscopic structures formed in tissue during the ontogeny of a mycetoma. These structures are firm aggregates of vegetative hyphae that are variable in shape. Sclerotia

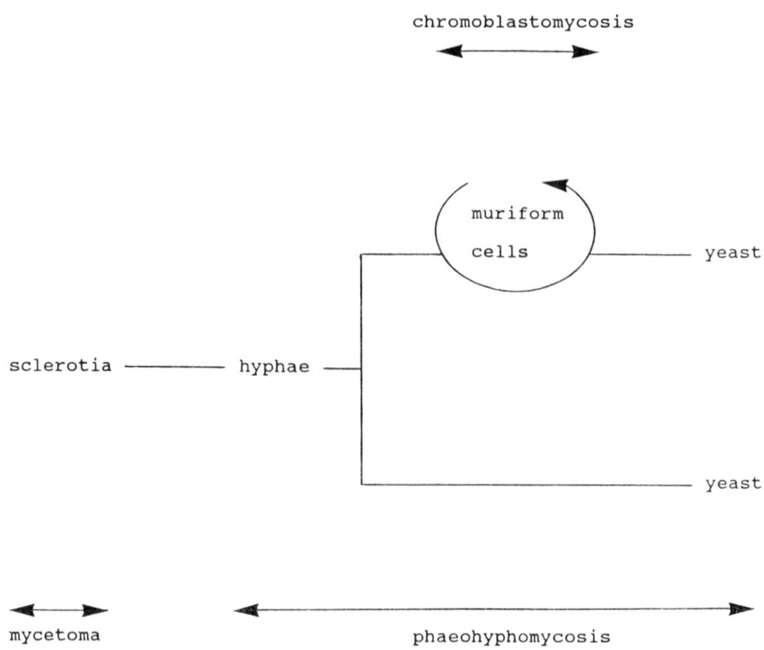

Fig. 1

have limited growth, and at maturity, they typically have an outer area of coalesced hyphal elements that are thickened and darkly colored. This outer region is called a rind, which encloses an inner portion known as the medulla. The hyphal elements enclosing the medulla are typically homogenous. During the development of a sclerotium, some host tissue may be enclosed, but at maturity the sclerotium is typically separated from the host tissue. The internal consolidation of the medulla may involve intrahyphal development (20, 21, 29, 75). In tissue, sclerotia proliferate by having small portions broken free from the parent sclerotium, which then increase in size and invade the surrounding tissue (44). An excellent discussion of sclerotium development has been presented by Tu et al. (71) for species classified in the *Rhizoctonia* complex. *Rhizoctonia* sp. (63) has been documented as an etiologic agent of mycotic keratitis in which the fungus produced only hyphae in corneal tissue.

The conditions that stimulate sclerotium formation in the pathogenic dematiaceous fungi are poorly understood. Because fungi like *M. mycetomatis* are not known to produce sclerotia in culture, it is safe to assume that the host-pathogen interaction and the environment of the traumatized tissue are extremely important. A fascinating question is: Why does a fungus like *Exophiala jeanselmei* form sclerotia in one patient and hyphae in a second patient when the fungus enters the subcutaneous tissue on a splinter in both patients?

Structures such as the fungoma (syn. fungus ball) superficially resemble sclerotia. A fungoma is a colony of a fungus growing in a cavity where there are space, nutrients, and aeration. For example, dematiaceous fungi like *Bipolaris spicifera* and *Exserohilum rostratum* occasionally form a fungoma in the nasal sinuses of some individuals (45). These vegetative mycelial structures consist of irregular hyphal masses and associated host tissue. Because they have neither rinds nor medulla and they do not consist of firm hyphal aggregates formed in response to a hostile environment for the fungus, they are distinct from sclerotia.

A number of dematiaceous fungi may form hyphae in tissue. The Fontana-Masson stain for melanin (78) may be used to demonstrate the presence of melanin in fungal cell walls when the hyphae appear hyaline. In tissue, dematiaceous hyphae are often moniliform, irregular, septate, branching and variable in size and length depending upon the fungus. Not infrequently, they appear distorted and swollen (Fig. 2). In addition to hyphal forms, dematiaceous fungi frequently produce pseudohyphae and yeast cells. All of these forms may co-exist in the same lesion at the same time. A heterogenous mixture of fungal elements in tissue with enormous morphological and size variation is characteristic of phaeohyphomycosis (19, 42).

Muriform cells (syn. sclerotic bodies) are specialized structures that are round, thick-walled, muriform, chestnut brown, and 5–12 um in diameter. Fungi like *Fonsecaea pedrosoi* (Fig. 3), *Phialophora verrucosa,* and *Cladosporium carrionii* form these structures in tissue when they are causing chromoblastomycosis. They originate from yeast cells when cessation of

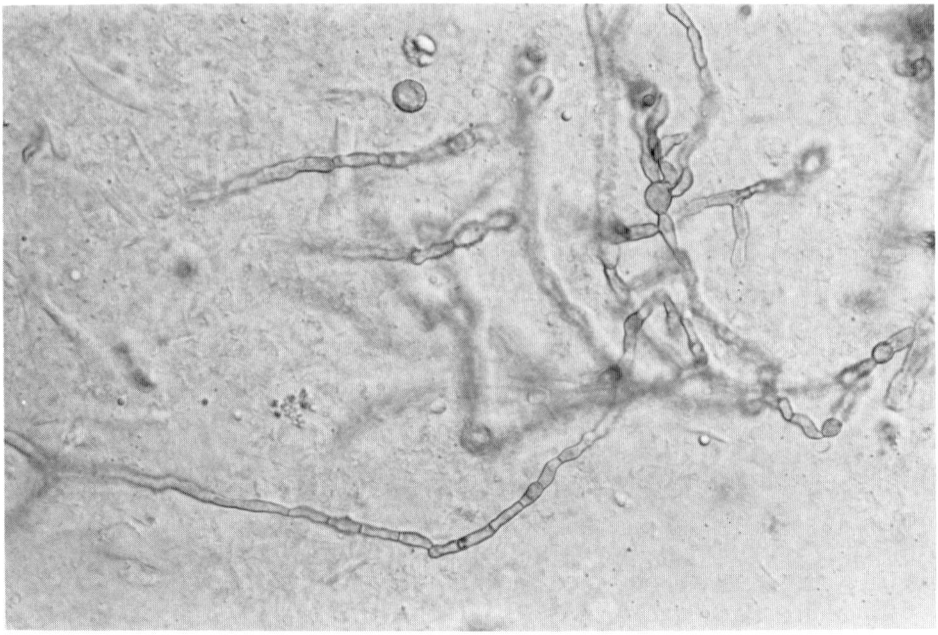

Fig. 2. Dematiaceous hyphae of *Xylohypha bantiana* in brain tissue. KOH, differential contrast microscopy, 630X

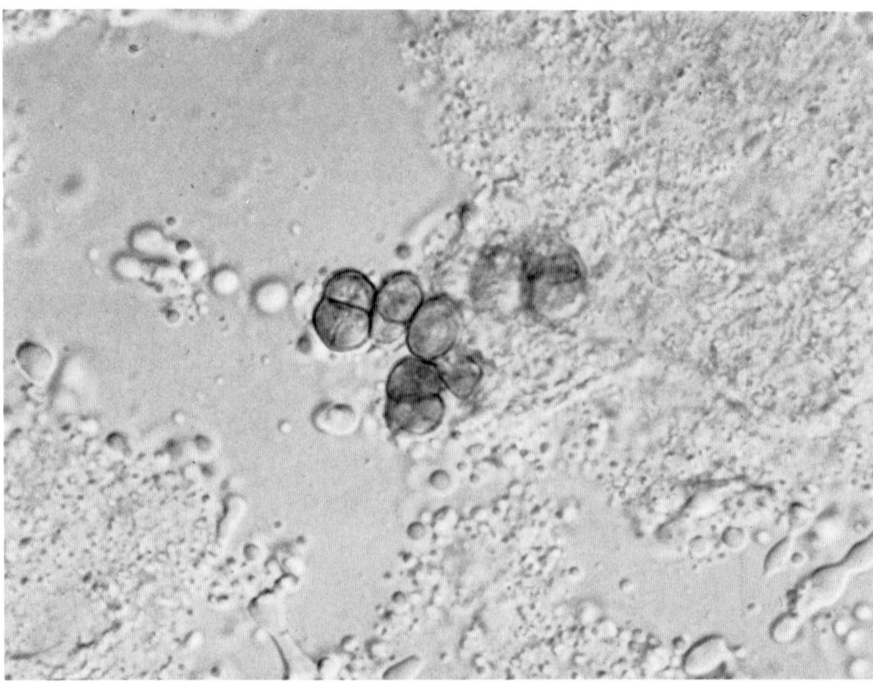

Fig. 3. Muriform cells produced by *Fonsecaea pedrosoi.* Skin biopsy, KOH, differential contrast microscopy, 400X

budding occurs. During their development, isotropic cell wall synthesis occurs, there is continued cellular growth and an increase in the size of the cells, repeated nuclear divisions result in new nuclei, cytokinesis continues, and transverse internal thickened septa form (24, 30, 68). Matsumoto et al. (41) have described a *Phaeotheca* synanamorph of *W. dermatitidis* characterized by the formation of endoconidia within large thick-walled cells that resemble muriform cells. Muriform cells have been formed *in vitro* under very acidic conditions (pH 2.5, 2–5 days, 25°C), on solid media following long term incubation, and in animal models. At pH 2.5, blastoconidium formation from the yeast cells is stopped without inhibition of growth, nuclear division, and cytokinesis. When the pH is above 3.5, muriform cells are not formed. Even at pH 2.5, muriform cells have not been formed by isolates of *Xylohypha bantiana* and *E. jeanselmei* (68), in contrast to isolates of *Phialophora verrucosa, F. pedrosoi,* and *C. carrionii* that were studied. It would be interesting to know whether the isolate of *E. jeanselmei* that was documented as an etiologic agent of chromoblastomycosis with muriform cells in human tissue (52) can produce muriform cells *in vitro* at pH 2.5. If so, valuable information regarding the importance of strain differences within a single taxon in determining whether mycetoma, chromoblastomycosis, or phaeohyphomycosis develops would be known.

Characterization of Dematiaceous Fungal Taxa

In addition to classical studies of morphogenesis and conidiogenesis, numerous new approaches are being taken as a means to better understand the biology of the dematiaceous fungi capable of causing human disease. Temperature growth studies (51, 54), exoantigens (18, 33, 55, 64), assimilation of carbon and nitrogen sources (17, 65), proteolytic activity (16), antigenicity (60), ultrastructure (49), DNA analysis (31), and coenzyme Q system study (79, 80) have provided a great deal of insight into this group of fungi. Unfortunately, the data obtained from these approaches have not adequately addressed issues such as why a particular isolate causes mycetoma in one patient and the same species causes chromoblastomycosis or phaeohyphomycosis in another.

Based upon DNA-DNA reassociation (28), Gueho and deHoog have concluded that *Pseudallescheria boydii* is genomically heterogeneous and phenotypically homogeneous. They were unable to distinguish isolates from patients having mycetomata from those originating from either phaeohyphomycosis or environmental sources such as wood pulp and soil. Mitochondrial DNA analysis of *Exophiala jeanselmei* and *W. dermatitidis* has yielded some interesting data (34). Of 45 isolates of *E. jeanselmei* studied, analysis of mitochondrial DNA by restriction enzyme digestion showed that they could be classified into 18 types. In a different study by Masuda et al. (40), where they employed DNA hybridizations using a dot blot method, the 14 isolates of *E. jeanselmei* could be divided into six groups. These two studies employing DNA analysis clearly show the potential for using DNA analysis to characterize strains of a particular taxon. Unfortunately, the absence of culture collection data describing the geographic origin and pathologic diagnosis of the isolates, limits the value of their data in addressing host-pathogen interactions resulting in specific types of infections.

Relationships among isolates, as well as their correlation to the types of diseases they cause may be approached by sequencing their 18S rDNA gene and then using the polymerase chain reaction (PCR) amplification procedure to compare isolates and their origins (77). Wang (46) compared nucleotide sequences of ribosomal RNA genes obtained from isolates identified as either *P. verrucosa* or *P. americana* (syn. of *P. verrucosa*), the latter being associated mostly with plant material and not disease. Her data suggested that PCR may have application in distinguishing isolates from human infections in comparison to isolates originating from environmental sources. At this time, it is too premature to characterize strain variation and its relationship to disease.

Mycoses Caused by Black Fungi

Mycetoma

A mycetoma (Fig. 4) is a localized infection involving cutaneous and subcutaneous tissue, fascia, and bone that is caused by either an actinomycete or fungus. Fungi that cause mycetoma are conveniently separated into two

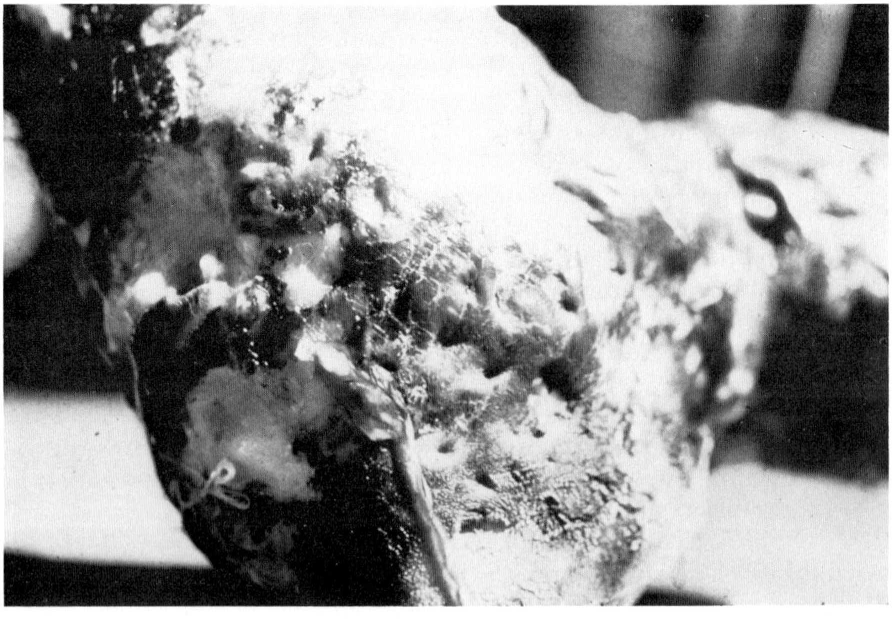

Fig. 4. A mycetoma is characterized by tumefaction, draining sinuses, and sclerotia. Draining sinuses are evident in the heel of this patient. Photograph courtesy Dr. Carlyn Halde

groups: dematiaceous or non-dematiaceous. Only mycetomata caused by dematiaceous fungi will be considered here.

Under the name *padavalmika*, mycetoma has been known since ancient times in India. In 1846, Godfrey (26) summarized four cases and named the disease morbus tuberculosis pedis. The first modern description may have been actually made in 1714 by French missionaries (62). Unfortunately, the descriptive terminology used by Kaempfer and the French missionary in Pondicherry is too vague to determine with certainty what was being described. The term madura foot was published by Colebrook in 1848 (8), although it was in common usage in the Madura District of India. Even though he described the disease, Colebrook was unaware that the infection was caused by a fungus. The term mycetoma, which means fungus tumor, was introduced in 1861 by Carter (9). As various actinomycetes and fungi were demonstrated to cause mycetoma, confusion was introduced. Subsequently, Pinoy (56) proposed the term actinomycosis for mycetomata having an actinomycete etiology, and later Chalmers and Archibald (10) coined the term maduromycosis for mycetomata caused by fungi.

The dematiaceous fungi that cause mycetoma are ascomycetous fungi that are normally associated with plants, plant debris, and occasionally soil. The reader is referred to the paper by McGinnis and Fader (44) for a listing of the currently known agents of mycetoma. Following the traumatic implantation of the etiological agent residing on a splinter or similar object into the subcutaneous tissue of an apparently healthy individual, a small, firm painless subcutaneous nodule that is attached to the skin forms. As the disease progresses, sinuses that communicate to the surface of the skin develop, in which, sclerotia are formed. The sclerotia are discharged through the sinuses and spread along the fascial planes to the adjacent tissue. The fungi do not spread by hematogenous means. With time, the fungus extends to bone and results in bone destruction accompanied by bone remodeling. Spontaneous fractures do not occur because the slow bone destruction is accompanied by remodeling which provides sufficient structural support to prevent spontaneous fractures. Secondary bacterial infections and osteomyelitis can result in total bone destruction. Depending upon the patient and etiologic agent involved, the incubation period for the disease is several months to several years (39, 44). Sinuses may appear in 2-to 6-months in approximately one-third of patients, but usually are present in nearly all patients within a year (38).

The sclerotia range from 0.1 mm to several millimeters in size (Fig. 5). Because the tissue response is not specific, the sclerotia become extremely important in making the diagnosis and determining the etiologic agent. The sclerotia can be readily used to distinguish between actinomycotic and eumycotic mycetoma. Surrounding the sclerotia, there is frequently a dense accumulation of neutrophils that is sometimes mixed with necrotic host debris. Chronic inflammation consisting of Iymphocytes, plasma cells, palisading epithelioid cells, and multinucleated giant cells occurs around the abscesses. Granulation tissue and dense fibrosis, which result in tumefaction and deformity, occurs as the mycetoma develops (11).

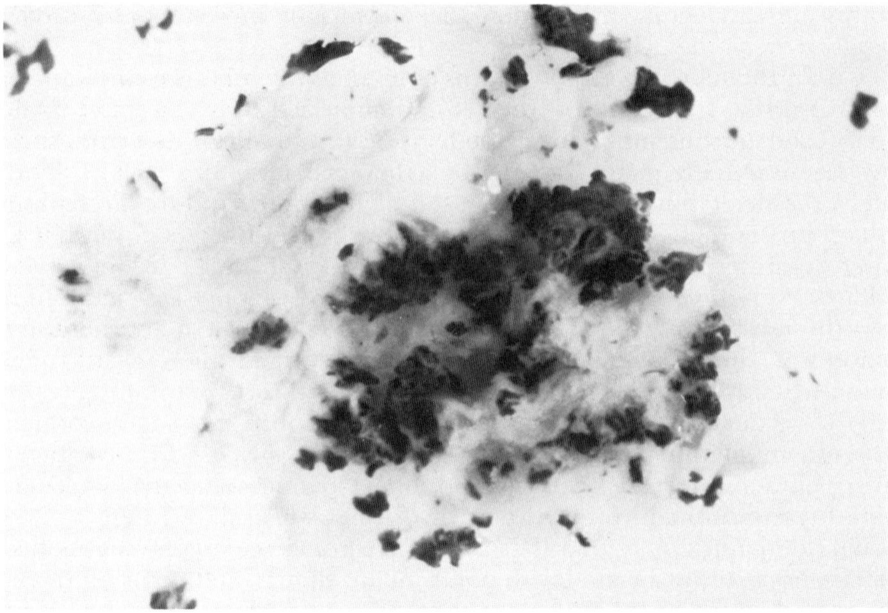

Fig. 5. Sclerotia, or granules, are organized vegetative structures 0.1 mm or larger in size. The darkly colored material in this tissue specimen mounted in KOH are sclerotia of *Madurella mycetomatis.* Photograph courtesy Mr. Wiley Schell

On a world wide basis (44), the major dematiaceous fungi causing mycetoma are *M. mycetomatis* (69%), *Pseudallescheria boydii* (11%), *Leptosphaeria senegalensis* (11%), *M. grisea* (6%), and *Pyrenochaeta romeroi* (1%). *Madurella grisea* and *P. romeroi* have been shown to be synanamorphs of the same fungus in most instances. Epidemiologically, mycetoma occurs predominantly in men with approximately 70% of the cases involving the foot, especially the dorsal side of the left foot. Approximately 12% of cases involve a hand; other infected sites include the arms, head and neck, knees, legs, and thighs. The greatest incidence of mycetoma occurs between the Tropics of Cancer and Capricorn where there are alternating dry and wet seasons. The infections are probably occupational rather than sexually or genetically based. The etiologic agents are fungi found throughout the world. In the United States, *P. boydii* is the most frequently reported dematiaceous fungus causing mycetoma (27).

Chromoblastomycosis

Chromoblastomycosis is a chronic, slowly progressing fungal infection that involves cutaneous and subcutaneous tissue, generally of the extremities (Fig. 6). The primary lesion often develops at a site where minor trauma has occurred, most frequently in males 20–50 years of age (6). Muriform cells are formed by the various etiologic agents in micro-abscesses in the subcutaneous tissue (42).

The term chromoblastomycosis was proposed in 1922 by Terra et al. (70) to distinguish a cutaneous infection that they were studying from an entity known as dermatitis verrucosa. The term chromoblastomycosis conveys an erroneous impression because it means a yeast infection having darkly colored yeast cells in tissue. Moore and Almeida (48) proposed the replacement term chromomycosis for chromoblastomycosis because they felt it was too misleading. The muriform cells (syn. sclerotic body, copper penny, Medlar body, fumagoid cell, sclerotium, chromo body, etc.) are arrested phenotypically between a hypha and yeast form. As time progressed, unfortunately and inappropriately, the concept of chromomycosis was expanded to include many new infections caused by a taxonomically disperse group of fungi. Ajello et al. (2) proposed the term phaeohyphomycosis to accommodate those infections that were clinically, pathologically, and mycologically different from the concept that Terra et al., Carrión, and others developed for classical chromoblastomycosis. McGinnis (42) has recently clarified much of the confusion surrounding the terms chromoblastomycosis and phaeohyphomycosis. To the list of accepted etiological agents (42), *E. jeanselmei* and *E. spinifera* must be added. The latter two taxa have been proven to be agents of chromoblastomycosis in humans.

Following the traumatic introduction of the fungus on a splinter or similar object, a small, pink, scaly papule develops that is frequently located on the foot or leg. A superficial nodule forms and increases in size to become a raised, purplish, superficial, irregular plaque. The central portion of the lesion may become scaly and cracked, or warty. Large, pruritic, papillomatous growths may form as the disease progresses. Satellite lesions

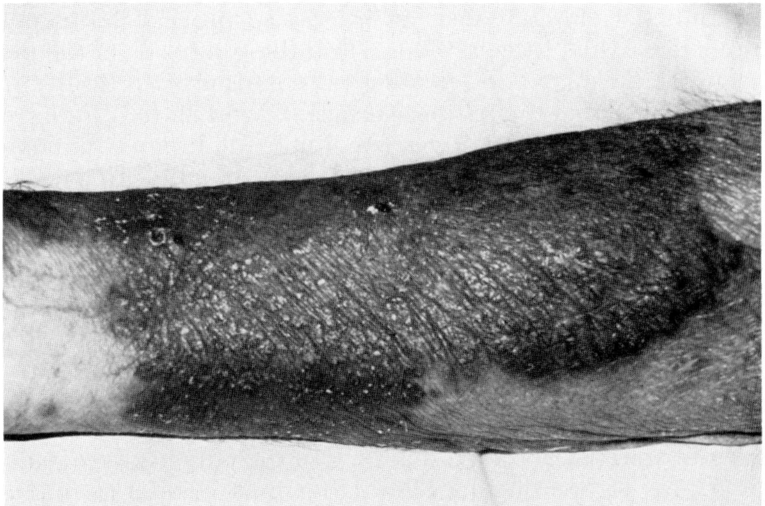

Fig. 6. Chromoblastomycosis on the arm of a patient that was caused by *Fonsecaea pedrosoi*

often develop as a result of either autoinoculation from the patient scratching the lesions, from lateral spread of the etiologic agent through the superficial lymphatics, or a combination of both methods. Hematogenous dissemination to the brain has been reported for *F. pedrosoi.* In brain tissue, the fungus produces hyphae without muriform cells; the disease in the brain is phaeohyphomycosis.

As the disease progresses, lesions may coalesce, and spread distally and centrifugally, with extensive fibrosis that contributes to lymph stasis because of blockage of the lymphatics. Edema, elephantiasis and deformity may occur in advanced infections. Patients living in Central and South America have lesions predominantly on the lower extremities, whereas patients living in Australia have a higher incidence of lesions on their upper limbs. In Australia, *Cladosporium carrionii* is the major agent of chromoblastomycosis. The reports of Carrión (5, 6, 7), McGinnis (42), and Fader and McGinnis (44) should be consulted for additional information regarding the clinical spectrum of chromoblastomycosis.

The host's tissue response to the etiological agents of chromoblastomycosis is not specific, even though it is classically described as showing hyperkeratotic pseudoepitheliomatous hyperplasia with microabscesses in the subcutaneous tissue (6, 42). The epidermis and dermis are involved. The stratum corneum is hyperkeratotic and distorted; the Malpighian layer is hyperplastic with epithelial downgrowths going into the dermis, with polymorphonuclear leukocyte infiltrates. Microabscesses containing muriform cells are usually present in abundance (6). The muriform cells (Fig. 3) are solitary or in groups, in the cellular infiltrates, in giant cells, in the central portion of granulomata and microabscesses, and sometimes within epithelial pearls in the epidermis. Hyphae and transition forms becoming muriform cells are not uncommon in the upper layers of the skin.

Transepithelial elimination is an important process that expels damaged connective tissue, foreign matter, and the fungus from the dermis to the skin surface during wound healing (42). This process results in "black dots" that are located at the lesion's surface. Oka et al. (53) have proposed that polymorphonuclear leukocytes encounter the fungus, microabscesses form, epithelioid granulomata form, some of the fungal cells are phagocytized by giant cells, epidermal pseudoepitheliomatous hyperplasia having projections into the dermis occurs, and the intraepidermal granulomata and microabscesses are then eliminated during epidermal turnover. Walter et al. (74) have recently reported that phagocytized muriform cells are damaged, but not killed. This finding may help explain why the disease is often difficult to manage.

Among 109 authentic cases of chromoblastomycosis reviewed by Carrión (5), 71% of the patients were between 20 and 50 years of age. In another study, Carrión observed that 96% of the patients were males. Race does not appear to be a factor. The higher male incidence might be explained by the fact that the majority of patients have been farm laborers (82%) working in the fields.

Phaeohyphomycosis

Phaeohyphomycosis encompasses a heterogenous group of mycotic infections that are caused by taxonomically diverse dematiaceous fungi. The presence of hyaline to pale brown hyphae that may be short or long, regular, distorted, or swollen, pseudohyphae, yeast, or any combination of these forms is characteristic of this disease. When hyaline hyphal or yeast cells are encountered in patients suspected of having phaeohyphomycosis, they should be stained with the Fontana-Masson stain to confirm the presence of melanin in the cell wall of the fungus.

Ajello et al. (2) proposed the name phaeohyphomycosis because the term chromomycosis had become superfluous. The purpose of the term phaeohyphomycosis is to provide an umbrella term for mycotic dematiaceous infections not classifiable as chromoblastomycosis. As new diseases were encountered, as well as a spectrum of taxonomically distinct fungi being recognized as new pathogens, it became evident that the diseases classifiable as phaeohyphomycosis needed to be better categorized. McGinnis (42) proposed that phaeohyphomycosis should be thought of as superficial, cutaneous and corneal, subcutaneous, and systemic infections. This concept is being expanded in this communication to include allergic processes as a fifth type of phaeohyphomycosis. This classification for phaeohyphomycosis negates the need for archaic terms to describe infections caused by dematiaceous fungi like systemic chromoblastomycosis, subcutaneous chromoblastomycosis, cerebral chromoblastomycosis, hypodermomycosis, encephalomycosis, chromomycosis, cystic chromomycosis, phaeomycosis, chromohyphomycosis, phaeomycotic cyst, keratochromomycosis, subcutaneous chromomycosis, cladsporiosis, cladosporoma, subcutaneous cystic granuloma, sporotrichosis (in part), phaeosporotrichoses, cerebral dematiomycosis, cerebral chromomycosis, and chromohyphomycosis. Phaeohyphomycosis, as well as mycetoma and chromoblastomycosis, are consistent, unifying, and unambiguous terms that clearly characterize the spectrum of diseases caused by the dematiaceous fungi. An example of each form of phaeohyphomycosis will now be used to illustrate the categories of phaeohyphomycosis.

Superficial phaeohyphomycoses consist of infections that are confined to the stratum corneum. There is little to no tissue response. If hair is involved, the fungus grows around the hair shaft. Tinea nigra and black piedra are examples of superficial phaeohyphomycosis. *Piedraia hortae,* which is a locule ascomycete, forms a hard, black, carbonaceous fruiting body known as an ascostroma around the hair shaft (Fig. 7). Cavities called locules are formed within the ascostroma, after which asci containing ascospores develop within the locules. The fungus forms ascostromata on a wide range of animals (32) living in tropical and subtropical regions of the world.

A series of studies dealing with people in Venezuela has revealed some interesting information. Two thousand eighty-seven ethnically heterogeneous dermatology patients were compared to 355 Indians living in nine

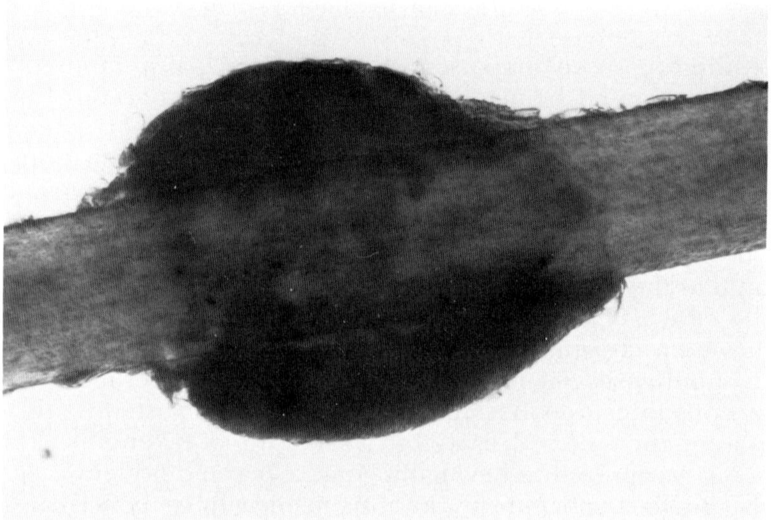

Fig. 7. Ascostroma of *Piedraia hortae* surrounding a hair shaft mounted in KOH

different villages in the same area as the dermatology patients. Only 2.3% of the ethnically diverse dermatology patients had *P. hortae* nodules on their hair, in contrast to 27.8% of the Indians living in the nine villages. Three of the dermatology clinic group patients with *P. hortae* nodules had Indian ancestry (47). In another study of the same Indian population, it was found that the male:female ratio was approximately 1:1, the incidence of colonization of hair increased post-pubertally, the number of ascostroma increased proportionally to the length of the hair, and a number of the affected Indians had marked Mongoloid features (73). In addition to population genetics, other factors such as the Indians resting their heads on the ground while sleeping and the application of oils and ashes to their hair are potentially important predisposing factors.

Cutaneous phaeohyphomycosis involves the keratinized tissues of the skin, nails and stratum corneum. Non-living skin layers are involved and often show extensive tissue damage. A cell-mediated immune response can typically be measured. *Scytalidium dimidiatum*, a synanamorph of *Nattrassia mangiferae* (syn. *Hendersonula toruloidea*), is a plant pathogen that occasionally infects humans living in tropical-to-subtropical regions, especially the Indian subcontinent. Clinically, *S. dimidiatum* infections are dry, scaling, chronic, and contain hyaline (occasionally dematiaceous in nails), septate hyphae. The clinical presentation resembles an infection caused by *Trichophyton rubrum*. Frankel and Tippon (22) reported that the chronicity, symptoms, and predilection for males is typical of dermatophytosis. Seventy-five percent of the infections have occurred in males, although females from non-endemic areas are more predisposed than males from the same area. The fungus attacks toenails (62% of patients), the foot (63% of patients), fingernails (33% of patients), nail folds (22% of patients), the palm, and rarely the scalp. *Scytalidium* infections are relatively refractory to antifungal agents.

Subcutaneous phaeohyphomycosis (Fig. 8) frequently occurs following the traumatic implantation of a fungus such as *Exophiala jeanselmei.* The lesion typically remains localized and can be managed with surgical excision without the need for antifungal agents. These localized, palpable, slightly elevated, solitary subcutaneous masses are frequently misdiagnosed as ganglion cyst, Baker's cyst, epidermal inclusion cyst, or foreign body granuloma. Histologically, the abscess is surrounded by dense collagenous connective tissue. The central portion of the abscess often contains necrotic debris mixed with polymorphonuclear leukocytes. The fungus is in both the wall and central portion of the abscess (42).

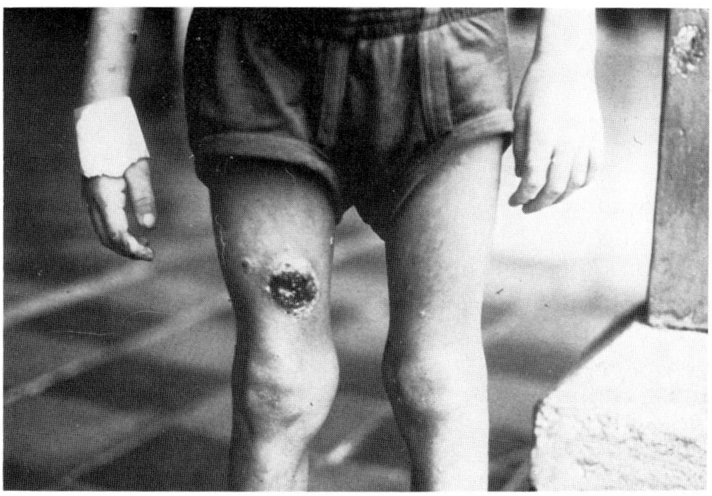

Fig. 8. Subcutaneous phaeohyphomycosis caused by *Exophiala spinifera*

Subcutaneous phaeohyphomycosis caused by *E. jeanselmei* occurs worldwide. A large number of the reported infections have occurred in women. Patients having this infection frequently have underlying problems such as diabetes, steroid therapy, systemic lupus erythematosus, and leukemia. Conversely, many individuals appear healthy without detectable underlying problems.

Systemic phaeohyphomycosis typically results from hematogenous dissemination from a primary site such as the lungs. When the brain is involved, the prognosis is often poor (Fig. 9). *Xylohypha bantiana* is a dematiaceous hyphomycete normally associated with wood that causes central nervous system infections characterized by chronic headache that is

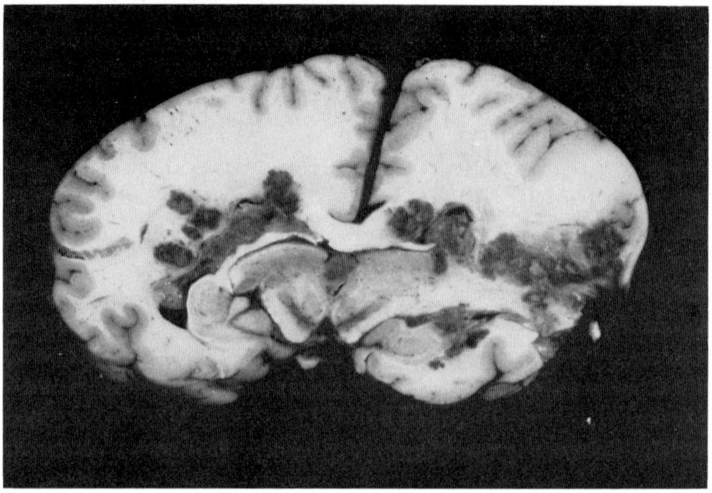

Fig. 9. Several abscesses are present that are darkly colored, partly due to the presence of large amounts of dematiaceous hyphae formed by *Xylohypha bantiana*

followed by fever and neurologic signs. In a study of 26 authentic infections caused by *X. bantiana* involving the brain, Dixon et al. (15) found that the male:female ratio was 2:1, that there was neither geographical nor racial predilection, and that pharmacologic immunosuppression was not important. Complete neurosurgical resection of the lesion was the single most important factor determining survival. Antifungal chemotherapy alone did not influence survival. Overall, the survival rate is 35%, and it is 45% when neurosurgery is employed.

Even though *X. bantiana* is associated with cerebral phaeohyphomycosis, the fungus has also been isolated from internal organs including the lungs. The lesions in brain tissue are a mixed purulent and granulomatous inflammatory reaction that most frequently occurs in the white matter of the frontal lobe of the cerebrum. The brain abscesses are either solitary or multiple and have a central zone of neutrophils and necrotic tissue that is surrounded by a thick wall of multinucleated giant cells, lymphocytes, epithelioid cells, and plasma cells, only if the patient survives long enough. Dematiaceous hyphae that are moniliform occur within the central purulent exudate and within the giant cells forming the wall of the abscess (11).

Allergic phaeohyphomycosis is a disease that is due solely to a hypersensitivity response to an inhaled fungus that non-allergic individuals would not respond too. The fungus is non-invasive and typically occurs as a fungoma (syn. fungus ball) in a cavity or anatomic air filled space such as the sinuses (43). Cosmopolitan fungi associated with plants such as *Bipolaris spicifera* and *Exserohilum rostratum* are not uncommon agents of allergic phaeohyphomycosis involving the nasal sinuses. Allergic rhinitis and nasal polyposis are two known predisposing factors to *Bipolaris* and *Exserohilum* sinusitis. Of the small number of cases reported, five occurred in males and two in females. Surgical debridement is the management approach of choice (1).

Fungomata often exhibit concentric zones of growth that can be readily seen in histological tissue sections. The respiratory mucosa has focally thickened broad zones of dense fibrosis containing a few lymphocytes and plasma cells. Clusters of small granulomata having cores of vacuolated histocytes surrounded by targetoid rims of concentric hyalinized collagen fibers occur throughout the fibrotic areas. The fungus forms hyphae and yeast-like cells in varying amounts and can be found in the centers of the granulomata. The Fontana-Masson stain for melanin may be needed to demonstrate the dematiaceous nature of the fungi in tissue (43).

Control and Prevention

Control and prevention are not practical for these opportunistic infections caused by the dematiaceous fungi. Owing to the cosmopolitan, ubiquous nature of these fungi, it is not feasible to attempt their eradication. Likewise, the incidence of infections does not justify the development of vaccines, assuming such an approach were to be plausible.

The incidence and severity of infections caused by the black fungi might be reduced through education, economic development, and early diagnosis and treatment. For example, wearing shoes could help to prevent mycetoma of the foot. If individuals do not have enough money to purchase shoes, this approach would not be successful. Health care delivery systems need money in order to purchase and provide antifungals. Surgical management is another approach, but again it requires money and facilities. Financial support for the family while the wage earner is unable to work will probably be necessary before individuals would be willing to accept treatment that would prevent them from working. Thus, the solution for control and prevention lies mainly in the areas of education and economic development.

Future Directions

Medical mycology is experiencing a tremendous growth involving the development of new antifungal agents that can be taken orally without toxic effects. Effective oral antifungal agents are important because they can be taken on an outpatient basis. Because the newer antifungal agents are known to be more effective against particular groups of fungi, it is becoming even more important to isolate and then identify the etiologic agents. The development of newer antifungal agents that are highly effective against the dematiaceous fungi via the oral route could have a major impact upon treating these mycoses. The design and development of new antifungal drugs must rely upon a clearer understanding of the basic biology of the fungi involved and their pathogenic mechanisms. Such information will have an important impact upon the management of mycetoma, chromoblastomycosis, and phaeohyphomycosis in the future.

Of the many diverse mycoses affecting persons in developing countries, virtually all would be classed as essentially opportunistic. Even the most highly prevalent infections such as coccidioidomycosis or histoplasmosis cause severe disease primarily in persons with altered host defenses. Like dematiaceous fungi, these normal mycotic inhabitants of the soil, decaying organic matter, and other niches in our environment cannot be eradicated. Although their cumulative burden as infectious diseases of tropical populations is substantial, our efforts at control must also rely at present on early diagnosis and treatment of individuals, education, and economic development.

References

1. Adam RD, Paquin ML, Petersen EA, Saubolle MA, Rinaldi MG, Corcoran JG, Galgiani JN, Sobonya RE (1986) Phaeohyphomycosis caused by the fungal genera *Bipolaris* and *Exserohilum*. A report of 9 cases and review of the literature. Medicine 65: 203–217
2. Ajello L, Georg LK, Steigbigel RT, Wang CJK (1974) A case of phaeohyphomycosis caused by a new species of *Phialophora*. Mycologia 66: 490–498
3. Bell AA (1981) Biochemical mechanisms of disease resistance. Ann. Rev Plant Pathol 32: 21–81
4. Beresky MA, Hall DW (1977) The influence of phenylthiourea on encapsulation, melanization, and survival in larvae of the mosquito *Aedes aegypti* parasitized by the nematode *Neoaplectana carpocapsae*. J Invert Pathol 29: 74–80
5. Carrión AL (1950) Chromoblastomycois. Ann NY Acad Sci 50: 1255–1282
6. Carrión AL (1977) Chromoblastomycosis. In: Graevenitz von A (ed) Clinical Microbiology, Vol 2, CRC Handbook Series in Clinical Laboratory Science. Cleveland, CRC Press, pp 3–11
7. Carrión AL (1975) Chromoblastomycosis and related infections. New concepts, differential diagnosis, and nomenclatural implications. Int J Dermatol 14: 27–32
8. Carter VD (1860) On a new and striking form of fungus disease, principally affecting the foot, and prevailing endemically in many parts of India. Trans Med Phys Soc Bombay 6: 104–142
9. Carter VD (1861) On "mycetoma" or the fungus-disease of India: Including notes of recent cases and new observations on the structure, and c. of the entophytic growth. Trans Med Phys Soc Bombay 7: 206–221
10. Chalmers AJ, Archibald RG (1918) The classification of the mycetomas. J Trop Med Hyg 21: 121–123
11. Chandler FW, Kaplan W, Ajello L 1980) A Colour Atlas and Textbook of the Histopathology of Mycotic Diseases. London, Wolfe Medical Publications
12. Day AW, Gardiner RB (1987) Fungal fimbriae. Stud Mycol 30: 333–349
13. Dixon DM, Polak A, Conner GW (1989) Mel-mutants of *Wangiella dermatitidis* in mice: Evaluation of multiple mouse and fungal strains. J Med Vet Mycol 27: 335–341
14. Dixon DM, Polak A, Szaniszlo PJ (1987) Pathogenicity and virulence of wild-type and melanin-deficient *Wangiella dermatitidis*. J Med Vet Mycol 25: 97–106
15. Dixon DM, Walsh TJ, Merz WG, McGinnis MR (1989) Infections due to *Xylohypha bantiana* (*Cladosporium trichoides*). Rev Infect Dis 11: 515–525
16. Espinel-Ingroff A, Goldson PR, McGinnis MR, Kerkering TM (1988) Evaluation of proteolytic activity to differentiate some dematiaceous fungi. J Clin Microbiol 26: 301–307

17. Espinel-Ingroff A, McGinnis MR, Pincus DH, Goldson PR, Kerkering TM (1989) Evaluation of the API 20C Yeast Identification System for the differentiation of some dematiaceous fungi. J Clin Microbiol 27: 2565–2569
18. Espinel-Ingroff A, Shadomy S, Dixon D, Goldson P (1986) Exoantigen test for *Cladosporium bantianum, Fonsecaea pedrosoi,* and *Phialophora verrucosa.* J Clin Microbiol 23: 305–310
19. Fader RC, McGinnis MR (1988) Infections caused by dematiaceous fungi: Chromoblastomycosis and phaeohyphomycosis. Infect Dis Clin N Am 2: 925–938
20. Findlay GH, Vismer HF (1974) Black grain mycetoma. A study of the chemistry, formation and significance of the tissue grain in *Madurella mycetomi* infection. Br J Dermatol 91: 297–303
21. Findlay GH, Vismer HF, Liebenberg NW (1979) Black grain mycetoma: The ultrastructure of *Madurella mycetomi.* Mycopathologia 67: 51–54
22. Frankel DH, Rippon JW (1989) *Hendersonula toruloidea* infection in man. Index cases in the non-endemic North American host and a review of the literature. Mycopathologia 105: 175–186
23. Friis J, Ottolenghi P (1969) Pigment formation by the "black yeast" *Phialophora jeanselmei.* Antonie van Leeuwenhoek Yeast Symp 35 [Suppl]: H 13–14
24. Geis PA, Jacobs CW (1985) Polymorphism of *Wangiella dermatitidis.* In: Szaniszlo PJ (ed) Fungal Dimorphism. New York, Plenum Publishing Corp, pp 205–233
25. Geis PA, Szaniszlo PJ (1984) Carotenoid pigments of the dematiaceous fungus *Wangiella dermatitidis.* Mycologia 76: 268–273
26. Godfrey J (1846) Disease of foot not hitherto described. Lancet 1: 593–594
27. Green WO, Adams TE (1964) Mycetoma in the United States. A review and report of seven additional cases. Am J Clin Pathol 42: 75–91
28. Gueho E, deHoog GS (1991) Taxonomy of the medical species of *Pseudallescheria* and *Scedosporium.* J Mycol Med i: 3–9
29. Hay RJ, Collins MJ (1983) An ultrastructural study of pale eumycetoma grains. Sabouraudia 21: 261–269
30. Jacobs CW, Szaniszlo PJ (1985) Altered development in a temperature-sensitive morphological mutant of *Wangiella dermatitidis.* Mycologia 77: 142–148
31. Jahnke KD (1987) Assessing natural relationships by DNA analysis. Techniques and applications. Stud Mycol 30: 227–246
32. Kaplan W (1959) The occurrence of black piedra in primate pelts. Trop Geograph Med 11: 115–126
33. Kaufman L, Standard PG, Padhye AA (1980) Serological relationship among isolates of *Exophiala jeanselmei* (*Phialophora jeanselmei, P. gougerotii*) and *Wangiella dermatitidis.* PAHO Sci Pub 396: 252–258
34. Kawasaki M, Ishizaki H, Nishimura K, Miyaji M (1990) Mitochondrial DNA analysis of *Exophiala jeanselmei* and *Exophiala dermatitidis.* Mycopathologia 110: 107–112
35. Kwon-Chung KH, Rhodes JC (1986) Encapsulation and melanin formation as indicators of virulence in *Cryptococcus neoformans.* Infect Immun 51: 218–223
36. Linderman RG, Toussoun TA (1966) Behavior of albino chlamydospores of *Thielaviopsis basicola.* Phytopathology 56: 887
37. Lockwood JL (1960) Lysis of mycelium of plant-pathogenic fungi by natural soil. Phytopathology 50: 787–789
38. Lynch JB (1964) Mycetoma in the Sudan. Ann R Coll Surg 35: 319–340
39. Mahgoub ES (1985) Mycetoma. Semin Dermatol 4: 230–239
40. Masuda M, Naka W, Tajima S, Harada T, Nishikawa T, Kaufman L, Standard P (1989) Deoxyribonucleic acid hydridization studies of *Exophiala dermatitidis* and *Exophiala jeanselmei.* Microbiol Immunol 33: 631–639
41. Matsumoto T, Matsuda T, McGinnis MR (1990) A previously undescribed synanamorph of *Wangiella dermatitidis.* J Med Vet Mycol 28: 437–444
42. McGinnis MR (1983) Chromoblastomycosis and phaeohyphomycosis: New concepts, diagnosis, and mycology. J Am Acad Dermatol 8: 1–16
43. McGinnis MR, Campbell G, Gourley WK, Lucia HL (1992) Phaeohyphomycosis caused by *Bipolaris spicifera:* An informative case. Eur J Epidemiol (in press)

44. McGinnis MR, Fader RC (1988) Mycetoma: A contemporary concept. Infect Dis Clin N Am 2: 939–954
45. McGinnis MR, Rinaldi MG, Winn R (1986) Emerging agents of phaeohyphomycosis: Pathogenic species of *Bipolaris* and *Exserohilum*. J Clin Microbiol 24: 250–259
46. McGinnis MR, Sigler L, Bowman BH, Masuda M, Wang CJK (1992) Impact of conidiogenesis, teleomorph connections, pleomorphism and molecular genetics on evolving Hyphomycete systematics. J Hum Vet Mycol (in press)
47. Molero B, Volcan GS, Medrano CE (1980) Differences in the prevalence of piedra between the mixed population of a city in Bolivar State, Venezuela and the Indian population of that region. PAHO Sci Pub 396: 77–81
48. Moore M, de Almeida F (1935) Etiologic agents of chromomycosis (chromoblastomycosis of Terra, Torres, Fonseca and Leão, 1922) of North and South America. Rev Biol Hyg 6: 94–97
49. Moore RT (1987) Micromorphology of yeasts and yeast-like fungi and its taxonomic implications. Stud Mycol 30: 203–226
50. Morganti L, Pozzuoli R, Strazzullo E (1980) Mycetoma granules: An electron microscopic study. Microbiologica 3: 349–362
51. Naka W, Harada T, Nishikawa T (1986) Growth temperature of pathogenic dematiaceous fungi and skin surface temperature with reference to local heat therapy. Jpn J Med Mycol 27: 245–250
52. Naka W, Harada T, Nishikawa T, Fukushiro R (1986) A case of chromoblastomycosis: With special reference to the mycology of the isolated *Exophiala jeanselmei*. Mykosen 29: 445–452
53. Oka K, Sato Y, Matsuo S, Okuda C (1981) Histopathology of chromomycosis: Especially on the elimination phenomenon. Jpn J Clin Dermatol 35: 1161–1166
54. Padhye AA, McGinnis MR, Ajello L (1978) Thermotolerance of *Wangiella dermatitidis*. J Clin Microbiol 8: 424–426
55. Pasarell L McGinnis MR, Standard PG (1990) Differentiation of medically important isolates of *Bipolaris* and *Exserohilum* with exoantigens. J Clin Microbiol 28: 1655–1657
56. Pinoy E (1913) Actinomycoses et mycetomes. Bull Inst Pasteur 11: 929–938
57. Polak A, Dixon DM (1989) Loss of melanin in *Wangiella dermatitidis* does not result in greater susceptibility to antifungal agents. Antimicrob Agents Chemother 33: 1639–1640
58. Polacheck I, Hearing VJ, Kwon-Chung KJ (1982) Biochemical studies of phenoloxidase and utilization of catecholamines in *Cryptococcus neoformans*. J Bacteriol 150: 1212–1220
59. Rhodes JC, Polacheck I, Kwon-Chung KJ (1982) Phenoloxidase activity and virulence in isogenic strains of *Cryptococcus neoformans*. Infect Immun 36: 1175–1184
60. Romero H, Mackenzie DWR (1989) Studies on antigens from agents causing black grain eumycetoma. J Med Vet Mycol 27: 303–311
61. Sorokin D Yu, Bab'eva IP (1982) Lysis of natural yeast populations by soil microorganisms. Microbiology USSR 51: 275–278
62. Sran HS, Narula IMS, Agarwal RK, Joshi KR (1972) History of mycetoma. Ind J Hist Med 17: 1–7
63. Srivastava OP, Lal B, Agrawal PK, Agarwal SC, Chandra B, Mathur IS (1977) Mycotic keratitis due to *Rhizoctonia* sp. Sabouraudia 15: 125–131
64. Standard PG, Kaufman L, Padhye AA (1988) An immunological procedure for the rapid identification of *Phaeoannellomyces werneckii*. Diag Clin Immunol 5: 367–370
65. Steadham JE, Geis PA, Simmonak JL (1989) Use of carbohydrate and nitrate assimilation in the identification of dematiaceous fungi. Diag Microbiol Infect Dis 5: 71–75
66. Sussman AS (1968) Longevity and survivability of fungi. In: Ainsworth GC, Sussman AS (eds) The Fungi, Vol. 3. New York, Academic Press, pp 447–486
67. Szaniszlo PJ, Geis PA, Jacobs CW, Cooper CR, Harris JL (1983) Cell wall changes associated with yeast-to-multicellular form conversion in *Wangiella dermatitidis*. In: Schlessinger D (ed) Microbiology 1983. Washington, ASM, pp 239–244
68. Szaniszlo PJ, Hsieh PH, Marlowe JD (1976) Induction and ultrastructure of the multicellular (sclerotic) morphology in *Phialophora dermatitidis*. Mycologia 68: 117–130
69. Taylor BE, Wheeler MH, Szaniszlo PJ (1987) Evidence for pentaketide melanin biosynthesis in dematiaceous human pathogenic fungi. Mycologia 79: 320–322

70. Terra F, Torres M, da Fonseca O, Area Leão AE (1922) Novo typo de dermatite verrucosa mycose por Acrotheca com associacao de leishmaniosa. Brasil Med 2: 363–368
71. Tu CC, Kimbrough JW (1975) Morphology, development, and cytochemistry of the hyphae and sclerotia of species in the *Rhizoctonia* complex. Can J Bot 53: 2286–2296
72. Uspenskaya GD, Reshetnikova IA, Kozlenko TN (1980) Some characteristics of the pycnidial mucus of fungi from the genera *Ascochyta* and *Phoma*. Mikol Filopatol 14: 21–23, 1980.
73. Volcan GS, Medrano CE, Molero B (1980) Notes on the *Piedraia hortai* cycle. PAHO Sci Publ 396: 63–69
74. Walter P, Garin Y, Richard-Lenoble D (1982) Chromoblastomycosis: A morphological investigation of the host-parasite interaction. Virchows Arch (Pathol Anat) 397: 203–214
75. Wethered DB, Markey MA, Hay RJ, Mahgoub ES, Gumaa SA (1987) Ultrastructural and immunogenic changes in the formation of mycetoma grains. J Med Vet Mycol 25: 39–46
76. Wheeler MH, Bell AA (1988) Melanins and their importance in pathogenic fungi. In: McGinnis MR (ed) Current topics in medical mycology Vol. 2. New York, Springer, pp 338–387
77. White TJ, Bruns T, Lee S, Taylor J (1990) Amplication and direct sequencing of fungal ribosomal RNA genes for phylogenetics. In: Innis M, Gelfand D, Snisky J, White T (eds) PCR protocols: a guide to methods and applications. Orlando, Academic Press, pp 315–322
78. Wood C, Russel-Bell B (1983) Characterization of pigmented fungi by melanin staining. Am J Dermatopathol 5: 77–81
79. Yamada Y, Banno I, von Arx JA, van der Walt JP (1987) Taxonomic significance of the coenzyme Q system in yeasts and yeast-like fungi. Stud Mycol 30: 299–308
80. Yamada Y, Sugihara K, van Eijk GW, Roeijmans HJ, de Hoog GS (1989) Coenzyme Q systems in ascomycetous black yeasts. Antonie van Leeuwenhoek 56: 349–356
81. Zhdanova NN, Gauryushina AI, Vasilevskaya AI (1973) Effect of γ- and UV-radiation on survival of *Cladosporium* sp. and *Oidiodendron cerealis*. Mikrobiol Zh Kiev 35: 449–451
82. Zhdanova NN, Melezhik AV, Vasilevskaya AI (1980) Thermostability of some melanin-containing fungi. Biol Bull Acad Sci USSR 7: 305–310
83. Zhdanova NN, Svishchuk AA, Shmygum MP, Bondar AI (1970) The protective effect of the pigment isolated from the fungus *Cladosporium* sp. Microbiology USSR 39: 520–524

Schistosomiasis – From Genes to Latrines[1]

Franz von Lichtenberg

Brigham and Women's Hospital, Harvard Medical School, Boston, Massachusetts

Introduction

Schistosoma mansoni, S. haematobium and *S. japonicum* are widely distributed throughout the tropics (Fig. 1). By the latest estimates, around 160 million people are infected and 550 million are at risk. In major endemic countries including Brazil, Egypt, the Phillipines and China, the toll of schistosomiasis is now well understood, and government sponsored control efforts are in progress. Effective drugs have become available, and the design of preventive campaigns has been rationalized and improved. Yet, in some of the least developed countries, e.g., around new water impoundments in Senegal and in Botswana (1), schistosomiasis continues spreading and international health organizations have given up the hope of halting transmission and are concentrating on the less ambitious task of lowering schistosomiasis morbidity.

Here we shall briefly review recent scientific advances applicable to the epidemiology, diagnosis, and chemotherapy of schistosomiasis and to vector control and vaccination. We shall also survey methodological and socioeconomic obstacles to their application and steps required for achieving long-lasting disease control.

Epidemiology

A large variety of new methods have been devised for detecting schistosome-specific antibodies. Most are modifications of enzyme linked- or radio- immunoassays and employ fractionated rather than crude schistosome egg and/or adult worm antigens; some of these antigens have already been characterized and sequenced and produced in recombinant form, e.g. schistosome glutathione-S-transferase (2). Intuitively, one would

---

[1] Title taken from: The Biology of Schistosomes: From Genes to Latrines, D Rollinson and AJB Simpson (eds) Academic Press, 1987

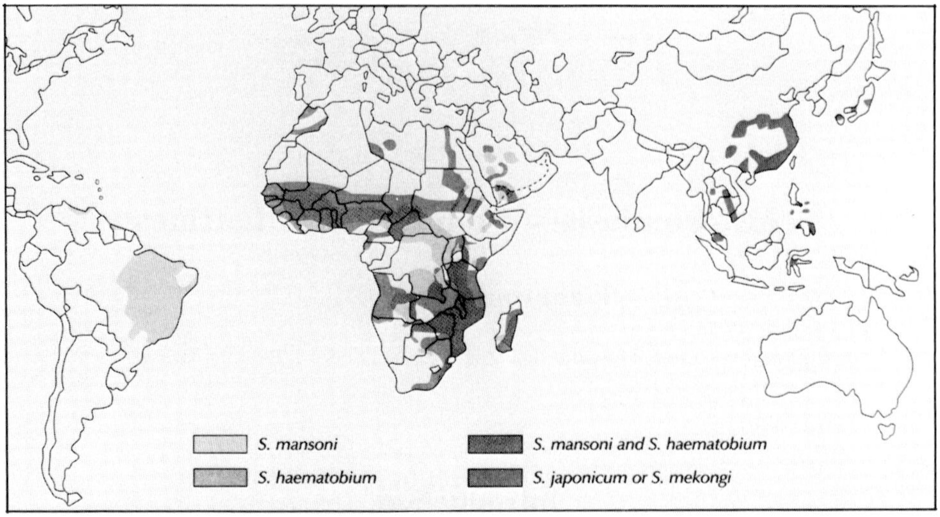

Fig. 1. Worldwide distribution of *Schistosoma mansoni, S. haematobium* and *S. japonicum*. From King CH (1991) Acute and chronic schistosomiasis. Hosp Practice 26: 95–106

expect defined antigens to outperform crude parasite fractions when assayed by sensitive ELISA or RIA techniques; they should also facilitate large-scale processing of finger stick blood samples in a central laboratory facility. Moreover, some egg antigen fractions might be sensitive enough to detect infections of minimal intensity. Thus, in mass treated communities with substantially lowered infection rates, ELISA tests for anti-egg antibodies might be preferable to labor-intensive stool examinations as a primary screening test since multiple negative stool samples result in observer fatigue and thus in false negative readings.

In a 1982 WHO collaborative study, various *S. mansoni* antigen fractions and serodiagnostic methods were tested against banked sera from endemic patients screened by repeated Kato smears. Several antigens showed >93% sensitivity and/or specificity in untreated individuals but none proved superior to crude egg antigens, e.g., to classical circumoval precipitation. Moreover, in sera of treated patients, the specificities of most tests fell below 70% (Table 1). Some of the post-treatment sera may have come from patients with false negative stool tests thus confounding the results (3), but, in other studies, patients with less than 25 eggs/gm of feces also sometimes proved to be ELISA negative. Thus, there is currently no consensus that serologic accuracy exceeds that of parasitologic examination; on the other hand, the final chapter on fractionated schistosome antigens has yet to be written. Recent studies have identified a 40 KD schistosome egg antigen which evokes antibody responses in >90% of infected persons; similarly, virtually all infected patients have been shown to form antibodies against two heat shock-like proteins (70 and 38 KD) which abound in the adult worm tegument (2).

Table 1. Specificity of *S. mansoni* and *S. japonicum* antigens. Sensitivities and specificities of the schistosome antigens used in the WHO/TDR collaboratory study. From ref. No. 3

Antigen	Antigen code	Test	Specificity (%)		
			Group 1[a]	Group 2[b]	Group 3[c]
Whole *S. mansoni* eggs	01	COPT	100	100	75.0
Fractionated SEA *S. mansoni*	07	ELISA	100	100	64.7
Fractionated SEA *S. japonicum*	08	ELISA	100	100	–
TCA-extracted *S. mansoni* adult worm	12	ELISA	100	100	75.0
CEF-6 *S. mansoni* egg	15	ISI	100	100	85.7
Crude SEA *S. mansoni*	05	ELISA	96.7	90	47.1
Purified glycoprotein fraction *S. mansoni*	09	MDD	96.7	95	64.7
Crude *S. mansoni* adult worm extract	10	IHA	96.7	94.7	58.8
Excretory-secretory *S. mansoni*	11	ELISA	96.7	100	31.2
S. mansoni GASP	13	IFA	96.7	94.7	25
Purified glycoprotein fraction *S. mansoni*	09	IHA	93.3	94.7	70.6
CEF-6 *S. mansoni* egg	15	ELISA	93.3	94.7	80
S. mansoni egg fraction	02	RIA	90.3	100	17.6
S japonicum egg glycoprotein	04	ELISA	90.3	90	–
Crude SEA *S. mansoni*	05	IHA	90.3	90	29.4
Crude SEA *S. japonicum*	06	ELISA	90.3	95	–
Crude saline extract *S. mansoni* adult worm	10	ELISA	87.1	80	41.2
S. mansoni gut	14	IFA	87.1	80	52.9
S. mansoni somatic	17	IFA	87.1	90	23.5
Crude SEA *S. japonicum*	06	IHA	83.9	95	–
Purified glycoprotein fraction *S. mansoni*	09	IgE RAST	83.9	75	35.3
Purified glycoprotein fraction *S. mansoni*	09	ELISA	77.4	65	64.7
Crude *S. mansoni* adult worm extract	10	IgE RAST	74.2	60	35.3
S. mansoni gut and somatic	14 & 17	IFA	74.2	–	–
Saline-extracted adult *S. mansoni*	10	MDD	67.7	65	11.6

[a] Combined results from a maximum of 11 sera from Europeans and 20 sera from Amazon Indians
[b] Results from a maximum of 20 sera from Amazon Indians
[c] Results from a maximum of 17 post-treatment sera from residents of *S. mansoni*-endemic areas with at least 15 negative Kato stool examinations

Even if an efficient seroepidemiologic screen for schistosomiasis were to emerge, in many developing countries the cost of equipping and operating modern central serodiagnostic facilities could run significantly higher than maintenance of a semi-skilled task force for field screening of stool or urine specimens. Moreover, the need for such a laboratory would become greatest toward the tail end of a successful control campaign, i.e., during a downward slope of the budget cycle. Also, among certain endemic population groups, blood samples are donated only with extreme reluctance. Serodiagnosis of schistosomiasis has therefore remained largely confined to urban laboratories, and it remains unclear whether large-scale seroepidemiologic screening could bring about a quantum leap in schistosomiasis control.

By contrast, large-scale dipstick urine testing for red cells and protein is clearly an important epidemiologic advance. Well controlled field studies have shown that these tests approximate the sensitivity and specificity of Nytrel filter concentration techniques for microscopic detection of *S. haematobium* ova and can greatly simplify definition of the local prevalence and geographic distribution of urinary schistosomiasis, an essential requisite for the success of chemotherapeutic campaigns (4). In addition, the dipstick method has been successfully used in conjunction with other laboratory tests in studying the effects of treatment on the anemia and nutritional deficiencies of endemically infected children (5). Great strides have also been made in measuring the morbidity caused by schistosomiasis in endemic communities by means of ultrasound imaging of target organs. As ultrasound equipment became available, first in urban hospitals and later in portable versions for field studies, it soon became apparent that the presence and intensity of liver pipestem fibrosis in Manson's schistosomiasis can be reliably and non-invasively determined by this method (6); it also became feasible to evaluate urinary tract pathology in *S. haematobium* infected children and to visualize bladder and ureteral deformities and hydronephrosis without performing intravenous pyelography (7). In *S. japonicum* infection, as well, ultrasound studies of endemic liver pathology are currently in progress. Thus, for the first time, an accurate, field-applicable method is now available for determining the morbidity of schistosomiasis in a given community and for monitoring the effect of chemotherapy on pathology in longitudinal and cohort studies. Several ambitious projects along these lines have begun to unveil serious pathology in ostensibly asymptomatic children with "red urine" or mild liver enlargement and are alerting previously complacent communities and government agencies to the need for attacking schistosomiasis at its roots. On the other hand, funds for the transfer of ultrasound technology into rural endemic communities have thus far emanated almost exclusively from donors in developed countries. Unfortunately, the large expenditures required for equipping rural health centers nationwide are beyond the means of third-world governments other than those of a few oil-rich countries.

In overview: the available tools for epidemiologic analysis of endemic schistosomiasis are now adequate and cost-effective. They include improved methods for schistosome egg counting, dipstick technology, and portable ultrasound equipment. Molecular biology has had no impact but may yet play a role in improving seroepidemiologic methods. Thus far, financial and organizational support for epidemiologic research has been limited to pilot studies, and, in the light of prevailing economic strictures in endemic countries, large scale support is unlikely to materialize soon.

Diagnosis

The above comments on seroepidemiology are also applicable to individual serodiagnosis. In the U.S., a sensitive rapid western blot assay is available through the CDC (8), but should not replace parasitological examination of stool or urine specimens or biopsy material, except during the earliest, prepatent stage of acute schistosomiasis. Antibody isotypes can be shown to switch during progression from acute to chronic schistosomiasis (9), but in the real world of medical practice, such studies will seldom be called for. More likely, clinical attention will be focussed on *schistosome antigen detection* in serum or body fluids. Several target antigens have already been identified, among them a macromolecular anodic glycoprotein, "CAA" (10, 11), and a thiol proteinase known as schistosome "hemoglobinase" whose entire 1390 base pair mRNA sequence has recently been determined (12). Both antigens originate in the gut of viable adult schistosomes and are regurgitated into the host bloodstream; their detection in serum or urine therefore signifies active infection and poses an indication for chemotherapy. Sandwich ELISA techniques and monoclonal reagents for that purpose have been developed. They will not be needed in patients excreting viable eggs, but, in treated patients, they could help determine whether male or sterile female schistosomes have survived therapy. Stage-specific antigen tests should also be particularly useful in the differential diagnosis of ectopic CNS schistosomiasis. It has even been suggested that quantitative antigen assays be used for measuring worm burdens (13); this could be helpful in late stage adult patients with "inactive" *S. haematobium* infection whose egg output has become erratic (14). Today's tests for schistosome antigen still lag in sensitivity compared to those for cryptococcal antigen and DNA probes have not yet been adapted to diagnostic laboratory use although they are widely employed in immunogenetic research and vaccine development (*vide infra*). Probes for schistosome DNA, when available, will likely be used for individual diagnostic purposes rather than for population studies for reasons to be discussed further below. As mentioned earlier, ultrasound has become the single most valuable imaging technique for visualizing schistosomiasis lesions but CAT, MRI and radionuclide scans as well as sophisticated angiographic methods are also being used in fully equipped hospital centers together with fiberoptic endoscopy of mucosal lesions. Simultaneously, the power and scope of laboratory tests have expanded, and urine cytology and fine needle biopsy have greatly improved, but the vast majority of endemic schistosomiasis patients never benefit from modern medical technology. In third world countries, up-to-date facilities are confined to only a few well staffed metropolitan medical centers. Local physicians are well versed in managing endemic schistosomiasis, but diagnostic facilities are scarce, and hospital care is often delayed and perfunctory. Conversely, physicians in developed countries make liberal use of specialized imaging methods and laboratory tests but often lack experience in assessing the intensity, morbidity and stage of schistosome infection and in monitoring therapy.

In conclusion, today's methods for diagnostic workup of schistosomiasis patients leave little to be desired. The principal remaining problems are patient access to modern medical care and physician education. Mercifully, for reasons to be discussed below, the number of patients with severe complications of schistosomiasis requiring tertiary hospital care has lately been decreasing (15).

Chemotherapy

Anti-schistosomal drug therapy has progressed greatly over the last two decades. Advances have also been made in schistosome molecular physiology and biochemistry, but Praziquantel (now FDA approved and widely used for all three major human schistosome infections), Metrifonate (active against *S. haematobium*) and Oxamniquin (active against *S. mansoni*) were all discovered by old-fashioned empirical drug testing rather than by rational design. The same is true of several seldom used alternate drugs, e.g., Niridazole (for *S. japonicum*). More recently some unique metabolic pathways and enzymes of schistosomes have been flagged as points of potential biochemical vulnerability. Thus, the enzymes of the purine salvage pathway of schistosomes were found to differ radically from those of humans (16) and have been successfully inactivated by synthetic analogs (17). Another potential target for rational drug design is trans-membrane calcium transport by schistosome calmodulin. It has also been shown that mevinolin, a potent inhibitor of HMG-CoA reductase, inhibits schistosome egg formation (18) and that two of the major schistosome GSH transferases (19) are coded for by unique mRNAs, but all "designer drugs" thus far are still too toxic for human application. Yet, prospects seem favorable and in view of rising drug resistance among the schistosomes, the search must continue.

Genetically mediated schistosome drug resistance was first reported against Hycanthone, a drug now abandoned because of its mutagenic potential (20). Cross-resistance and increasing primary resistance has since also been observed against Oxamniquin, but there is as yet no convincing evidence of resistance to Praziquantel. The latter two drugs can be given in a single oral dose, a great advantage under rural endemic conditions. Metrifonate is usually given in three divided doses. As of today, praziquantel is acclaimed as first in line against all human schistosome infections, and its cost has recently fallen to between \$0.50 and \$1.00 per treatment; in addition to the original Bayer product, it is now locally fabricated in China and Egypt for government-sponsored control campaigns. If chemotherapeutic programs were instituted in all endemic areas, the global need for praziquantel by WHO estimate would be of the order of 427 million tablets (21). The least expensive drug is metrifonate which has proven safe and effective against *S. haematobium* in African children. Yet, there is still need for alternative compounds that can be inexpensively substituted if drug resistance should spread further afield.

The benefits of large-scale drug therapy are largely due to the simple fact that the morbidity of schistosomiasis is directly related to worm and egg burden. When infection intensity falls below a threshhold level, pipestem fibrosis (Fig. 2) or life-threatening uropathy (Fig. 3) are unlikely to develop (14, 22); however, this correlation does not apply to acute schistosomiasis or to ectopic neural manifestations (23). There is therefore a growing consensus that all patients bearing egg-laying schistosome worm pairs should be treated, regardless of whether their lesions are mild or severe and barring only specific contraindications (e.g., pregnancy). If initial treatment does not result in complete cure, it usually reduces egg excretion to a fraction of the prior level. Parasitological follow-up can then determine whether additional drug courses are needed. Patients with heavy infections may suffer a transitory hypereosinophilic febrile reaction related to massive worm death, but even in patients with established pipestem liver fibrosis or with obstructive uropathy the benefits of treatment outweigh the risks.

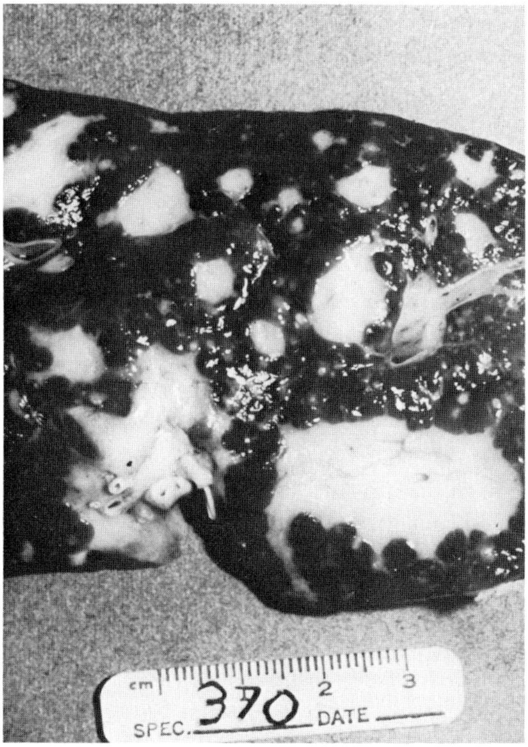

Fig. 2. Advanced pipestem fibrosis of liver

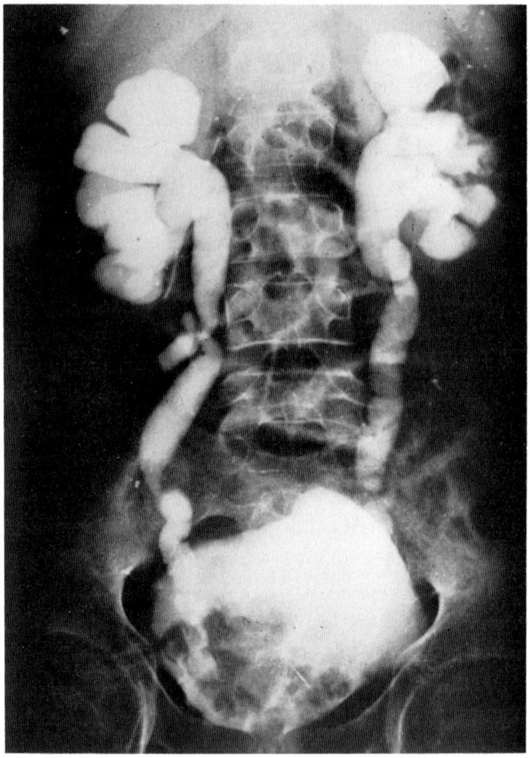

Fig. 3. Bilateral hydronephrosis due to *S. haematobium* infection. Ascending pyelogram

There is, however, no advantage to be gained from treating patients with burned out, inactive schistosomiasis whose lesions require surgical rather than medical correction (14).

Sterile cure is a reasonable aim in office practice but not in mass treatment campaigns where the goal is to reduce rather than abolish schistosome egg excretion. In fact, a few residual schistosomes may serve to maintain acquired host resistance in endemic patients still at risk of reinfection. On the other hand, given the enormous multiplication of schistosomes during the snail portion of their cycle, even small numbers of eggs deposited in local waters may suffice to maintain the transmission cycle and eventually restore it to its former level. Thus, unless vector snails are exterminated, or water sources are made safe, drug treatments may have to be repeated periodically *ad infinitum*, making their cost prohibitive. There has been considerable variation between community-wide chemotherapy projects as regards rates of reinfection during follow-up; some projects in the least-developed African locations have shown discouragingly high rates, e.g., in Burundi (24). In other studies, e.g., in Kenya and Gambia (25), mean egg outputs have remained much below pre-treatment levels consistent with age-related acquired resistance to cercarial exposure (*vide infra*).

Chemotherapy campaigns have varied in target populations, drugs, dosages and monitoring methods. Some have aimed at the least costly method for lowering schistosomiasis morbidity, others at achieving the greatest possible reduction of transmission. Some teams, following a household census, have treated all reachable and compliant community members; others have concentrated on the group responsible for the largest egg output namely school age children. With respect to follow-up, small scale control projects limited to a single community have breen meticulous and quantitative, while countrywide control efforts, such as took place in Egypt, Brazil or China could not afford comprehensive monitoring. Comparisons are further complicated by projects in which mass chemotherapy was combined or contrasted with other interventions, e.g., molluscidide application, sanitary engineering or community educational efforts. Despite these disparities, in all communities and countries in which chemotherapeutic campaigns have been instituted, schistosome morbidity has declined as evidenced by a drop in the number of patients hospitalized with severe pathology and/or complications. This decline is at least partly attributable to a shift of the mean worm burden below the threshhold level for severe pathology (26) and has been observed even after chemotherapy campaigns which fell short of their stated objectives (14). Moreover, during the Saint Lucia project of the Rockefeller Foundation, reductions in egg output also followed other interventions, e.g., application of molluscicide or construction of sanitary water facilities (27). Thus, part of the improvement observed after mass chemotherapy is certainly attributable to the drug treatment itself while part may represent a collective "placebo effect" resulting from other unspecified interactions between the preventive task force and its community beneficiaries; nor can coincidental improvement in the local economy be discounted as a possible factor. By the same token, poverty and lack of education have been common denominators in community chemotherapeutic projects with relatively poor results. Distributing drugs to indentured African plantation workers or Brazilian favela families without weaning them from contact with their polluted, snail-infested waters has yielded only aleatory results with prevalence climbing back to pretreatment levels (28). The principal lesson has been that endemic foci differ in their biological, environmental and socio-economic features and that control procedures must be adjusted to these local conditions rather than copied from schemes that may have been successful elsewhere. Epidemiologists, vector biologists and anthropologists must team together, and it is critically important to secure the voluntary participation of the target community at every step of the campaign, including its design.

Vector Control

Over the last two decades, the manpower pool of trained malakologists has begun to dry out even while the vector snails for each of the schistosome species continue prospering and expanding their habitat. The most important long-term goal of vector research is biologic control either by introduction of natural snail predators or pests or of refractory snail competitors. These could either be snails of a different species adaptable to the vectors' ecological niche or refractory strains raised from vector stock by selective breeding or genetic engineering. Failing these attempts, the aim would then be improved chemical molluscicides that are inexpensive, biodegradable and manufactured in endemic countries from local plant materials. Finally, in communities with sufficient resources, construction of hygienic privies and of safe, vector-free water supplies is the definitive solution.

Voracious sweet water fish (e.g., *Astatoreochromis alluadi*) and crayfish (e.g., *Procambarus clarkii*) have successfully suppressed *Biomphalaria* populations in small-scale experiments involving water tanks and impoundments, but there is understandable reluctance to undertake large scale predator studies whose ecological effects are, in essence, unpredictable (29). Ducks bred for sport and consumption are known to feed on snails and, in some countries, duck breeding has been recommended for schistosomiasis control, but results are unknown. Experiments with competitor snails such as *Marisa cornuaretaris* were initially quite promising. This large, voracious black snail efficiently starved out *Biomphalaria glabrata* populations (30), but several seasons later the *Marisa* snails in turn began thinning out as vector populations resurged. Since studies of mollusc genetics are still in their infancy, the obstacles to breeding refractory vector snails loom large; however, natural susceptibility to miracidial development is known to vary by strain within a single vector species and, in theory, refractory snails should enjoy a selective advantage. There are also numerous natural snail pathogens, e.g., acid-fast bacilli, predatory protozoa and trematodes which compete with schistosomes for snail host tissue (31); these pathogens presumably keep vector snails from overpopulating their home waters, but thus far none of them has shown realistic potential for biologic control.

Mollusciciding with niclosamide is costly and has proven beneficial only in those communities whose points of water contact are well known and few; even under optimal conditions, benefit is usually transitory and regular reapplication is required. Endod, an extract of the common tropical plant, *Phytolacca dodecandra*, is the only alternative molluscicide developed thus far. It is cheap to produce locally and field tests in Ethiopia have been favorable (32), but it, too, offers only temporary vector control. Other plant molluscicides have thus far either been too weak or have caused unacceptable ecologic damage, but research is bound to continue (33).

Construction of dams, impoundments and irrigation canals for agricultural development frequently creates new snail breeding grounds which can make a smoldering endemic situation far worse (34). Conversely, provision of safe, snail-free water is the definitive solution for controlling endemic schistosomiasis. Safe water puts an end to schistosome transmission regardless of whether sanitation is undertaken for that purpose alone or for other reasons. Thus, in Japan's Katayama area, all agricultural irrigation channels were lined with cement and monitored for *Oncomelania* infestation in order to eliminate the world's most notorious focus of *S. japonicum* infection; by contrast, in Kurume city the snails responsible for most of the local infections were displaced from their riverbank habitat by the construction of a golf course. Similarly, the waning prevalence of *S. mansoni* in Puerto Rico over the last three decades is largely attributable to construction, cementing and water channeling for developments, shopping centers and parking lots. Thus, in areas of rapid economic-industrial development, schistosomiasis control can be achieved as an almost involuntary by-product; by contrast, in undeveloped rural areas a conscious community effort is certainly required. Some highly effective rural water sanitation projects have, in fact, been carried out under local leadership, using unpaid labor and simple sanitary engineering, but these have been few and far between. Wider progress can be expected only when government and/or international agencies begin to lend higher priority and funding to rural community development and water sanitation. In China, for instance, soil and water contamination with human excreta had been pervasive for centuries, but a vast campaign of sanitary privy contruction and health education was mounted about 30 years ago. This effort substantially reduced *S. japonicum* morbidity, but the disease has since reemerged in China's lake areas and around expanded irrigation projects, spread in part by infected water buffalo. A pilot project of cattle vaccination against *S. japonicum* is therefore being tried (35).

In summary, current snail control methods are limited in efficacy and high in cost, and future prospects remain problematic; breakthroughs in molecular snail genetics and biological vector control will certainly be needed. Schistosomiasis tends to rise with irrigational agriculture, but efforts at water sanitation and health education have proven effective in reducing schistosome transmission. However, many endemic communities lack the necessary leadership and resources, and the corps of skilled personnel for assisting rural communities in their sanitary efforts remains pitifully small.

Vaccination

In this last section, we return from latrines to genes. Since the advent of molecular biology, progress in immunoprotection against the schistosomes has been fast and exciting. One recombinant antigen for vaccination against *S. mansoni* has already been tested for human safety and is under consideration for a phase II field trial. It consists of a cloned polypeptide derived from schistosome p28 glutathione^{S} transferase, a secretory product of adult worms with protective efficacy of up to 59% in animal experiments. A similar glutathione transferase has been cloned from *S. japonicum*, and two more antigens are also under consideration for vaccine trials, namely schistosome paramyosin genetically engineered into BCG, and recombinant schistosome triose phosphate isomerase (36). The genes encoding all four polypeptides have been sequenced, and their metabolic functions in schistosomes are known. Indeed, we have come a long way since the first vaccination attempts by percutaneous exposure to live or irradiated cercariae which were begun in the 1950s (37, 38). On the other hand, 30 years of labor have been consumed and the verdict on human vaccination is not yet in.

Even under optimal experimental conditions, sterile immunity against schistosome challenge is seldom if ever induced; instead, experimental animals manifest only partial, concomitant immunity, characterized by the survival of resident adult worms during the elimination of immature worms ("schistosomula") introduced by challenge exposure. A number of ingenious mechanisms have been uncovered by which the maturing and fully mature worms are able to counteract and evade immune host aggression, as summarized in a recent review (39). When hosts are immunized with radiated cercariae which die during their early development, challenge attrition ranges between 35% and 80% depending upon experimental conditions. The locations and mechanisms of challenge reduction in immune hosts have been under debate for many years and seem to vary between animal species and research laboratories. Part of the reduction is clearly due to extrusion of schistosomula into lung alveoli (40).

Workers from two continents have reported acquired resistance to reinfection by *S. mansoni* or *S. haematobium* in older endemic children and adults, manifested by dramatic reductions in egg output after chemotherapy despite continuing cercarial exposures. In that respect, human acquired resistance resembles experimental concomitant immunity, but its development is slower and less consistent. Even among 12–14 year old children resistance to challenge ranges from nil to almost complete (25). The lagging development of human resistance has been attributed to the generation of blocking antibodies of the IgG class directed against worm epitopes which are the target sites for protective antibodies of the IgE and IgA isotypes (41). Alternatively, young children may be handicapped by predominant stimulation of Th-2 type lymphocytes with deficient cytokine production by their Thl counterparts (42). No one expects human anti-schistosomal vaccination to elicit sterile immunity; indeed, a 50% challenge reduction would be satisfactory since it would measurably reduce chronic morbidity.

Vaccines composed of live, radiated cercariae or schistosomula were protective in cattle (35) and in non-human primates (43), but cannot be mass-produced or -delivered; moreover injected schistosomula or repeated cercarial skin exposures can induce severe local inflammation (44). It became necessary to turn to defined-antigen vaccines and the advent of molecular technology fortuitously relieved investigators from large-scale parasite breeding and antigen partitioning and has enormously facilitated the characterization and recombinant production of the immunogens already cited as current vaccine candidates. However, several imponderables must still be faced and cannot be resolved by studies *in vitro* or in experimental animals: How much human protection will be gained from injection of a single recombinant antigen versus a combination of several products? Will BCG-associated antigen boost T-cell help or cytokine production? Should vaccine trials be undertaken in praziquantel-treated or in untreated populations? How long will vaccine protection last? How will it measure up against the benefits of chemotherapy? This list of questions is far from exhaustive; it only illustrates the complexities faced by the human vaccine trials still to come (45).

Many of us are aware of the disappointments which have dampened the initial enthusiasm about the prospects of a malaria vaccine and have shifted emphasis from empirical vaccine trials to basic malaria research. By contrast, schistosomiasis research started out with basic immunobiology and has only recently turned toward vaccine trials. Even if human vaccination should come to naught, our understanding of the mechanisms underlying acquired resistance to tissue helminths will have deepened. Moreover, while a malaria vaccines must aim for sterile immunity against a self-replicating parasite, our hopes for an anti-schistosome vaccine are limited to a reduction of morbidity equivalent to that effected by available antihelminthics. Hopefully, the vaccine will lack serious side effects and provide durable protection, but fulfillment of these desiderata is far from guaranteed.

Epilogue

It should be clear from this brief review that endemic schistosomiasis is deeply rooted in agriculture and human life in the tropics and that schistosomes are biologically versatile parasites, well adapted to man, and will be formidable foes to overcome. Considering the scarce resources and serious socio-political problems handicapping countries of the third world today, it would have been foolhardy to proclaim elimination of human infection as an attainable goal. Even the more limited aim of reducing schistosomiasis morbidity will require larger, costlier, better planned efforts than are currently being marshalled. The resources of poor tropical communities will have to be steadily supplemented by donors, researchers and public health volunteers from the developed countries, acting as helpers and advisors, but the core problem of water contamination must ultimately be solved by the dedicated labor and educational effort of the affected people themselves (46). If no new tools are added to our armamentarium, these efforts must take the long and arduous routes of mass chemotherapy and of water sanitation. Our best hope resides in the open hearts and minds of the school children growing up in developing countries. Disease control could of course materialize much more quickly if immunoprophylaxis proves feasible. Regarding that prospect, the optimists of today's tropical disease fraternity are still outnumbered by the skeptics, but past experience has taught all of us never to say "It can't be done".

References

1. Cook, JA (1990) The Edna McConnell Clark Foundation Annual Report. Philadelphia, WM Fell Co, pp 50–52
2. Newport GR, Agabian N (1990) Molecular biology of schistosomes and filariae. In: Wyler DJ, (ed) Modern parasite biology, cellular, immunological and molecular aspects. New York, WH Freeman and Co, pp 362–383

3. Mott KE, Dixon H (1982) Collaborative study on antigens for immunodiagnosis of schistosomiasis. Bull WHO 60: 729–753,1982
4. Mott KE, Dixon H, Osei-Tutu E, England EC, Ekue K, Tekle A (1985) Indirect screening for *Schistosoma haematobium* infection: a comparative study in Ghana and Zambia. Bull WHO 63: 135–142
5. Stephenson LS Latham MC, Kinoti SN, Oduori ML (1984) Sensitivity and specificity of reagent strips in screening of Kenyan children for *Schistosoma haematobium* infection. Am J Trop Med Hyg 33: 862–871
6. Doehring-Schwerdtfeger E, Mohamed-Ali G, Abdel-Rahim IM, Kardorff R, Franke D, Kaiser C, Elsheik M, Ehrich JH (1989) Sonomorphological abnormalities in Sudanese children with *Schistosoma mansoni* infection. A proposed staging-system for field diagnosis of periportal fibrosis. AmJ Trop Med Hyg 41: 63–69
7. Degremont A, Burki A, Burnier E, Schweizer W, Meudt R, Tanner M (1985) Value of ultrasonography in investigating morbidity due to *Schistosoma haematobium* infection. Lancet 1: 662–665
8. Brand JA, Tsang VC (1989) A rapid immunoblot assay (Western blot) to detect specific antibodies for human immunodeficiency virus, *Schistosoma mansoni* and *Taenia solium* (Cysticercosis). J Immunoassay 10: 237–255
9. Gazzinelli G, Lambertucci JR, Katz N, Rocha RS, Lima MS, Colley DG (1985)Immune responses during human schistosomiasis mansoni. XI.-Immunologic status of patients with acute infections and after treatment. J Immunol 135: 2121–2127
10. Nash, TE (1974) Localization of the circulating antigen within the gut of *Schistosoma mansoni.* Am J Trop Med Hyg 23: 1085–1087
11. Deelder AM, Kornelis D, Van Marck EAE, Eveleigh PC, Van Egmond JG (1980) *Schistosoma mansoni:* characterization of two circulating polysaccharide antigens and the immunoglobulin response to these antigens in mouse, hamster and human infection. Exp Parasitol 50: 16–32
12. El Meanawy MA, Aji T, Phillips NFB, Davis RE, Salata RA, Malhotra I, McClain D, Aikawa M, Davis AH (1990) Definition of the complete *Schistosoma mansoni* hemoglobinase mRNA sequence and gene expression in developing parasites. Am J Trop Med Hyg 43: 67–78
13. De Jonge N, Gryseels B, Hilberath GW, Polderman AM, Deelder AM (1988) Detection of circulating anodic antigen by ELISA for seroepidemiology of schistosomiasis mansoni. Trans R Soc Trop Med Hyg 82: 591–594
14. Smith JH, Christie JD (1986) The pathobiology of *Schistosoma haematobium* infection in humans. Human Pathol 17: 333–345
15. Andrade ZA (1988) Schisto in Brazil ... and how it was fought. World Health, pp 26–27
16. Craig III SP,McKerrow JH, Wang CC (1988) Analysis of DNA encoding the hypoxanthine-guanine phosphoribosyltransferase of *Schistosoma mansoni:* A putative target for chemotherapy. Nucleic Acids Res 16: 7087–7101
17. el Kouni MH, Messier NJ, Cha S (1987) Treatment of schistosomiasis by purine nucleoside analogues in combination with nucleoside transport inhibitors. Biochem Pharmacol 36: 3815–3821
18. Chen GZ, Foster L, Bennett JL (1990) Antischistosomal action of menivolin: evidence that 3-hydroxy-methylglutaryl-coenzyme A reductase activity in *Schistosoma mansoni* is vital for parasite survival. Naunyn Schmiedeberg Arch Pharmacol 324: 477–482
19. Holy JM, O'Leary KA,Oaks JA, Tracy JW (1989) Immunocytochemical localization of the major glutathione S-transferases in adult *Schistosoma mansoni.* J Parasitol 75: 181–190
20. Archer, S (1985) The chemotherapy of schistosomiasis. Ann Rev Pharmacol Toxicol 25: 485–508
21. Utroska JA, Chen MG, Dixon H, Yoon S, Helling-Borda M, Hogerzeil HV, Mott KE (1989) An estimate of global needs for praziquantel within schistosomiasis control programmes. Document WHO/Schisto/89.102 (Distr. Limited). Geneva, WHO
22. von Lichtenberg F, Sadun EH, Cheever AW, Erickson DG, Johnson AJ, Boyce HW (1971) Experimental infection with *Schistosoma japonicum* in chimpanzees. Parasitologic, clinical, serologic and pathologic observations. Am J Trop Med Hyg 20: 850–893
23. Scrimgeour EM, Gajdusek DC (1985) Involvement of the central nervous system in *Schistosoma mansoni* and *S. haematobium* infection, a review. Brain 108: 1023–1038

24. Gryseels B (1990) Morbidity and Morbidity Control of Schistosomiasis mansoni in Subsaharan Africa. Thesis, U of Leiden. CIP – Gegevens Koninklije Bibliotheek den Haag, pp 150–151
25. Butterworth AE, Hagan P (1987) Immunity in human schistosomiasis. Parasitol Today 3: 11–16
26. Butterworth AE (1990) Immunology of Schistosomiasis. In: Wyler DJ (ed) Modern parasite biology. Cellular, immunological and molecular aspects. New York, WH Freeman & Co, p 263
27. Jordan P (1985) "Schistosomiasis: The St. Lucia Project". Cambridge, University Press, p 442
28. Polderman AM, Manshande JP (1981) Failure of targeted mass treatment to control schistosomiasis. Lancet 1: 27–28
29. Hobbs III HH, Jass JP, Huner JV (1989) A review of global crayfish introductions with particular emphasis on two North American species (*Decapoda, Cambaridae*). Crustaceana 56: 299–316
30. McCullough FS (1981) Biological control of the snail intermediate hosts of human *Schistosoma* sp.: A review of its present status and future prospects. Acta Trop 38: 5–13
31. Pan CT (1956) Studies on the biological control of schistosome-bearing snails; a preliminary report on micro-organisms found in *Australorbis glabrata.* J Parasitol 42: 33
32. Lemma A, Goll P, Duncan J, Mazengia B (1978) Control of schistosomiasis with use of endod in Adwa, Ethiopia: Results of a five-year study. In: Proceedings of the International Conference on Schistosomiasis, Vol. 1, 415–136, Cairo, Ministry of Health
33. Mott KE (1987) (ed) Plant molluscicides. Chichester, John Wiley & Sons Ltd, p 325
34. Mobarak AB (1982) The schistosomiasis problem in Egypt. Am J Trop Med Hyg 31: 87–91
35. Shi YE, Jiang CF, Han JJ, Li YL, Ruppel A (1990) *Schistosoma japonicum:* an ultraviolet-attenuated cercarial vaccine applicable in the field for water buffalo. Exper Parasitol 71: 100–106
36. Cherfas J (1991) New hope for vaccine against schistosomiasis. Science 251: 630–631
37. Vogel H, Minning W (1953) Über die erworbene Resistenz von Macaca rhesus gegenüber Schistosoma japonicum. Zeitschr Tropenmed Parasitol 4: 418–505
38. Villela JB, Gomberg HJ, Gould SE (1961) Immunization of *Schistosoma mansoni* in mice inoculated with irradioated cercariae. Science 134: 1073–1075
39. Sher FA, Colley DG (1989) Immunoparasitology. In: Paul WE (ed) Fundamental immunology. New York, Raven Press, pp 957–983
40. Dean DA, Mangold BL, Kassim OO, von Lichtenberg F (1987) Sites and mechanisms of schistosome elimination. Mem Inst Oswaldo Cruz, Rio de Janeiro 82 [Suppl IV]: 31–37
41. Butterworth AE, Bensted-Smith R, Capron A, Capron M, Dalton PR, Dunne DW, Grzych JM, Kariuki HC, Khalife J, Koech D, Mugambi M, Ouma JH, Arap-Siongok TK, Sturrock RF (1987) Immunity in human schistosomiasis mansoni. Prevention by blocking antibodies of the expression of immunity in young children. Parasitology 94: 269–280
42. Pearce EJ, Caspar P, Grzych JM, Lewis FA, Sher A (1991) Down regulation of Th1 cytokine production accompanies induction of Th2 responses by a parasite helminth, *Schistosoma mansoni.* J Exp Med 173: 159–166
43. Webbe G, Sturrock RF, James ER, James C (1982) *Schistosoma haematobium* in the baboon (*Papio anubis*): effect of vaccination with irradiated larvae on the subsequent infection with percutaneously applied cercariae. Trans R Soc Trop Med Hyg 76: 354–361
44. Byram JE, Harrison RA, von Lichtenberg F, Webbe G, Sturrock RF (1989) Pathology resulting from the administration of a live attenuated anti-*Schistosoma haematobium* vaccine in baboons. Am J Trop Med Hyg 40: 55–65
45. WHO (1991) Meeting on strategies for the development of a schistosomiasis vaccine, 15–16 January 1991, Geneva. Doc. TDR/SCH/VAC-DEV/91.3
46. Health Education in the Control of Schistosomiasis (1990) Geneva, WHO, pp 13–55

Filariasis: Present Status and Future Challenges

Eric A. Ottesen

Laboratory of Parasitic Diseases, National Institute of Allergy and Infectious Diseases, National Institutes of Health, Bethesda, Maryland, U.S.A.

Introduction

There are seven filarial parasites affecting over 100,000,000 individuals worldwide (Table 1) (1). Despite these impressive statistics as recently as 15 years ago, filariasis was still considered to be a "primitive" discipline. The initiation of the UNDP/World Bank/WHO Special Programme in Tropical Disease Research (TDR) has highlighted the importance of filariases, and advances in immunology have led to an increased awareness of many issues of great practical significance. While the prospects for further advances are promising, there still remain a number of significant hindrances. From a positive perspective, these will become challenges for future work. The purposes of this review are to summarize our understanding of the filariases, to identify why we have not progressed further, and to suggest a direction for future research on filarial infections and disease.

Animal Models

Current Status

The lack of adequate animal models is a major handicap that impedes our understanding of filariasis. As seen in Table 2, for most of the seven filarial parasites of humans, there are no animal models for study. *Brugia malayi,* which occurs naturally in felines as well as humans, can be studied in animals such as cats, dogs, jirds, and rats. The sophisticated immunological tools available for the study of mice are largely unavailable to those interested in *Brugia* infections because mice cannot serve as a natural host. For the other filarial parasites, it is evident that the situation is even worse (Table 2).

The absence of animal models leads to many difficulties in understanding the pathogenesis of these diseases. It is more surprising to realize that the lack of such models inhibits our ability to understand the parasites' basic development within the vertebrate host. Although the life cycles of these

Table 1. Filarial Parasites of Humans

Parasite	Distribution	No. affected
Wuchereria bancrofti	Tropics Worldwide	80 million
Brugia malayi	Asia	10 million
Onchocerca volvulus	Africa, Americas	20 million
Loa loa	Africa	13 million
Mansonella streptocerca	Africa	?
Mansonella perstans	Africa, S. America	?
Mansonella ozzardi	Americas	?

parasites are confidently portrayed (Fig. 1), only the stages found in the insect vectors are well understood (2). For mammalian hosts, there have been various *in vitro* and *in vivo* studies defining the L3 to L4 moult as requiring 6–14 days, but the time estimates for the L4 to L5 moult are much more vague. Furthermore, the published estimates of the period from infection to maturation of the adult worm (ie., pre-patent period) seem reasonable for *Onchocerca volvulus, Wuchereria bancrofti, B. malayi,* and *Loa loa,* but for the other three filarial pathogens of humans, the published estimates are only speculative. Similarly, the life span of adult worms is poorly documented except for onchocerciasis, where intensive studies by the Onchocerciasis Control Program in West Africa have provided estimates of approximately 12–15 years (3). For the other filarial parasites, estimates are much less certain even though we assume that they are similar. The microfilarial stage of the parasite has been estimated to survive 3 to 6 months, but such estimates are difficult to prove because little experimental evidence is available. Thus, it is clear that even understanding of the basic biology of the parasite and its life cycle remains a significant and important challenge for the future.

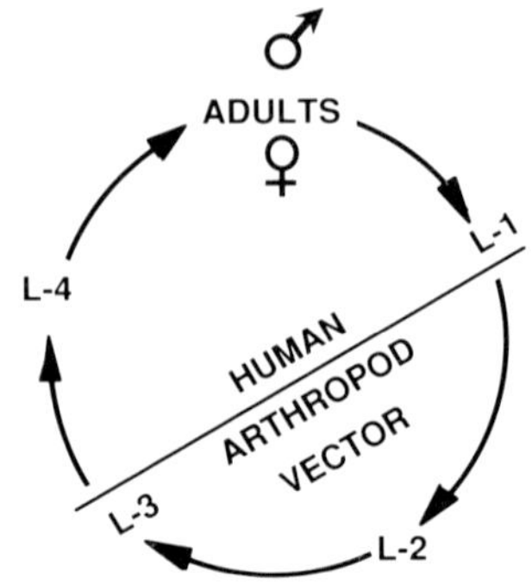

Fig. 1. A generalized life cycle of the filariae depicts the adult forms with sexual production of first stage larvae (microfilariae) in the human host and the subsequent larval development in the arthropod and human hosts

Table 2. Animal Models Available for Study

Parasite	Rodent models	Other Models
Wuchereria bancrofti	–	–
Brugia malayi	jird, rat	cat, dog, ferret
Onchocerca volvulus	–	chimpanzee
Loa loa	–	monkey
Mansonella streptocerca	–	–
Mansonella perstans	–	–
Mansonella ozzardi	–	–

Because of constraints imposed by the lack of animal models for studying these infections, obtaining parasite material either to study or to serve as a source for antigens has been difficult. This material is needed to investigate problems involving diagnosis, pathogenesis, and protective immunity. Not only has the lack of parasite material limited our progress in these areas, but it has also limited the number of investigators interested in undertaking such studies. Perhaps more than in most fields, the development of recombinant DNA expression libraries (now available for *B. malayi, W. bancrofti, L. loa,* and *O. volvulus*) has been of particular importance as a means to overcome some of the seemingly intractable problems, finally making them addressable through experimental investigations.

The Future

The future is affected by the lack of animal models. Unfortunately, it appears that there will be little opportunity of developing new 'complete' animal models better than those already existence. The major challenge will be to synthesize our knowledge of the life cycle from data obtained from *in vitro* studies or, for observations, at least some stages, *in vivo,* in normal or immunodeficient animals. The important questions of functional and biological relevance to the host and parasite can then be asked, and the parasite material for further analytic study can be produced. Another important challenge will be to develop cDNA expression libraries for the different stages of the parasite (particularly the L2, L3, and L4 stages). These tools can be used for "differential screening" of humoral, and later cellular, immune responses of immunopathogenic importance to the host, or for the identification of molecules of functional importance to the developing parasite that might become targets for future vaccine or chemotherapeutic strategies. It is important to note that molecular studies of the major filarial parasites are progressing.

Clinical Filariasis: Current and Future

For most of the common filariases, the clinical syndromes presented by individuals living in endemic areas have been reasonably well described (4). In lymphatic filariasis, these clinical manifestations include the most recognizable sequelae of lymphatic tract obstruction (elephantiasis and hydrocele), the hyperresponsive tropical pulmonary eosinophilia syndrome, and the more difficult to diagnose syndrome of episodic adenolymphangitis (ADL), as well as the extremely common, though impossible to diagnose clinically, presentation of asymptomatic microfilaremia. In onchocerciasis, the most common manifestation is onchocercal dermatitis, with pruritus, excoriation, and atrophy being frequently observed. The most dramatic presentation is blindness resulting from both anterior and posterior ocular damage caused by the presence of microfilariae in the eye. For loiasis, calabar swellings (recurrent episodes of localized angioedema) and the presentation of an adult worm (approximately 0.5 x 70 mm in size) crawling across the eye just beneath the conjunctiva are the characteristic clinical manifestations.

While there is much discussion and description of the important clinical manifestations of these three filarial infections, for other filariases (Table 1) the clinical information is minimal or almost non-existent. One of the most important challenges for the future with regard to clinical filariasis is the basic definition of the most common clinical presentations of the less common filarial infections.

The diagram in Fig. 2 summarizes the major clinical syndromes associated with lymphatic filariasis. Unfortunately, the specific relationships of these syndromes to one another is poorly understood. The natural history of the clinical course of filarial infections must be determined. Observations need to be made that will shed light on whether the asymptomatic state of microfilaremia progresses to the clinically symptomatic state, or whether disease develops without having to go through a preceding period of asymptomatic microfilaremia. Such observations will be particularly difficult to make, because treatment of diagnosed patients will certainly alter the natural history of the infection. Indirect assessments may have to be relied upon almost exclusively as a means to enhance our understanding of these critical issues.

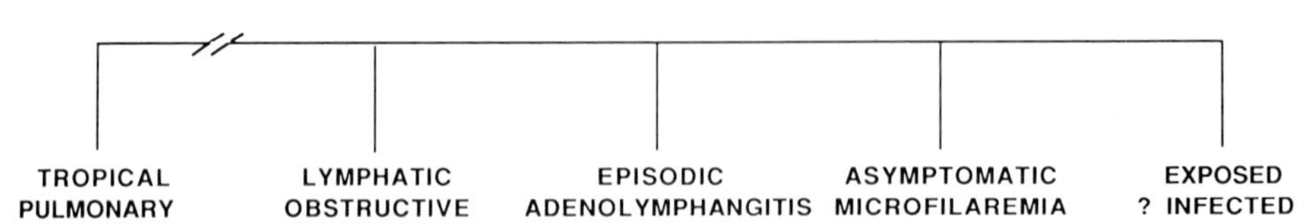

Fig. 2. The spectrum of clinical manifestations of lymphatic filarial infection in endemic populations

A third future challenge involves the clinical aspects of new or previously unrecognized syndromes associated with infections caused by these organisms. For example, although hinted at earlier, only in the past year have clear descriptions of the renal abnormalities associated with asymptomatic microfilaremia been fully described in patients with bancroftian filariasis (5). Similarly, a new syndrome seen in expatriate visitors to regions endemic for loiasis has been described recently (6). The syndrome, of course, is not actually new since similar clinical descriptions not only with loiasis, but also with onchocerciasis, lymphatic filariasis, and other filarial infections have been made. This clinical presentation might well be called the "expatriate syndrome." Rather than developing the common, classical clinical manifestations of endemic filarial infections, individuals who live outside of the endemic regions and then enter one of these regions and acquire filarial infection manifest prominent signs and symptoms of inflammatory (including allergic) reactions to their mature or maturing parasites. In loiasis, these manifestations have included calabar swellings, hives, rashes and occasionally asthma (6). In contrast, bancroftian filariasis, especially in migrants to endemic areas who acquire these infections, is usually characterized by lymphangitis, lymphadenitis, and genital pain from inflammation of the associated lymphatics, as well as hives, rashes, and other "allergic-like" manifestations (7). Although the "expatriate syndrome" is certainly not new, its recognition and the emphasis on its importance have increased. In all likelihood, there are numerous other clinical syndromes in patients with filarial infections that will be described following additional clinical investigations.

Pathogenesis

Current Status

The contrast between clinical outcomes following exposure to infection in expatriate individuals and in endemic residents provides an excellent example of what is assumed to be the most important underlying concept in the pathogenesis of filarial disease: different clinical presentations are the result of different individual immunological responses to the parasite (8). Figure 3 schematically illustrates that the most common outcome of infection depends upon the geographic origin of the apparently normal individuals exposed to the filariae. The most frequent outcome of exposure to infection in endemic populations is becoming microfilaria positive. In most circumstances, this finding is not associated with inflammatory reactivity. Thus, the infected individuals remain asymptomatic and free of overt pathology. Less often seen in most endemic populations are individuals manifestating disease as a result of inflammatory responses to the adult parasite or its developmental stages. For lymphatic filariasis, this pathology includes the lymphatic obstructive manifestations of adenolymphangitis, elephantiasis, hydrocele, and chyluria, as well as tropical pulmonary eosinophilia. For onchocerciasis, it includes dermal and ocular lesions. The

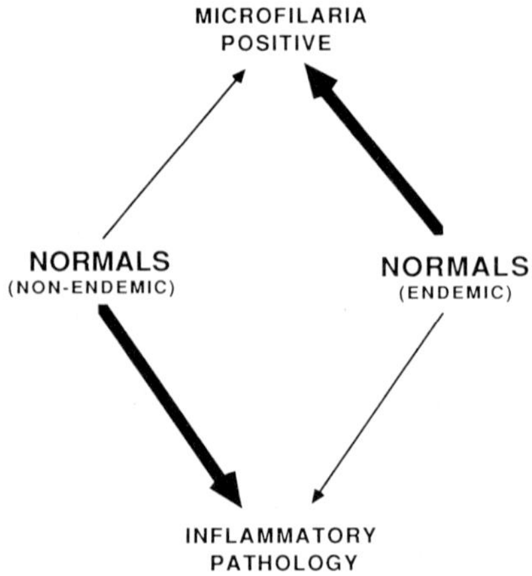

Fig. 3. Patients from endemic and non-endemic areas differ in the proportions with disease and with asymptomatic microfilaremia

predominant prevalence of asymptomatic microfilaria positive individuals in endemic populations when relatively few individuals develop inflammatory responses contrasts remarkably with the situation of expatriates in whom the most frequent manifestations of infection are inflammatory, with very few individuals developing microfilaria positivity. Why people who are exposed to the same filariae develop one clinical presentation rather than another is not understood completely, but almost certainly the character of the host's immune response must be involved.

In support of this contention, data from many studies in lymphatic filariasis have led to the generalization that asymptomatic microfilaremic individuals have meager or potentially suppressed immune responses to parasite antigens, ie., they are hyporesponsive. Those with the pathologic residua of inflammatory reactions respond relatively vigorously to such antigens (7). This generalization has been documented with respect to lymphocyte proliferation, serum antifilarial antibody levels, *in vitro* studies of immunoglobulin production induced by filarial antigens, and *in vitro* cytokine production in response to filarial antigens. While the generalization has been validated for many of the immune response parameters examined, suppression probably plays an important role in protecting the parasites from immune attack *in vivo.* It is now realized that this generalization is not entirely true. In fact, hyporesponsive microfilaremic patients can be extremely hyperresponsive when particular parameters are investigated – namely, those that serve to down-regulate the host's inflammatory mechanisms rather than to promote them. For example, recent studies have shown that the seemingly hyporesponsive, asymptomatic microfilaremic patients who make relatively low levels of anti-parasite IgG_1, IgG_2, and IgG_3, actually make extremely large amounts of anti-filarial IgG_4 antibody (9), the IgG subclass most prominently associated with blocking the allergic responsiveness of patients. These asymptomatic individuals make very high levels of IL-4 in response to parasite antigen stimulation but relatively low levels of γ-interferon, in comparison with patients having one of the inflammatory syndromes (Mahanty, King, Ottesen, Jayaraman, and Nutman, unpublished). Thus, it appears that the pro-inflammatory elements are held in check by a number of molecules secreted by components of the immune system. Asymptomatic microfilaremic individuals appear to be those whose lymphocytes, upon activation by parasite antigens, secrete these anti-inflammatory molecules. This condition is in contrast to that of patients having inflammatory pathology whose response to parasite antigens is the production of pro-inflammatory immune mediators.

Our recent understanding of the importance of the host immune response in the pathogenesis of filarial disease has not sufficiently taken into account earlier concepts that emphasize the importance of the parasites themselves in initiating pathology, nor do they completely account for the clinically overlapping syndromes where microfilaremia is found in the presence of localized pathology, e.g., lymphatic filariasis patients with both microfilaremia and lymphedema/elephantiasis. The major difficulty in determining the relative contributions of the host's immune response and the parasite itself to disease development has been derived primarily from the fact that in humans, as well as in animal models using cats, dogs, and ferrets, infections coexist with intact immune systems. With the development of animal models involving immunodeficient mice infected with brugian parasites (10, 11), it has been possible to separate these effects. In such immunodeficient animals, it can be shown that infection alone initiates lymphatic dilatation and endothelial proliferation with resultant lymphedema and gross elephantiasis. When the mice are reconstituted with immune cells, they become capable of initiating inflammatory reactions around the parasites, which result in local tissue damage, lymphatic obstruction, and lymphedema/elephantiasis (12). There appear to be two forces at work capable of inducing lymphatic damage: one dependent on the host immune system and the other entirely independent of it.

The Future

Distinguishing the relative roles of the parasite and the host immune system is one of the many interesting challenges for understanding the pathogenesis of filarial disease. The importance is that different therapeutic strategies may be required that depend upon which of the two fundamental factors is causing the pathology in question, ie., lymphatic, pulmonary, ocular, or dermal. Insight may be gained on these questions by detailed histologic and immunohistologic studies using patient tissues. Such studies are extremely scarce, and a great deal of basic work must be done in this area.

Second, since the immune system of patients with microfilaremic or microfilaridermic forms of the various filarial infections is markedly immunosuppressed with respect to generating effector responses to filarial antigens but is actually very hyperresponsive to these antigens in terms of generating inflammatory-control molecules, it is very important to identify the mediators of this immunological down-regulation and to assess the effects of such down-regulation. The down-regulatory activity might affect not only responses to the parasite antigens but also responses to other non-parasite-directed immunity such as those following routine vaccinations and exposure to other microorganisms.

Control of Filarial Infections

Current Status

An ideal strategy for controlling filariasis is vaccination, especially if the vaccine is as effective and safe as the common anti-viral vaccines in current use. The difficulty in filariasis involves knowing what target molecules the vaccines should be directed against. Study in this area has been hindered by the lack of satisfactory animal models for human filarial parasites (Table 2) and by the difficulty in obtaining parasite antigens. Using currently available animal models, it is difficult to determine the actual mechanism of immunity. Partial immunity can be induced by immunizing animals with irradiated larvae. A great deal of work has been carried out to identify those components of the host's response that are responsible for protection (13). Eosinophils appear to be important, but the relative contributions of various humoral and cellular immune components for protective immunity have not been established.

Attempts to define the molecules responsible for inducing protective immunity to filarial infections in humans have relied primarily upon differential screening between the immune responses of infected individuals and repeatedly exposed persons who live in the same endemic area but appear not to be infected. These latter individuals have been referred to as being putatively immune, since there is no way to determine with certainty whether or not they really are immune (14). The challenge of detecting protective immune responses using such approaches is formidable, not only because of the number of possible molecules and immune responses that could be subjected to this differential screening, but also due to the fact that there is no current way to determine whether or not putatively immune individuals are really immune or are only maintaining a cryptic infection that cannot be detected with current diagnostic tools.

The Future

Despite these limitations, the strategy of differential screening has already identified molecules both in lymphatic filariasis and in onchocerciasis that may have protective potential (14,15). The likelihood for success of such a strategy carried out both in humans and in animal models should be increased by screening potentially protective antigens through the cooperation of a number of researchers supported by organizations such as the Edna McConnell Clark Foundation.

Immunodiagnosis

Current Status

Figure 4 illustrates the same problems concerning the immunodiagnosis of filariasis. A useful serodiagnostic test is one that will be negative in individuals not exposed to the filariae and positive in those who are currently infected. In the filariases, exposure is prolonged in endemic areas, a situation which makes it extremely difficult to distinguish between uninfected, antigenically stimulated individuals and those with past infection or current cryptic infection. Most diagnostic tests based on the detection of antibodies can be positive in currently-infected individuals, individuals with past infections, and individuals with antigenic exposure but no current or past infection. Such serologic tests have relatively little use in studies in endemic areas except for diagnosing individuals with hyperresponsive syndromes such as tropical pulmonary eosinophilia. They have proven useful in diagnosing infections in expatriates, who are initially seronegative before they develop an infection and concurrent seropositivity.

Recently, diagnosis based on the detection of parasite antigens in blood or other body fluids has been proposed as a means for distinguishing between active infections and early exposure or past infection (16). Four such antigen assays are currently under intensive study in multi-center trials coordinated through the TDR Programme at WHO. These assays show great promise for future diagnostic usefulness, particularly in lymphatic filariasis (17, 18) and onchocerciasis (19).

Despite the seeming lack of promise for antibody-based immunodiagnostic assays, there have been two recent observations that demon-

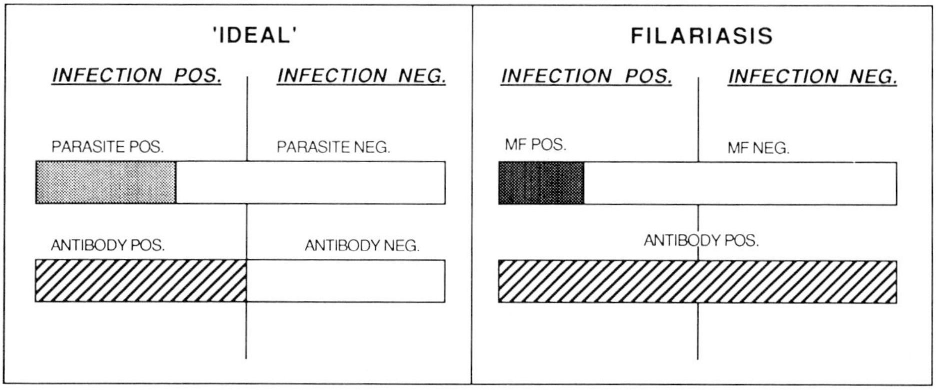

Fig. 4. The ideal laboratory diagnostic situation differs from the current situation in filariasis. Many uninfected persons have antibodies, and many infected persons have no detectable parasites

strate the potential usefulness of assays that detect IgG_4 antibody responses. The first observation showed that IgG_4 antibody assays were more specific than other IgG-based assays in detecting filarial infection, i.e., fewer problems with cross-reactivity, because this immunoglobulin subclass in humans fails to recognize the phosphorylcholine epitope common to many organisms throughout nature (20). In fact, IgG_4 recognizes few carbohydrate antigens at all and, therefore, appears to be more specific in its diagnostic capabilities. This occurs because it recognizes a restricted set of protein antigens. The second feature of IgG_4 responses with diagnostic implications is that such responses appear to require chronic antigenic stimulation before they are induced, as well as to sustain them. There is evidence that these antibodies may be useful in distinguishing between active infection and past infection, a goal previously thought to be reachable only with antigen detection assays (21).

The Future

For the future, there is a need to improve the serodiagnostic assays. There are major initiatives underway in this regard that are sponsored largely by the Special Programme in Tropical Disease Research of the UNDP/World Bank/WHO. Hopefully, this impetus should lead to a solution for this problem.

Chemotherapy: Current and Future

Individual Patients

For more than forty years, there has been essentially only one chemotherapeutic agent used for filariases, ie., diethylcarbamazine. Although it rapidly kills microfilariae of *W. bancrofti, B. malayi, B. timori, O. volvulus, L. loa,* and *Mansonella streptocerca,* it affects neither the microfilariae of *M. perstans* nor of *M. ozzardi* (Table 3). It induces destruction of the microfilariae so rapidly that a vigorous host response to the dying parasites often leads to severe, sometimes fatal, side reactions (22). Thus, diethylcarbamazine is contraindicated for use in *O. volvulus* infections and is extremely difficult to use in control programs with other filarial infections. Recently, ivermectin has undergone clinical trials involving a number of different filarial infections, as well as in onchocerciasis where it has shown superiority to diethylcarbamazine in its ability to kill microfilariae without inducing severe side reactions. It has completely replaced diethylcarbamazine as the drug of choice. Moreover, its use as a single oral dose microfilaricidal agent has entirely transformed control strategies for onchocerciasis wherever the infection exists (23).

Table 3. Tteatment of Choice for Filariasis

Parasite	Individual patients	Population
Wuchereria bancrofti	Diethylcarbamazine	? Diethylcarbamazine, ? Ivermectin
Brugia malayi	Diethylcarbamazine	? Diethylcarbamazine, ? Ivermectin
Onchocerca volvulus	Ivermectin	Ivermectin
Loa loa	Diethylcarbamazine	?
Mansonella streptocerca	Diethylcarbamazine	?
Mansonella perstans	?	?
Mansonella ozzardi	Ivermectin	?

Studies comparing ivermectin to diethylcarbamazine for treating lymphatic filarial infections are currently in progress. Trials comparing single oral doses of ivermectin to diethylcarbamazine suggest the superiority of ivermectin in decreasing microfilaremia in both *W. bancrofti* and *B. malayi* infections.

One advantage that diethylcarbamazine might have over ivermectin in lymphatic filarial infections is diethylcarbamazine's recognized microfilaricidal effect, ie., the killing of adult worms as well as microfilariae (24). Long-term treatment is required before the microfilaricidal effect of diethylcarbamazine is seen, but it has yet to be demonstrated whether or not ivermectin has a macrofilaricidal effect. There has been little use of ivermectin for treating filarial infections other than onchocerciasis and the lymphatic filariases. The effectiveness of this new drug for treating other filariases remains to be seen.

In the future, additional trials with ivermectin and diethylcarbamazine will be needed to define the range of infections for which they are useful and to learn how to maximize their effectiveness. Greater experience is needed for treating filarial infections with albendazole, other benzimidazoles, and certain amoscanate-related compounds such as amocarzine.

Chemoprophylaxis

Two recent studies have shown that diethylcarbamazine, when given either weekly or monthly, can have a prophylactic effect in preventing the development of infection caused by *W. bancrofti* (25) and *L. loa* (26). Even though these studies were conducted in different settings using different techniques, the results support observations made in animal models regarding the effectiveness of diethylcarbamazine in killing developing third- and fourth-stage larvae of *W. bancrofti, B. malayi,* and *L. loa.* Although there have been no studies to indicate the most effective dosage regimen for prophylaxis, the regimens used in each of the two studies are feasible.

Mass Treatment Programs

Filarial infections are widespread in both rural and urban areas. The most common treatment strategies are aimed at populations rather than individuals. Massive control efforts based on elimination of the vector have been carried out for many years in areas of mosquito-borne lymphatic filariasis. They have usually been effective only during periods when the operations were continued with diligence and constant effort. The feasibility for long-term success of such strategies to control transmission does not appear great. On the other hand, with respect to onchocerciasis, the massive effort to rid wide regions in eleven countries of West Africa of the Simulium black fly vector by a combination of vector control conducted with aircraft, entomologists and field workers has proven to be an enormous success. Unfortunately, massive amounts of money have been required in order to initiate and sustain these operations. This program has been successful in controlling infection in a large area. However, because of the longevity of the parasites in the human host, the difficulty in sustaining this degree of effort for the 15 years or more required to achieve eradication is obvious. When ivermectin was used as a single-oral-dose-administered drug as a means to clear microfilariae from the skin for periods of up to one year, the onchocerciasis control program strategy shifted to a combined approach using single yearly doses of ivermectin and vector control. In other parts of Africa and in the Americas where vector control is not as achievable as in the West Africa area, control strategies based simply on the use of yearly doses of ivermectin have been formulated.

As with any drug-based control strategy, the cost of the medication to treat onchocerciasis is an important factor in deciding whether or not it is feasible to treat the 20,000,000 people estimated to be infected in endemic countries. Fortunately, it was decided by the developers of the drug (Merck, Sharp and Dohme) that it was possible for them to provide the drug at no cost for as long as needed to eradicate onchocerciasis completely (27). This extraordinarily generous offer has been received with great enthusiasm by ministries of health and private foundations who are working with public health agencies to use this strategy as a means to control onchocerciasis in their endemic regions.

For lymphatic filariasis, the usefulness of ivermectin is still being assessed, and no control strategies have been formulated. For these infections, control strategies based on single doses of diethylcarbamazine given at annual or semiannual intervals have been studied in Polynesia for years with appreciable success. Whether these strategies will be effective in the heavily endemic areas of India, Indonesia, and elsewhere remains to be determined. Control strategies based on the distribution of diethylcarbamazine-medicated salt, which also has been shown to be an effective control method in numerous small demonstration projects, as well as in very large regions in China, are still being evaluated (24).

Conclusion

While it is obvious that there are many gaps in our current understanding of the different filarial infections, it should be clear that there are numerous advances being made on several different fronts. Perhaps even more importantly, there has been additional emphasis placed on these diseases during the past two decades that has allowed us to better understand the issues that need to be addressed, as well as formulate concretely the questions that need to be asked. The filariases and the study of these diseases and their etiologic agents are finally recognized as being scientifically important.

References

1. WHO (1984) Filariasis-Report of the Fourth Expert Committee, Technical Report Series No. 702. Geneva, World Health Organization,
2. Sasa M (1976) Human filariasis. Baltimore, University Park Press
3. WHO (1987) Expert Committee on Onchocerciasis – Third Report, Technical Report Series No. 752. Geneva: World Health Organization
4. Ottesen EA (1990) The filariases and tropical pulmonary eosinophilia. In: Warren KS, Mahmoud AAF (eds) Tropical and geographical medicine. New York, McGraw-Hill, pp 407–428
5. Dreyer G, Ottesen EA, Galdino E, Andrade L, Rocha A, Medeiros Z, Moura I, Casimiro I, Beliz F, Coutinho A (1992) Renal abnormalities in microfilaremic patients with bancroftian filariasis. Am J Trop Med Hyg (in press)
6. Nutman TB, Miller KD, Mulligan M, Ottesen EA (1986) *Loa loa* infection in temporary residents of endemic regions: recognition of a hyperresponsive syndrome with characteristic clinical manifestations. J Infect Dis 154: 10–18
7. Ottesen EA (1989) Filariasis now. Am J Trop Med Hyg 41: 9–17
8. Ottesen EA (1980) Immunopathology of lymphatic filariasis in man. Springer Semin Immunopathol 2: 373–385
9. Ottesen EA, Skvaril F, Tripathy SP, Poindexter RW, Hussain R (1985) Prominence of IgG_4 in the IgG antibody response to human filariasis. J Immunol 134: 2707–2712
10. Suswillo RR, Doenhoff MJ, Denham DA (1981) Successful development of *Brugia pahangi* in T-cell deprived CBA mice. Acta Trop 1981 38: 305–308
11. Vincent AL, Vickery AC, Lotz MJ, Desai U (1984) The lymphatic pathology of *Brugia pahangi* in nude (athymic) and thymic mice C3H/HeN. J Parasitol 70: 48–56
12. Vickery AC, Albertine KH, Nayar JK, Kwa BH (1991) Histopathology of *Brugia malayi* infected nude mice after immune-reconstitution. Acta Trop 49: 45–55
13. Philipp M, Davis TB, Storey N, Carlow CKS (1988) Immunity in filariasis: perspectives for vaccine development. Ann Rev Microbiol 42: 685–716
14. Ward DJ, Nutman TB, Zea-Flores G, Portocarrero C, Lujan A, Ottesen EA (1988) Onchocerciasis and immunity in humans: enhanced T cell responsiveness to parasite antigen in putatively immune individuals. J Infect Dis 157: 536–543
15. Freedman DO, Nutman TB, Ottesen EA (1989) Protective immunity in bancroftian filariasis. Selective recognition of a 43-kD larval stage antigen by infection-free individuals in an endemic area. J Clin Invest 83: 14–22
16. Weil GJ (1990) Parasite antigenemia in lymphatic filariasis. Exp Parasitol 71: 353–356
17. Forsyth KP, Spark R, Kazura J, Brown GV, Peters P, Heywood P, Dissanayake S, Mitchell GF (1985) A monoclonal antibody-based immunoradiometric assay for detection of circulating antigen in bancroftian filariasis. J Immunol5 134: 1172–1177
18. More SJ, Copeman DB (1990) A highly specific and sensitive monoclonal antibody-based ELISA for the detection of circulating antigen in bancroftian filariasis. Trop Med Parasitol 41: 403–406

19. Chandrashekar R, Ogunrinade AF, Alvarez RM, Kale OO, Weil GJ (1990) Circulating immune complex-associated parasite antigens in human onchocerciasis. J Infect Dis 162: 1159–1164
20. Lal RB, Ottesen EA (1988) Enhanced diagnostic specificity in human filariasis by IgG4 antibody assessment. J Infect Dis 158: 1034–1037
21. Kwan-Lim G-E, Forsyth KP, Maizels RM (1990) Filarial-specific IgG_4 response correlates with active *Wuchereria bancrofti* infection. J Immunol 145: 4298–4305
22. Ottesen EA (1987) Description, mechanisms and control of reactions to treatment in the human filariases. Ciba Fndn Symp 127: 265–283
23. Remme J, De Sole G, Dadzie KY, Alley ES, Baker RHA, Habbema DJF, Plaisier AP, van Oort-Marssen GJ, Samba EM (1990) Large scale ivermectin distribution and its epidemiological consequences. Acta Leidensia 59: 177–192
24. Ottesen EA (1985) Efficacy of diethylcarbamazine in eradicating infection with lymphatic-dwelling filariae in humans. Rev Infect Dis 7: 341–356
25. Chakravertty RK, Srivastav VK, Srivastava SP, Chand P, Rao CK (1987) Prophylactic effect of diethylcarbamazine on *Wuchereria bancrofti* filariasis. J Commun Dis 19: 128–135
26. Nutman TB, Miller KD, Mulligan M, Reinhardt GN, Currie BJ, Steel C, Ottesen EA (1988) Diethylcarbamazine prophylaxis for human loiasis. Results of a double-blind study. N Engl J Med 319: 752–756
27. Dull HB (1990) Mectizan donation and the Mectizan expert committee. Acta Leidensia, 1990 59: 399–404

Current Issues in Cysticercosis: Proteins, Proglottids, Pigs, and Privies

Ralph T. Bryan

Division of Parasitic Diseases, National Center for Infectious Diseases,
Centers for Disease Control, Atlanta, Georgia, U.S.A.

Abstract

Cysticercosis has existed since ancient times. The life cycle of the cestode responsible for this condition (*Taenia solium*) is often misunderstood. It is important to distinguish between taeniasis, an intestinal infection with the adult tapeworm, and cysticercosis, a tissue infection with larval *T. solium*. Humans are suseptible to both conditions. Clinically, cysticercosis exhibits great diversity. Neurocysticercosis is the most clinically significant form of the disease, but cysts can occur in almost any anatomic location. Geographic and age/gender-related differences in clinical manifestations also occur. Diagnosis depends on the appropriate use of radiologic, immunologic, and histopathologic techniques. Both surgical and medical treatments are available. The *T. solium* taeniasis/cysticercosis complex is endemic throughout the developing world where human consumption of inadequately cooked pork and swine husbandry practices favor transmission. The importance of person-to-person transmission is being increasingly recognized. Recent advances include the use of magnetic resonance imaging and improved immunologic techniques for diagnosis; alternative medical treatment with the new antiparasitic agent, albendazole; and recent epidemiologic insights into risk factors and transmission dynamics in both endemic and nonendemic areas.

Despite considerable progress, many unanswered questions remain. Future efforts should focus on controlled clinical trials, wider application of available technology, and expanded epidemiologic studies. Intervention efforts should emphasize education and social determinants of disease. Finally, better utilization of existing data to foster prevention is crucial. Despite a wide range of clinical and epidemiologic variables, the single most consistent and important aspect of this disease is that it is preventable.

Introduction

Cysticercosis has probably existed as long as man has shared his environment with his atriodactylous companion, the pig. Aristotle (384–322 BC), in his "History of Animals", described this condition in pigs when he wrote, "... pigs whose meat is tender have bladders which are like hailstones ...". He also noted that cysticercosis is easily recognized in pigs by examining the under surface of their tongues. The first historical account of cysticercosis in humans is attributed to Paranoli in 1550. Laennec subsequently named these bladders, "cysticercus", derived from the Greek words "kystic", meaning bladder and "kercos", meaning tail. Their life cycle and relationship to taeniasis were finally demonstrated in 1855 (1).

Overview and Current Status of Cysticercosis

Life Cycle of T. solium (Fig. 1)

Before proceeding further, it is important to emphasize the distinction between cysticercosis and taeniasis. The former condition is a host tissue infection with the metacestode, or larval, stage of the Cyclophyllidean tapeworm, *Taenia solium,* commonly known as the pork tapeworm. Taeniasis, on the other hand, is an intestinal infection with the adult *T. solium,* a tapeworm composed of a scolex (or head) and a 2–7 meter strobila (body) containing 800–1000 proglottids or segments. Although several animal species can harbor cysticerci (intermediate hosts), man is the only known, natural definitive host for the adult tapeworm. The *T. solium* life cycle is often misunderstood because humans are susceptible to both cysticercosis and taeniasis (2, 3).

Gravid *T. solium* proglottids, containing up to 50,000 eggs each, detach from the main body of the adult tapeworm and are passed with the feces of human hosts. Once passed, proglottids rupture and eggs are released into the environment where they may remain viable for up to a year. In areas of the world with primitive sanitary facilities and free-roaming swine husbandry practices, coprophagic pigs have ready access to human feces laden with eggs of *T. solium.* Upon ingestion by a suitable intermediate host such as the pig, exposure to intestinal fluids induces egg hatching which allows taenia embryos (onchospheres) to penetrate the intestinal mucosa and disseminate to various tissues. After reaching a preferred tissue site (most commonly skeletal muscle), onchospheres develop over the next 60–70 days into typical cysticerci (larvae): fluid-filled bladders containing invaginated protoscolices. The cycle is completed when the definitive host, man, consumes inadequately cooked pork containing cysticerci. In the jejunum of man, the protoscolex evaginates and attaches to the intestinal mucosa where it develops into a mature worm over the next 5 to 12 weeks. Adults can survive for long periods in the human intestine, persisting for up to 25 years in some cases (2–4).

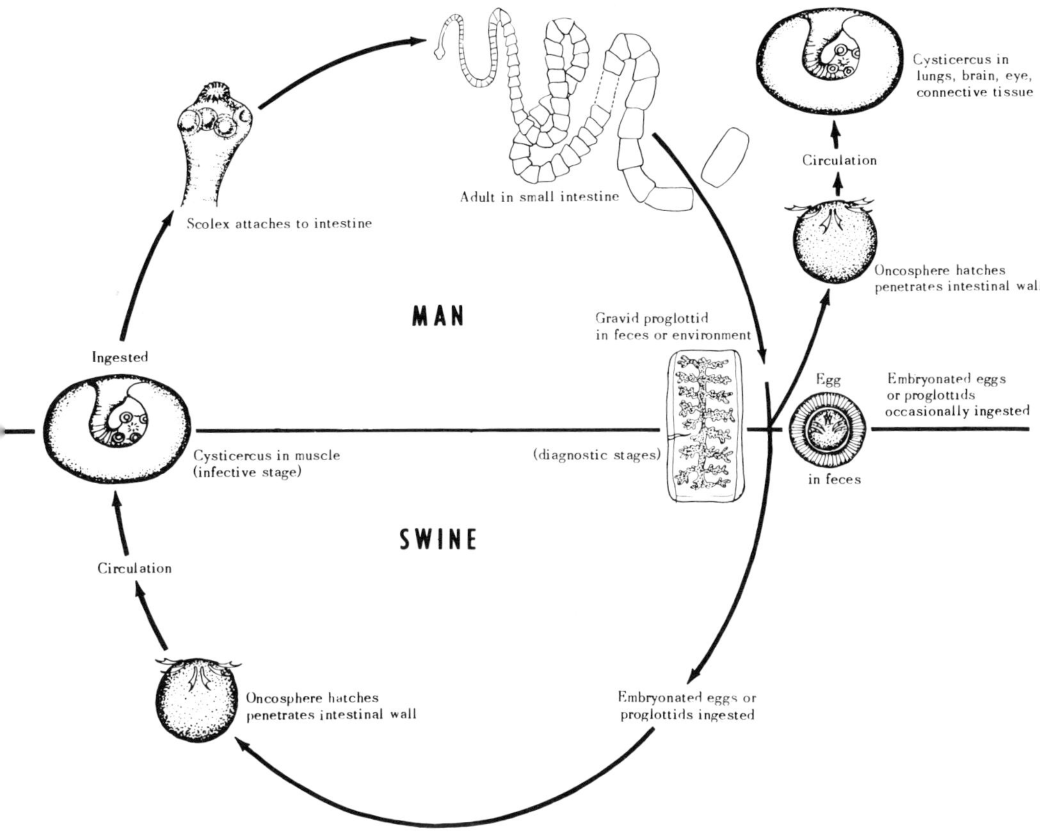

Fig. 1. Life cycle of *Taenia solium*

Humans contract cysticercosis in the same manner as pigs – by the direct or indirect consumption of taeniid eggs. Internal autoinfection via reverse peristalsis has been postulated, but never confirmed (2).

Clinical Manifestations in Man

Nash has stated that the hallmark of cysticercosis is the diversity of its clinical findings (5). Others have compared it to multiple sclerosis (6,7) and syphilis (8) because of its propensity to confuse clinicians. The clinical manifestations of cysticercosis vary according to the number, location, size, and morphology of cysts as well as the presence or absence of associated inflammatory response (2, 5, 9). Neurocysticercosis is the most commonly recognized and clinically significant form of the disease. Subcutaneous cysts are also common in some populations. Although percentages vary widely, most published series report seizures or signs/symptoms of increased intracranial pressure (ICP) as the most common clinical presentations among patients with neurocysticercosis; personality changes and focal neurologic deficits also occur (2, 6–13). In addition to discrete intraparenchymal and intraventricular lesions, neurocysticercosis can also manifest as acute encephalitis and chronic arachnoiditis (meningitis). Except in cases of acute cysticercotic encephalitis, increased ICP is generally associated with subarachnoid and intraventricular cysts; whereas, seizures, focal neurologic deficits, and personality changes occur more commonly with intraparenchymal cysts (9).

Another form of neurocysticercosis results from the formation of racemose cysts. The word "racemose" derives from the Latin "racemosus," meaning "full of clusters," and the lesion of racemose cysticercosis is often compared to a cluster of grapes. Racemose cysts are somewhat amorphous and are thought to result from an aberrant proliferation of larval membranes. Scolices are generally absent from these cysts which display dramatic variations in size and form. Racemose cysticercosis has been noted in 10–33% of cases and occurs most frequently in the ventricles, basal cisterns, and subarachnoid space (4, 5, 14). An intermediate or "pre-racemous" form has also been described (15).

Ocular or periocular involvement occurs in approximately 13%–20% of cysticercosis cases, with cysts located primarily in the vitreous humor, subretinal space, and anterior chamber. Orbital and extraocular structures may also be affected. Patients' presenting symptoms commonly include unilateral ocular pain and decreased visual acuity. Both intraocular and intraparenchymal cysticerci may result in blindness (2, 16–19).

Cysticerci can occur in almost any other imaginable anatomic location. Examples include the spine, breast, myocardium, lung, thyroid, pancreas, parotid, and tongue (6, 11, 12, 20–22). Several cases of disseminated disease and generalized muscular pseudohypertrophy have also been reported (23).

To date, cysticercosis has been rarely recognized in association with infection with the human immunodeficiency virus (HIV). One case in an HIV-positive Rwandan male was diagnosed in New York state and successfully treated with praziquantel (DL Borenstein, personal communication; CDC, unpublished data). A second case, this one fatal, was identified in California in 1990 (24).

Although cysticercosis occurs with similar frequency in males and females (7, 8, 12, 26–30), some studies have suggested that host inflammatory reactions may be more intense in women, particularly in cases of chronic cysticercotic arachnoiditis and acute cysticercotic encephalitis (26, 31, 32). All ages are affected, but the disease is most often recognized in the 20 to 50 year age group. Children, however, may be more susceptible to an encephalitic syndrome. Cysticercotic encephalitis is thought to result from massive exposure to taenia eggs with subsequent diffuse parenchymal infection. An intense inflammatory response and reactive edema give rise to increased intracranial pressure, which is commonly accompanied by headaches, seizures, vomiting, and fever. Mortality can be high, but survivors generally show improvement by 6 weeks (6, 9, 31, 33).

Clinical manifestations may also exhibit some degree of geographic variation. Muscular and subcutaneous cysticercosis, for example, is recognized more frequently in Asian and African patients than in Latin Americans (3, 9, 21). There is also evidence to suggest that children living in the United States at the time of diagnosis may have less severe manifestations of neurocysticercosis than children who reside in endemic areas (34, 35). The reasons for this difference are unclear, but Earnest et al. have suggested that smaller infective doses of *T. solium* eggs may play a role (12). Also, children with early or more benign manifestations of the disease may be more likely to seek and receive medical care in the United States.

Diagnosis of Cysticercosis and Taeniasis

Cysticercosis

The diagnosis of cysticercosis depends on the clinician's "index of suspicion", assessment of the patient's clinical manifestations, and the application of appropriate radiologic, immunologic, and histopathologic techniques. Other routine clinical laboratory studies are generally not helpful. Peripheral eosinophilia, for example, is not a common feature of this disease. Although evaluation of cerebrospinal fluid (CSF) may help support the diagnosis, abnormalities, when present, are usually nonspecific (3).

Radiologic imaging procedures form the foundation for the diagnosis of neurocysticercosis and have also proven helpful in cases of disseminated and/or musculocutaneous disease (3, 12, 20, 23, 36). In recent years, computed tomography (CT) has been the most common and most successful radiologic technique used in the diagnosis of cysticercosis (5, 9,10, 12, 14, 25, 28, 37). It is important to point out, however, that CT images are rarely, if ever, pathognomonic for cysticercosis and that negative scans do not necessarily rule out the presence of cysticerci. Moreover, the appearance of cysticercal lesions on CT will vary according to location, viability, and size of the cysts, and whether or not intravenous contrast material is used.

Although popular in the pre-CT era, routine skull X-rays, pneumoencephalography, ventriculography, and cerebral angiography have little to offer the modern clinician in the assessment of cysticercosis. "Plain" or "soft tissue" films of the upper arms, thighs, or calves may still be helpful in demonstrating calcified cysts in cases of late-stage or chronic disseminated and/or musculocutaneous disease (36). The impact of magnetic resonance imaging (MRI) on the diagnosis and management of this disease will be discussed below.

Immunologic testing for cysticercosis will likely always be used as an adjunct to, rather than a replacement for, radiologic diagnosis – particularly when evaluating patients in modern facilities in industrialized nations. In the developing world, however, reliance on immunologic testing may be greater due to the expense and limited availability of sophisticated radiologic equipment. Certainly, immunologic tests are essential for conducting epidemiologic field investigations in such settings. Recent advances in serologic techniques and antigen purification have greatly enhanced the laboratory diagnosis of cysticercosis (3, 38–40). Techniques for the detection of human anticysticercal antibodies such as immunoelectrophoresis, indirect hemagglutination, indirect immunofluorescence, and complement fixation have generally been replaced by more sensitive and specific enzyme-linked immunosorbent assays (ELISAs) and the enzyme-linked immunoelectrotransfer blot (EITB, immunoblot or "western blot") (41–43). The EITB assay represents a particularly significant advance for several reasons. The assay is easily performed and reproducible, and its reagents are very stable (3). Moreover, when first reported, the EITB showed a sensitivity of 98% and a specificity of 100%, making it clearly superior to any other currently available assay (39). More recent evaluations, however, suggest that the EITB may be somewhat less sensitive than originally reported (see below) (44). The diagnostic accuracy of all currently available immunologic tests will vary depending on the specimen source (e.g., serum/plasma, CSF, or saliva), the patient's exposure history (resident of endemic versus nonendemic area), and the stage or extent of infection. Also, the value of immunologic testing will vary according to its intended use (e.g., clinical evaluation of a specific patient versus epidemiologic field surveys).

The histopathologic evaluation of appropriate tissue specimens can often provide rapid and accurate diagnosis of cysticercosis. This is particularly true in cases with musculocutaneous lesions which can be excised with relative ease and minimal risk to the patient. In addition to complete excisional biopsy of such lesions, fine needle aspiration has also been used (22, 45). Numerous excellent and detailed descriptions of the histopathologic appearance of cysticercal lesions have appeared in previous publications (3, 9–11, 46, 47).

Although uncertainty regarding a diagnosis of neurocysticercosis not infrequently leads to craniotomies (48, 49), biopsies of CNS lesions are unnecessary in most cases of uncomplicated intraparenchymal cysts. Empiric therapeutic trials with praziquantel, for example, can be an effective alternative to brain biopsy (48). Surgical intervention will continue to have a role in the management of neurocysticercosis, but the availability of reliable serologic assays and safe, effective medical therapy obviates the need for invasive diagnostic procedures in most cases.

Taeniasis

Patients with taeniasis due to *T. solium* are rarely symptomatic. Diagnosis of this condtion, however, is crucial because tapeworm carriers serve as a constant source of reinfection for patients, their immediate families, and, in the appropriate setting, other community members and any free-roaming pigs in the area. Despite the potentially large numbers of taeniid eggs passed daily by a carrier, the diagnosis of taeniasis is often difficult to confirm. Most eggs remain inside intermittently shed proglottids, and those eggs that are released prior to defecation are not evenly distributed within feces (3). Although most techniques used for routine ova and parasite examinations are capable of detecting taeniid eggs, they are generally insensitive. Perianal cellophane tape tests, such as those used to detect pinworm infections, appear to be more sensitive and are the preferred method for detection of taeniid eggs (3). Unfortunately, once identified in fecal specimens, eggs of the two *Taenia* species infecting man *(T. solium* and *T. saginata*) cannot be differentiated microscopically. Speciation currently depends on the examination of intact proglottids, which can be difficult to recover (4).

Treatment

Prior to 1980, most cases of cysticercosis were managed with anticonvulsants, antiinflammatory agents, and/or surgery (11, 47). In the past decade, however, large numbers of patients have been treated (orally) with the pyrazinoisoquinoline derivative, praziquantel, alone or in combination with steroids (6, 9, 12, 14, 28–30, 50–54). Despite this vast experience and its reputation as both a "major advance" and "new hope", much controversy continues to surround the use of this medication (14, 53, 55, 56). Foremost among the arguments in favor of its use is the observation that the majority of patients treated with praziquantel show clinical improvement (14). Perhaps the most dramatic examples of such improvement are the visible resolution of subcutaneous cysts and/or muscular pseudohypertrophy (50, 57) and the rapid improvement of lost neurologic function such as that seen in a 5 year old child whose total blindness resolved after treatment with praziquantel (18).

Many other authors, however, advise caution regarding the use of praziquantel and note that this drug may not be a panacea or "magic bullet" (14, 56, 58). These authors, and others, correctly point out that there have been no prospective, double-blind, placebo-controlled trials with this medication. Hence, clear, objective documentation of its efficacy is lacking. Treatment trials conducted to date have varied in terms of drug dosage, clinical status of patients treated, criteria for drug response, and concommitant use of steroids, to name a few. In addition, many studies examining the natural history of cysticercosis in untreated (no specific anticysticercal medications) patients have demonstrated a relatively benign course in some patient populations (11, 34, 35). Finally, adverse reactions are very common in patients treated with praziquantel (28–30). Reactions are thought to result from the host inflammatory response to degenerating cysticerci and often include headache, nausea/vomiting and other evidence of increased ICP, as well as CSF pleocytosis (5). This combination of signs and symptoms has been referred to as the CSF reaction syndrome and occurs in 90–100% of patients on praziquantel alone (59). The severity and sequelae of this syndrome vary from mild, transient symptoms, to significant neurologic impairment due to cerebral infarcts (60), to death (6, 59). A delayed reaction may also be seen in patients treated concomitantly with steroids (61). Steroids, such as dexamethasone and prednisone, have been used for both prophylaxis and treatment of adverse reactions with generally good results (6, 52, 62). However, their use is also controversial, particularly in view of the aforementioned delayed reactions and recent data suggesting that dexamethasone decreases plasma levels of praziquantel (63).

In general, it can be said that praziquantel appears to be relatively safe and effective in many cases of intraparenchymal neurocysticercosis and in patients with multiple subcutaneous cysts and/or muscular pseudohypertrophy. It is less effective in patients with intra-ventricular, racemose or disseminated cysts, chronic meningitis, and acute encephalitis (6, 23, 29, 31, 64). Its safety and efficacy in spinal and ocular cysticercosis is unknown and may actually be contraindicated in the latter (9, 16, 65). Appropriate treatment for most cases of intraventricular, spinal, and ocular cysticercosis is surgical; shunting procedures to relieve hydrocephalus and intracranial hypertension are often required in patients with obstruction due to intraventricular cysts or chronic meningitis/arachnoiditis (26, 29).

Other agents used in the nonsurgical treatment of cysticercosis have included metrifonate, flubendazole, and indium 113-labeled anticysticercus antibodies. Experience with these therapeutic regimens is limited, and their potential role in the management of human cysticercosis remains uncertain (66–68). Recent experience with the drug, albendazole, will be discussed below.

T. solium taeniasis is safely and effectively treated with a single dose of niclosamide (3, 58, 65). Praziquantel in a single dose is equally effective, but may elicit adverse reactions in persons co-infected with both taeniasis and cysticercosis (58, 69).

Epidemiology (Fig. 2)

The *T. solium* taeniasis/cysticercosis complex is endemic throughout most of the developing world. Geographic distribution is influenced by local hygienic conditions, swine husbandry practices, and other sociocultural factors. Infection with *T. solium* is rare, for example, in many Moslem and Jewish population groups where pork is excluded from the diet (2). Other examples of potential sociocultural influences include the use of taeniid proglottids in the traditional healing practices of certain Bantu groups in southern Africa (65) and the combination pigsty-privy structures used on Cheju Island in South Korea (70). Similarly, in some remote regions of Mexico, latrines have been built so that pigs have easy access to human excrement. Also in Mexico, pork highly infested with cysticerci ("measled") is sometimes preferred for its superior flavor (71).

Two primary conditions are necessary for ongoing transmission of taeniasis/cysticercosis to occur: human consumption of raw or inadequately cooked pork and swine husbandry practices that favor pig consumption of human feces (Fig. 3). Inadequate disposal of human fecal waste with subsequent contamination of water and food sources facilitates the transmission of taeniid eggs to both humans and pigs. Environmental contamination with eggs not only fosters foodborne and waterborne transmission, but possibly airborne and insectborne as well (3, 65). In addition,

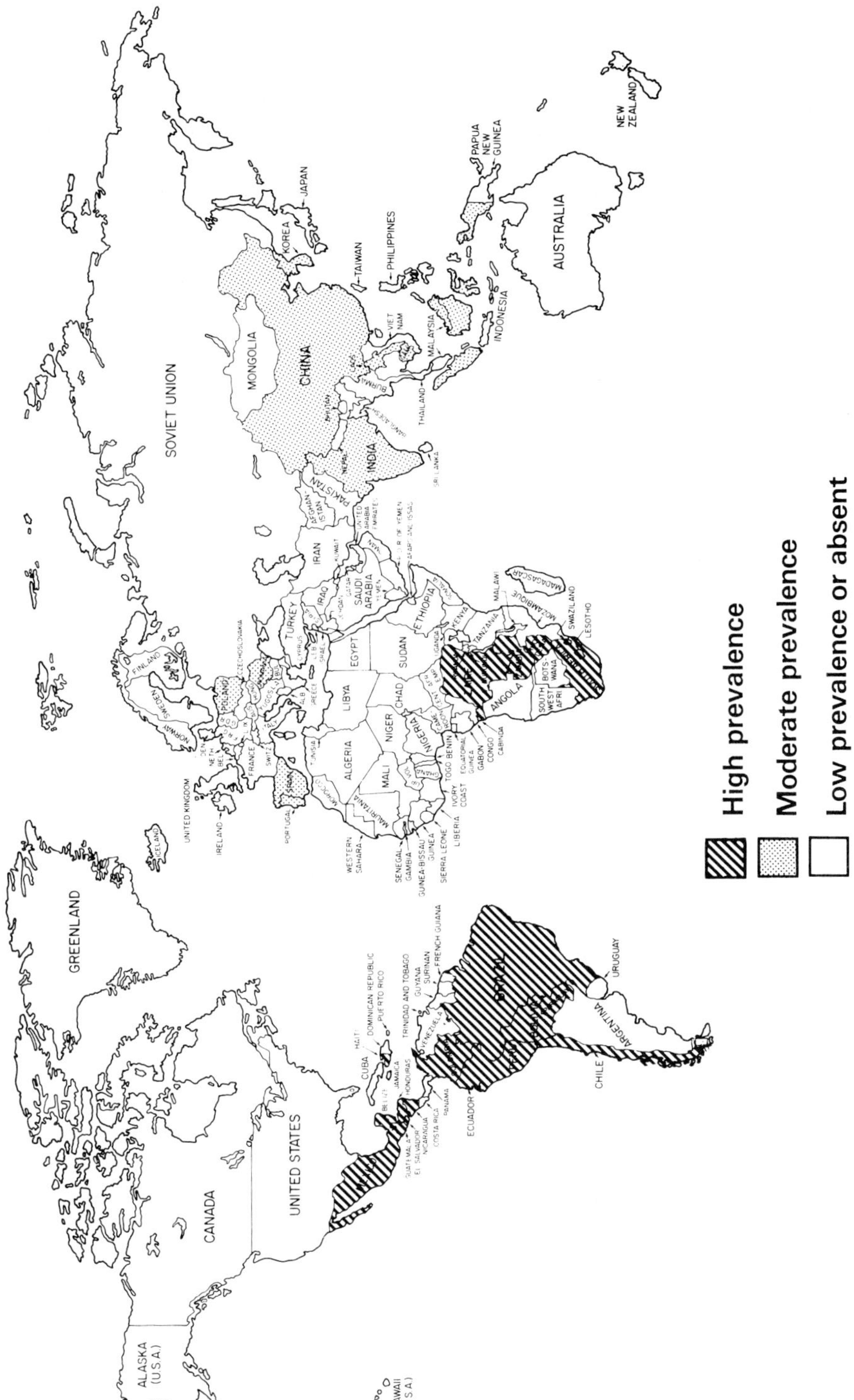

Fig. 2. Geographic distribution of *Taenia solium*

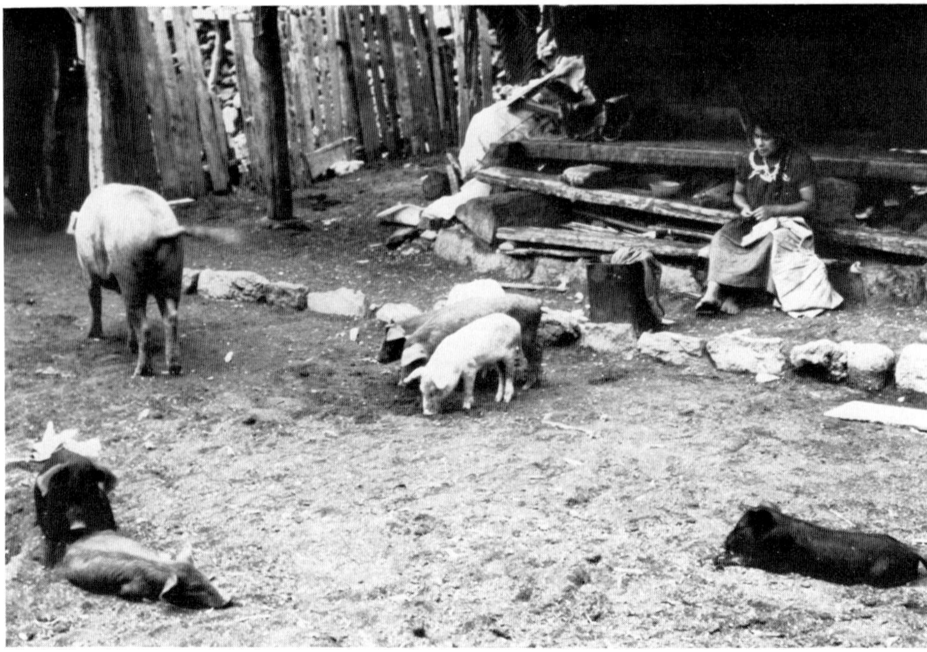

Fig. 3. Scene from a Mexican village where free-roaming swine husbandry practices provide coprophagic pigs with ready access to human waste (photograph courtesy of Peter M. Schantz and Elsa Sarti)

person-to-person transmission likely occurs because infectious eggs may be found on the clothing, under the fingernails, and elsewhere on the body of tapeworm carriers (72). Indeed, recent epidemiologic studies in Mexico and Panama suggest that household clustering of taeniasis/cysticercosis is occurring in endemic areas (73–75). Epidemiologic data also suggest that tapeworm carriers themselves are at increased risk for cysticercosis. In their classic study of British soldiers returning from India, Dixon and Lipscomb found that taeniasis was approximately 8 times more common among persons with cysticercosis than among noninfected individuals from the same military population (11). More recently, Sacks and Berkowitz noted that a history of tapeworm was the only significant risk factor for cysticercosis that they could identify in the South African population they studied (76). Similar findings have been reported from Columbia, China, the United States, and elsewhere in South Africa, with rates of taeniasis/cysticercosis coinfection ranging from 14–53% (25, 30, 50, 51).

Despite numerous clinical and epidemiologic studies, reliable statistics regarding the prevalence of taeniasis/cysticercosis are rare. Available data have come from varied sources including hospital admission and discharge records, autopsy series, serologic and intestinal parasite surveys, and swine slaughterhouse inspections (77). Unfortunately, these data are often limited by biased sampling and insensitive or nonspecific diagnostic techniques. Existing estimates, nevertheless, suggest that the prevalence of cysticercosis is high in many areas. Figures frequently quoted in the literature include reports from Mexico City noting that neurocysticercosis accounts for 9% of admissions to neurological and neurosurgical wards, 11–25% of craniotomies performed for brain tumors, and 50% of cases of adult-onset epilepsy (3, 73, 77, 78).

In Africa, cysticercosis was detected in 0.45% of 2,148 autopsies performed in Zimbabwe and has been identified in up to 8.1% of pigs slaughtered in Zaire (79). Clinical descriptions of cysticercosis are also frequently reported from medical centers in Pretoria and Durban, South Africa, where the disease is considered to be one of the "major health hazards" of the region (30, 52, 64). In another South African study, the seroprevalence of cysticercosis was 7.4% in an urban black population (76).

Cysticercosis is also being reported with increasing frequency from several Asian countries. Wei et al., for example, described the characteristics of 1400 cases of neurocysticercosis from one hospital in Beijing, China (13). In Korea, cysticercosis accounted for 73% of the parasitic diseases encountered in tissue specimens at the Seoul National University Hospital from 1968–1977 (21). Case reports from India are also common, where cerebral cysticercosis has been reported to be the second most important cause of intracranial space-occupying lesions (after tuberculomas) (79).

Cysticercosis also occurs in Taiwan, Thailand, Vietnam, the Philippines, and Indonesia (65). Epidemics of epilepsy and burns attributed to neurocysticercosis have been reported from Irian Jaya where Muller et al. found subcutaneous cysts in approximately 17% of a random sample of 242 persons (79, 80).

It is difficult to assess the overall public health and socioeconomic impact of cysticercosis. Flisser has emphasized that 75% of patients with neurocysticercosis fall within productive age groups, thereby making a significant socioeconomic impact due to inability to work. Flisser also estimates that in 1986 over 14.5 million US dollars were spent in Mexico alone to treat approximately 2700 newly hospitalized patients with neurocysticercosis. Moreover, significant economic losses occur due to condemnation of pig carcasses, which in Mexico in 1980 resulted in a loss of over 43 million US dollars (74).

Recent Developments and Latest Advances

Diagnostics

Radiology

The recent introduction of magnetic resonance imaging (MRI) has greatly expanded diagnostic capabilities in many fields of medicine. MRI has proven to be particularly efficacious, and superior to CT, for the detection and characterization of posterior fossa lesions, spinal cord myelopathies, and lesions related to seizure foci. MRI is also notable for its versatility in providing images in different cross-sectional orientations and for its safety (81). Experience with MRI in the evaluation of cysticercosis is growing rapidly, and the latest reports suggest that this imaging modality offers various advantages over traditional CT.

Perhaps the most important contribution MRI has made to the care of patients with cysticercosis is its superior ability to detect intraventricular and cisternal cysts (82–85). This capability is important because intraventricular cysts are potentially life-threatening, but amenable to early surgical intervention (82, 83). MRI is also superior to CT in the detection of superficial intracranial cysts and in demonstrating the extent of pericystic edematous changes (82, 84). MRI may also be useful for preoperative reconfirmation of potentially mobile intraventricular and subarachnoid cysts (83). Moreover, there is increasing evidence that MRI is generally more sensitive than CT in detecting most noncalcified cysts, regardless of their location. Martinez et al. found MRI to be 4 times (85% vs 21%) more sensitive than CT in the detection of multiple intracranial cysts. They attributed this observation to the ability of MRI to detect cysts in the brainstem, cerebellum, subarachnoid space, and ventricles (85).

Finally, MRI has provided clinicians with their first truly pathognomonic radiographic sign for cysticercosis. Several authors have described the characteristic appearance of viable cysticerci when viewed with MRI. Typically, a 2–4 mm high-intensity "mural nodule" corresponding to the protoscolex is seen within an approximately 1 cm area of low-intensity, the so-called "bladder." These lesions have been described in intra- as well as extracranial sites, and histopathologic correlation has been well documented (20, 82–86).

Immunology

Several important developments relevant to the immunologic diagnosis of cysticercosis have occurred in the past 5 years. The EITB assay described above has been in use at the Reference Immunodiagnostic Laboratory of the Parasitic Diseases Branch at the Centers for Disease Control (CDC) for over 3 years. During that time, clinical information has been collected on patients whose serum and/or CSF was submitted for cysticercosis antibody testing. Comparison of EITB and radiographic findings confirmed earlier reports of this test's high sensitivity (94%) in patients with 2 or more intracranial cysticerci. This sensitivity, however, was significantly lower in patients with single intracranial cysts (28%) or with only calcified (single or multiple) cysts (64%). In addition, comparison of paired serum and CSF specimens showed that serum specimens were consistently more sensitive than CSF, and no case in which the CSF tested positive, but serum negative, has been encountered (44). It appears, therefore, that the EITB assay will continue to be a useful clinical and epidemiologic tool in most situations, but that results should be interpreted with caution in patients whose disease involvement is limited to single and/or calcified cysts. The advantages of preferentially testing serum over CSF are obvious in that the need for lumbar puncture is obviated. The usefulness of the EITB in epidemiologic field situations has recently been demonstrated in Mexico (43, 87), Panama (75), and Peru (88, 89). In addition, the EITB assay has been shown to be 100% sensitive and specific in field tests of porcine cysticercosis in Peru (90).

Another recent EITB development has been the demonstration of sequential immunologic responses with different immunoglobulin classes in experimentally infected pigs. Tsang et al. have shown an early (prepatent) antigen-specific IgM response that declines to undetectable levels by 6–9 weeks postinfection. The IgG response began within 5–8 weeks postinfection and rose as IgM levels fell. The authors suggest that, if similar responses occur in human cysticercosis, detection of anticysticercal IgM antibodies may help to distinguish early from chronic infections (40).

Other advances in the field of cysticercosis immunodiagnosis include recent developments in the testing for anticysticercal antibodies in saliva. Feldman et al. compared ELISA and EITB in both serum and saliva from 28 patients with "confirmed" (by surgery or CT) neurocysticercosis. Their results verified that EITB is more sensitive (100% vs 74%) when testing serum, but that ELISA is the better test for saliva (82% vs 70%). When both techniques were applied to saliva, sensitivity rose to 89%. The specificity for both tests when using saliva was reported as 100% because no cross-reactions with their control groups were observed (43). In a similar study that compared ELISA testing of CSF, serum, and saliva from 29 patients with neurocysticercosis, Acosta reported positive results in 21(72%) saliva and 20 (69%) serum specimens (91).

Although it is not likely to have a significant impact on the clinical management of individual patients, the use of saliva for epidemiologic purposes appears promising. In addition to the relative ease of specimen collection and improved patient compliance, the use of saliva makes the handling and disposal of needles and syringes unnecessary. The technique has reasonable sensitivity and should be widely applicable to many field situations. It should be noted, however, that the testing of saliva may be less sensitive in patients with few or no teeth because the gingival sources of plasma-derived proteins (crevicular fluid) are reduced. Also, high background values may confound results in patients with extensive periodontal disease (91).

The detection of *T. solium* antigens in CSF has been the topic of several recent publications (92, 93). Various investigators have employed different combinations of techniques to detect and characterize *T. solium* larval antigens in human CSF. Reported sensitivities have generally been disappointing, ranging from 56% to 78%. Although these studies have confirmed that larval *T. solium* antigens are present and detectable in the CSF of selected patients with neurocysticercosis, CSF antigen detection is not yet practical for clinical and/or epidemiologic applications. Detection of circulating antigen in serum specimens would be more widely applicable, but few studies have addressed this possibility.

The last topic in cysticercosis immunodiagnostics that warrants brief discussion is the specific detection of *T. solium* eggs and/or adult stage proteins in human stool specimens. Flisser and others have applied DNA hybridization techniques to demonstrate sensitive and specific detection of eggs of both *T. solium* and *T. saginata* in human fecal specimens (94,95). More recently, Flisser et al. report that these hybridization techniques, as well as an ELISA for detection of adult proteins, are undergoing standardization and should soon be ready for clinical and epidemiologic field trials (96).

Treatment

Since the intial reports of successful medical therapy with praziquantel in the early 1980s, further advances have been limited. Recently, however, a relatively new antiparasitic drug, albendazole, has been evaluated for use in patients with cysticercosis. Albendazole is an oral benzimidazole with broad anthelminthic activity (97). The majority of clinical trials with this drug have been reported from one group of investigators in Mexico City (27, 97–99), but rare reports have also come from China (50), Ecuador (100), Brazil (101), and India (102). With few exceptions (102), results of therapy with albendazole have been very favorable. In their first report in 1987, Escobedo et al. documented an 86% reduction in the total number of CT-visualized cysts in 7 patients enrolled in an open trial (97). A subsequent study comparing albendazole to praziquantel demonstrated comparable efficacy between these two agents (76% reduction with albendazole vs 73% reduction with praziquantel) (98). Several cases of praziquantel "failures" which subsequently responded to albendazole have also been described (97, 99). More recently, the Mexican investigators have completed a randomized, four-arm study comparing praziquantel and albendazole in different dosages. Their results (again based on the reduction of CT-visualized intracranial cysts) suggest that albendazole (15 mg/kg/day for 8 or 30 days) is actually more effective than praziquantel (50 mg/kg/day for 8 or 15 days) for all regimens tested (85% vs 60%, and 85% vs 48%). They also noted that reducing the course of praziquantel from 15 to 8 days resulted in a 12% decrease in efficacy (60% vs 48%); whereas, a reduction in the duration of albendazole therapy from 30 to 8 days showed no change (85% vs 85%) (27). Other studies, also from Mexico, have documented cases of remarkable recoveries in patients with forms of cysticercosis that are usually considered to be refractory to medical therapy. These include two cases of subarachnoid cysticercosis, one with an accompanying intraventricular cyst which disappeared after therapy (103) and another which demonstrated almost immediate full recovery of significant, bilateral visual field loss (17).

Similar to praziquantel, plasma and CSF levels of albendazole demonstrate fairly wide interpatient variability that appears to result from individual differences in pharmacokinetics. Also, there has been no documentation of any correlation between drug efficacy and plasma or CSF drug levels for either medication. Unlike praziquantel, however, plasma levels of albendazole have been shown to increase by 50% in patients taking dexamethasone (104).

Finally, albendazole is also advantageous in terms of cost. Although not commercially available in the United States, the cost of one 30 day course of treatment in Mexico is approximately US$ 25.00. A 15 day course of praziquantel costs about US$ 250.00 (105). This cost differential would be even greater if the aforementioned 8 day regimen of albendazole were used.

Immunoprophylaxis

The scientific literature is replete with studies of parasite antigens and host immune response, and these will not be reviewed here. There is currently no human vaccine for any parasitic infection and research in this area, although intense, has been frustrating. One recent development in veterinary science, however, may have potentially significant application to human disease due to larval cestode infections. Johnson et al. have reported the successful identification of a protective antigen of *T. ovis* produced by recombinant DNA technology (106). *T. ovis* causes cysticercosis of sheep, or "sheep measles" and is a major economic problem in areas such as Australia and New Zealand. Although their product does not produce complete protection, levels of protection were adequate enough that commercial vaccine development is underway (107).

Also pertinent to the potential development of vaccines for cysticercosis is the recent identification by Tsang et al. of a specific glycoprotein (GP97) associated with a transient rise in IgM in acutely infected pigs. The authors suggest that, if made to persist, antibodies against this glycoprotein might be protective (40).

Epidemiology

Some of the limitations of existing epidemiologic data have been discussed above. In addition, it should be stressed that too few community-based field studies have been carried out in endemic areas. Surveys recently completed in Mexico and Peru, however, have provided new and important epidemiologic information regarding human and porcine cysticercosis. In Mexico, Sarti-Gutierrez and colleagues conducted a comprehensive epidemiologic survey in a village in Morelos State. In addition to an overall cysticercosis seroprevalence of 10.8% (EITB assay), these investigators also identified significant associations between seropositivity and a history of tapeworm infection, frequent pork consumption, infrequent bathing, and poor household hygienic conditions. Moreover, as in a previous survey of another Mexican village (73), household clustering of seropositive persons was noted. A history of having passed tapeworm proglottids and a history of convulsions, both of which also correlated significantly with seropositivity, also demonstrated familial clustering (87).

This study also assessed certain epidemiologic factors relevant to porcine cysticercosis and performed environmental surveys for taeniid eggs.

Water sampling revealed no eggs and only one soil sample collected near a latrine was positive for *Taenia* sp. Eggs of other human intestinal helminths, however, were detected in 2.5% of 424 soil samples. The prevalence of cysticercosis in pigs, based on tongue examinations, was 4% and 30% of pig owners admitted to the deliberate feeding of human fecal waste to their pigs (87; PM Schantz, personal communication).

Data from the Cysticercosis Working Group in Peru have provided additional insights into the epidemiologic characteristics of cysticercosis in Latin America. A community-based survey has just been completed in a village located in a tropical forest region of Peru. In this community, 8% of its human inhabitants were seropositive for cysticercosis by the EITB assay, as were 43% of its pig population. A limited number of soil and water samples were also collected, all of which were negative for taeniid eggs. In contrast to the Mexican study, however, neither household clustering nor specific risk factors for infection were identified in humans or pigs. Reasons for this discrepancy are uncertain, but may relate to sample size, sampling methodology, and/or as yet undefined sociocultural differences. In another village survey done on the Peruvian altiplano (high plain), household clustering of seropositive humans *was* observed, but complete data from that study are not yet available (88).

Also from Peru are recent data indicating that neurocysticercosis is a significant cause of neurologic morbidity in that country. Another study from the Cysticercosis Working Group has shown that 11% of neurologic admissions in a major hospital in Lima are seropositive by EITB. This figure contrasts to 2% of patients attending a public clinic and 1% of patients seen at a private endoscopy clinic, both also in Lima. All but one of the 21 seropositive patients had abnormal CT scans; that patient had both ocular cysticercosis and an adult tapeworm (89).

Taken together, these recent data from Mexico, Peru, and elsewhere in Latin American suggest certain trends and permit some tentative generalizations. First, the seroprevalence of cysticercosis in some rural areas is high. Both of the studies described above demonstrated seroprevalences in the 10% range. Preliminary data from other Peruvian villages (Tsang, personal communication) suggest similar figures, and we have found the same in two villages on the Bolivian altiplano (CDC, unpublished data). Secondly, the evidence for household clustering in the face of consistently negative environmental sampling suggests that person-to-person transmission of taeniid eggs is a major source of human cysticercosis in endemic areas. Data of this sort are crucial for planning appropriate control measures. Finally, the Peruvian finding of high seroprevalence among neurological patients is consistent with earlier, similar studies from Mexico and helps to demonstrate the public health impact of neurocysticercosis. The Peruvian Cysticercosis Working Group has examined this problem a step further by showing that nearly 50% of the seropositive patients in their study were misdiagnosed on admission. They go on to point out that cysticercosis is 10–20 times more common in that hospital population than syphilis, a condition that is routinely screened for with VDRL. They conclude that serologic screening for cysticercosis in neurological hospitals in endemic areas is practical, cost-effective, and capable of identifying patients with potentially severe, but highly treatable disease (89).

In closing this discussion of recent developments, a brief update on cysticercosis in the United States is appropriate. Since the early 1970s, cysticercosis has been increasingly recognized in patients in the United States (8, 12, 25, 108). This trend has been particularly apparent in areas with large numbers of Latin American immigrants such as Los Angeles. The majority of cases are diagnosed in immigrants (particularly from Mexico), but an increasing number of travel-related and autochthonous cases are being recognized (24, 109). Since surveillance was initiated in January, 1988, the LA County Health Department has identified nine travel-associated cases in US-born persons, one of which was fatal, and ten autochthonous cases. Investigation into one of these US-acquired cases revealed 3 close personal contacts with taeniasis who were thought to the likely source of this patient's cysticercal infection (109). Additionally, in the past year, the CDC has assisted in the evaluation of two other autochthonous cases, one in Boston and the other in South Carolina. Three other household contacts of the Boston case, a 16 month old girl, were also seropositive for cysticercosis, and taeniasis was confirmed in the patient's father. In the South Carolina investigation, although no tapeworm carrier was identified, three close personal contacts of the 8 year old female patient were seropositive. These cases serve to emphasize the fact that transmission of cysticercosis is indeed occurring in the US and that autochthonous cases are being recognized in diverse geographic locations within this country (110).

Unanswered Questions

These recent developments and latest advances indicate that progress in understanding various clinical and epidemiologic aspects of cysticercosis is taking place. Nevertheless, many unanswered questions remain. In terms of caring for patients currently afflicted with cysticercosis, the best therapy has yet to be determined definitively. The answer may lie with praziquantel, albendazole, or some other, thus far untested, medication. Although albendazole appears promising, the number of patients treated is relatively small, and the results have rarely been reproduced outside of Mexico City. The question of when, and whether or not, to use steroids simultaneously with either praziquantel or albendazole also remains unanswered. Heated discussions over this issue continue, with some investigators insisting on their use throughout anticysticercal therapy while others start steroids only after adverse reactions reactions develop. The issue of who to treat is also unsettled. There is mounting evidence that some patient populations, such as children seen at certain Los Angeles area hospitals, require nothing more than symptomatic treatment. On the other hand, progressive neurologic impairment in untreated patients has been well documented elsewhere. A related question is how best to determine prognosis in different population groups and in different forms or stages of disease.

From an epidemiologic perspective, the complexities of the taeniasis/cysticercosis complex are just beginning to be understood. What is the true geographic distribution of this disease? Is its impact on public health in the US much greater than currently realized? It is known that, at least focally, the prevalence of cysticercosis in some developing countries is high, but the actual extent or magnitude of this problem in endemic areas is uncertain. Similarly, uncertainty remains as to what are the best intervention strategies in endemic areas. Is attacking taeniasis by mass treatment with low dose praziquantel or some other intestinal anthelmintic agent the most efficacious and cost-effective method for controlling cysticercosis? Or, should research dollars be directed toward the development of porcine and/or human vaccines?

Conclusions and Directions for the 21st Century

In order to address these and other questions adequately, much remains to be done. The need for controlled clinical trials seems obvious. It will be important that such trials be conducted not only by the experienced investigators of areas such as Mexico City, but also by researchers in other endemic regions. Multicenter trials with standard protocols would seem to be a reasonable approach. Collaboration and pooling of patient data between medical centers in the developed and developing worlds should also be encouraged. Clinical risk assessment studies are needed to address the issues of who to treat and how to assess prognosis, as well as to identify risk factors for progression to severe disease.

In those areas where it is available, new technology should be used to its full advantage. New diagnostic assays such as the EITB need to be more widely utilized, and physicians must be made aware of its availability and its limitations. Consideration should be also given to the more frequent use of MRI as perhaps the radiologic imaging technique of choice for the evaluation of neurocysticercosis. In addition, newer, more sensitive diagnostic tests would be helpful. Antigen detection would facilitate treatment decisions in patients with cysticercosis and greatly enhance our ability to detect tape worm carriers who constitute a constant threat to themselves and those with whom they have close contact.

Much work will need to be done regarding the epidemiology of taeniasis/cysticercosis. Several new survey tools are available, or near ready, for use in epidemiologic field studies. Even ancient techniques such as the pig tongue examination have found new application. Modern techniques like the testing of saliva for anticysticercal antibodies or the detection of taeniid antigens in stool need to be standardized for use in the field. In addition, recent epidemiologic insights such as the familial clustering and risk factors identified in community-level surveys should be utilized in the design of control strategies. Comparative intervention trials should be preceded by appropriate baseline studies so that impact can be adequately assessed. In comparisons of different control strategies, cost and, particularly, sociocultural factors must also be taken into account. As Leonardo Mata has written, "social determinants of disease are the most important factors to identify when planning intervention programs" (111).

Finally, better utilization of existing data to foster prevention should begin now. In the developing world, this means that current knowledge could be imparted to the residents of studied villages in the form of basic educational campaigns. In developed countries such as the US, better use of existing knoweldge means taking the time to investigate the households of patients with cysticercosis in order to identify and treat tapeworm carriers, thereby preventing further transmission in that home. Even serologic screening of other family or household members may be appropriate in order to avert adverse clinical outcomes in family members who may also be unknowingly afflicted with cysticercosis. Indeed, despite a wide range of clinical and epidemiologic variables, the single most consistent, and crucially important, aspect of this disease is that it is preventable.

References

1. Nieto D (1982) Historical notes on cysticercosis. In: Flisser A, Willms K, Laclette JP, Larralde C, Ridaura C, Beltran F (eds) Cysticercosis: present state of knowledge and perspectives. New York, Academic Press, Inc, pp 1–2
2. Acha PD, Szyfres B (1987) Zoonoses and communicable diseases common to man and animals. 2nd ed. Washington, DC, Pan American Health Organization, pp 749–760
3. Richards F, Schantz PM (1991) Laboratory diagnosis of cysticercosis. Clin Lab Med 11: 1011–1028
4. Beaver PC, Jung RC, Cupp EW (1948) Clinical parasitology. 9th ed. Philadelphia, Lee and Febiger, pp 512–519
5. Nash TE (1986) Diagnosis and treatment of cysticercosis. In: Remington JS, Swartz MN (eds) Current clinical topics in infectious diseases. New York, McGraw Hill 7: 297–310
6. Sotelo J, Guerrero V, Rubio F (1985) Neurocysticercosis: a new classification based on active and inactive forms. A study of 753 cases. Arch Intern Med 145: 442–445
7. Bittencourt PRM, Costa AJ, Oliveira TV, et al (1990) Clinical, radiological and cerebrospinal fluid presentation of neurocysticercosis, a prospective study. Arq Neuropsiquiatr (Sao Paulo) 48: 286–295
8. Scharf D (1988) Neurocysticercosis: two hundred thirty-eight cases from a California hospital. Arch Neurol 45: 777–780
9. Del Brutto OH, Sotelo J (1988) Neurocysticercosis: an update. Rev Infect Dis 10: 1075–1087
10. Flisser A, Larralde C (1986) Cysticercosis. In: Walls KW, Schantz PM (eds) Immunodiagnosis of parasitic diseases. Helminthic diseases. Florida, Academic Press, Inc, pp 109–161
11. Dixon HBF, Lipscomb FM (1961) Cysticercosis: An analysis and follow-up of 450 cases. In: Medical Research Council Special Report Series No. 299. London, Her Majesty's Stationary Office
12. Earnest MP, Reller LB, Filley CM, Grek AJ (1987) Neurocysticercosis in the United States: 35 cases and a review. Rev Infect Dis 9: 961–979
13. Wei GZ, Li CJ, Meng JM, Ding MC (1988) Cysticercosis of the central nervous system. A clinical study of 1400 cases. Chin Med J 101: 493–500
14. Nash TE, Neva FA (1984) Recent advances in the diagnosis and treatment of cerebral cysticercosis. N Engl J Med 311: 1492–1496
15. Rabiela MT, Rivas A, Flisser A (1989) Morphological types of *T. solium* cysticerci. Parasitol Today 5: 357–358
16. Welsh NH, Peters AL, Crewe-Brown W, Blignaut P, Donnoli P, Da Souza BS, Javary Y (1987) Ocular cysticercosis. A report of 13 cases. S Afr Med J 71: 719–722

17. Santayo H, Corona R, Sotelo J (1991) Total recovery of visual function after treatment for cerebral cysticercosis. N Engl J Med 324: 1137–1139
18. Pansey BK, Basra KS, Pasricha R (1989) Medically treated cysticercosis in a blind child. A case report. Surg Neurol 32: 56–58
19. DiLoreto DA, Kennedy RA, Neigel JM, Rootman J (1990) Infestation of extraocular muscle by cysticercus cellulosae. Br J Ophthalmol 74: 751–752
20. Cheung YY, Steinbaum S, Yuh W, Chiu L (1987) MR findings in extracranial cysticercosis: case report. J Assist Tomography 11: 179–181
21. Chi JG, Sung RH, Cho SY (1988) Tissue parasitic diseases in Korea. J Korean Med Sci 3: 51–62
22. Vuong PN (1989) Fine needle aspiration cytology of subcutaneous cysticercosis of the breast: case report and pathogenic discussion. Acta Cyto 33: 659–662
23. Wadia N, Desai S, Bhatt M (1988) Disseminated cysticercosis. New observations, including CT scan findings and experience with treatment by praziquantel. Brain 111: 597–614
24. California Morbidity (1990) Cysticercosis in California. June 15, 1990, #23/#24.
25. Loo L, Braude A (1982) Cerebral cysticercosis in San Diego: a report of 23 cases and a review of the literature. Medicine (Baltimore) 61: 341–359
26. Sotelo J, Marin C (1987) Hydrocephalus secondary to cysticercotic arachnoiditis. A long-term follow-up of 92 cases. J Neurosurg 66: 686–689
27. Sotelo J, Del Brutto OH, Penagos P, Escobedo F, Torres B, Rodriguez-Carbajal J, Rubio-Donnadieu F (1990) Comparison of therapeutic regimen of anticysticercal drugs for parenchymal brain cysticercosis. J Neurol 237: 69–72
28. Sotelo J, Escobedo F, Rodriguez-Carbajal J, Torres B, Rubio-Donnadieu F (1984) Therapy of parenchymal brain cysticercosis with praziquantel. N Engl J Med 310: 1001–1007
29. Robles C, Sedano AM, Vargas-Tentori N, Galindo-Virgen S (1987) Long-term results of praziquantel therapy in neurocysticercosis. J Neurosurgery 66: 359–363
30. Van Dellen JR, McKeon CP (1988) Praziquantel in active cerebral cysticercosis. Neurosurgery 22: 92–96
31. Rangel R, Torres B, Del Brutto O, Sotelo J (1987) Cysticercotic encephalitis: a severe form in young females. Am J Trop Med Hyg 36: 387–392
32. Del Brutto OH, Garcia E, Talarnas O, Sotelo J (1988) Sex-related severity of inflamation in parenchymal brain cysticercosis. Arch Intern Med 148: 544–546
33. Lopez-Hernandez A (1983) Clinical manifestations and sequential computed tomography scans of cerebral cysticercosis in childhood. Brain Dev 6: 269–277
34. Mitchell WG, Snodgrass SR (1985) Intraparenchymal cerebral cysticercosis in children: a benign prognosis. Neurol 1: 151–156
35. Mitchell WG, Crawford TO (1988) Intraparenchymal cerebral cysticercosis in children: diagnosis and treatment. Pediatr 82: 76–82
36. Reeder MM, Palmer PES (1981) The radiology of tropical diseases with epidemiogical, pathological and clinical correlation. Baltimore, The Williams and Wilkins Co, pp 911–931
37. Byrd SE, Daryabagi J, Thompson R, Zant J, Locke GE, Biggers S (1985) The computed tomographic spectrum of cerebral cysticercosis. J Natl Med Assoc 78: 553–560
38. Gottstein B, Zini D, Schantz PM (1987) Species-specific immunodiagnosis of *Taenia solium* cysticercosis by ELISA and immunoblotting. Trop Med Parasitol 38: 299–303
39. Tsang VCW, Brand JA, Boyer AE (1989) An enzyme-linked immunoelectrotransfer blot assay and glycoprotein antigens for diagnosing human cysticercosis (*Taenia solium*). J Infect Dis 159: 50–59
40. Tsang VCW, Pilcher JA, Zhou W, et al (1991) Efficacy of the immunoblot assay for cysticercosis in pigs and modulated expression of distinct IgM/IgG activities to *Taenia solium* antigens in experimental infections. Vet Immunol Immunopathol 29: 69–78
41. Nuñez R, Muñoz A, Nuñez C, Gomez B (1989) A micro ELISA for the diagnosis of cerebral cysticercosis. J Immunoassay 10: 169–178
42. Schantz PM, Sarti-Gutierrez E (1989) Diagnostic methods and epidemiologic surveillance of *Taenia solium* infection. Acta Leidensia 57: 153–163

43. Feldman M, Plancarte A, Sandoval M, Wilson M, Flisser A (1990) Comparison of two assays (EIA and EITB) and two samples (saliva and serum) for the diagnosis of neurocysticercosis. Trans R Soc Trop Med Hyg 84 :559–562
44. Wilson M, Bryan RT, Fried JA, et al (1991) Clinical evaluation of the cysticercosis enzyme-linked immunoelectrotransfer blot (EITB)) in patients with neurocysticercosis. J Inf Dis 164: 1007–1009
45. Kung ITM, Lee D, Yu HC (1989) Soft tissue cysticercosis: diagnosis by fine-needle aspiration. Am J Clin Pathol 92: 834–835
46. Sparks AK, Neahe RC, Connor DH (1976) Cysticercosis. In: Binford CH, Connor DH (eds) Pathology of tropical and extraordinary diseases. Washington, DC, Armed Forces Institute of Pathology, pp 539–542
47. Trenes JO, Trelles L (1979) Cysticercosis of the nervous system. In: Vinken PJ, Bruyn GW (eds) Handbook of clinical neurology. Amsterdam, NY, North Holland, pp 291–320
48. Case Records of the Massachusetts General Hospital (Case 20-1990) (1990) N Engl J Med 322: 1446–1457
49. Binstock PD, Azimi PH, Williams RA (1987) Cerebral cysticercosis in a 22-month-old infant. Am J Clin Pathol 88: 655–658
50. Zhi-biao X Wen-kai C, Hui-lan Z, et al (1985) Praziquantel in treatment of cysticercosis cellulosae: report of 200 cases. Chin Med J 98: 489–494
51. Castano S, Botero D (1985) Treatment of neurocysticercosis with praziquantel in Columbia. Progress in Clinical Neurosciences 2: 220–321
52. Joubert J, Joubert MJ, Lombaard CM (1985) Neurocysticercosis: a comprehensive approach to medical treatment. South Afr Med J 68: 11–14
53. King CH, Mahmoud AAF (1989) Drugs five years later: praziquantel. Ann Intern Med 110: 290–296
54. Spina-Franca A, Nobrega JPS, Machado LR, Livramento JA (1989) Neurocisticercose e praziquantel: evolucao a longo prazo de 100 pacientes (Portugese with English Abstract). Arq Neuropsiquiat 47: 444–448
55. Pearson RD, Guerrant RL (1983) Praziquantel: a major advance in antihelminthic therapy. Ann Intern Med 99: 195–198
56. Moodley M, Moosa A (1989) Treatment of neurocysticercosis: is praziquantel the new hope? Lancet 1: 262
57. Baranski MC (1984) Treatment of dermal cysticercosis with praziquantel. A new cestocidal agent. Rev Inst Med Trop Sao Paulo 26: 259–266
58. Richards F (1986) Praziquantel in the treatment of cysticercosis (Letter). JAMA 256: 349–50
59. Richards F (1986) Diagnosis and treatment of neurocysticercosis. IM 7: 1–11
60. Woo E, Yu YL Huang CY (1988) Cerebral infarct precipitated by praziquantel in neurocysticercosis: a cautionary note. Trop Geogr Med 40: 143–146
61. Ciferri F (1988) Delayed CSF reaction to praziquantel (Letter). Lancet
62. DeGhetaldi LD, Norman RM, Douville AW (1983) Cerebral cysticercosis treated biphasically with dexamethasone and praziquantel. Ann Intern Med 99: 179–181
63. Vasquez ML Helgi J, Sotelo J (1987) Plasma levels of praziquantel decrease when dexamethasone is given simultaneously. Neurology 37: 1561–1562
64. Joubert J (1990) Cysticercal meningitis: a pernicious form of neurocysticercosis which responds poorly to praziquantel. S Afr Med J 77: 528–530
65. Pawlowski ZS (1990) Cestodiases: taeniasis, cysticercosis, diphyllobothriasis, hymenolepiasis and others. In: Warrren KS, Mahmoud AAF (ed) Tropical and geographic medicine, 2nd ed. New York, McGraw Hill, pp 490–504
66. Trujillo-Valdes VM, Gonzalez-Barranco D, Orozco-Bohne R, et al (1981) Experimental treatment of cysticercosis with metrifonate. Arch Invest Med 12: 15–28
67. Skromme-Kadlubik G, Celis C (1981) Cysticercosis of the nervous system: treatment by means of specific internal radiation. Arch Neurol 38: 288
68. Tellez-Giron E, Ramos MC, Dufour L, et al (1984) Treatment of neurocysticercosis with flubendazole. Am J Trop Med Hyg 33: 627–631
69. Torres JR (1989) Use of praziquantel in populations at risk of neurocysticercosis (Letter). Rev Inst Med Trop Sao Paulo 31: 290

70. Nemeth DJ (1989) Commentary: a study of the interactions of human, pig and the human pork tapeworm. Anthrozoos 3: 4–13
71. Salazar-Schettino PM (1983) Customs which predispose to Chagas' disease and cysticercosis in Mexico. Am J Trop Med Hyg. 1983;32:1179-80.
72. Richards F, Schantz PM (1984) Cysticercosis and taeniasis (Letter). N Engl J Med 312: 787
73. Sarti-Gutierrez EJ, Schantz PM, Lara-Aquilera R, et al (1988) *Taenia solium* taeniasis and cysticercosis in a Mexican village. Trop Med Parasitol 39: 194–198
74. Flisser A (1988) Neurocysticercosis in Mexico. Parasitol Today 4: 131–136
75. Gracia F, Chavarria R, Archibold C, et al (1990) Neurocysticercosis in Panama: preliminary epidemiologic study in the Azuero region. Am J Trop Med Hyg 42: 67–69
76. Sacks LV, Berkowitz I (1990) Cysticercosis in an urban black South African community: prevalence and risk factors. Trop Gastroenterol 11: 30–33
77. Schantz PM (1989) Surveillance and control programs for cestode diseases. In: Miller MJ, Love EJ (eds) Parasitic diseases: treatment and control. Florida, CRC Press, Inc, pp 275–290
78. Medina MT, Rosas E, Rubio-Donnadieu F, Sotelo J(1990) Neurocysticercosis as the main cause of late-onset epilepsy in Mexico. Arch Intern Med 150: 325–327
79. Gernmen M, Matayas Z, Pawlowski Z, et al (eds) (1983) Guidelines for Surveillance, Prevention and Control of Taeniasis/Cysticercosis. VPH/83.49. Geneva, WHO, pp 69–75
80. Muller R, Linywhite J, Bending JJ, Catford JC (1987) Human cysticercosis and intestinal parasitism amongst the Ekari people of Irian Jaya. J Trop Med Hyg 90: 291–296
81. Kent DL, Larson EB (1988) Magnetic resonance imaging of the brain and spine. Ann Intern Med 108: 402–424
82. Suss RA, Maravilla KR, Thompson J (1986) MR imaging of intracranial cysticercosis: comparison with CT and anatomopathologic features. AJNR 7: 235–242
83. Zee CS, Segall HD, Boswell W, et al (1988) MR imaging of neurocysticercosis. J Comp Assist Tomography 12: 927–934
84. Teitelbaum GP, Otto RJ, Lin M, et al (1989) MR imaging of neurocysticercosis. AJR 153: 857–866
85. Martinez HR, Rangel-Guerra R, Elizondo G, et al (1989) MR imaging in neurocysticercosis. AJNR 10: 1011–1019
86. Lotz J, Hewlett R, Alheit B, Bowen R (1988) Neurocysticercosis: correlative pathomorphology and MR imaging. Neuroradiol 30: 35–41
87. Sarti-Gutierrez E, Schantz PM, Plancarte A, et al (1991) Prevalence and risk factors for *Taenia solium* taeniasis and cysticercosis in humans and pigs in a village in Morelos, Mexico. Am J Trop Med Hyg (in press)
88. Diaz F, Garcia HH, Gilman R, et al (1991) Epidemiology of taeniasis and cysticercosis in a Peruvian tropical village. Am J Epidemiol (in press)
89. Garcia HH, Martinez M, Gilman R, et al (1991) Diagnosis of cysticercosis in endemic regions. Lancet 338: 549–551
90. Gonzalez AE, Cama V, Gilman RH, et al (1990) Prevalence and comparison of serologic assays, necropsy, and tongue examination for the diagnosis of porcine cysticercosis in Peru. Am J Trop Med Hyg 43: 194–199
91. Acosta E (1990) Antibodies to the metacestode of *Taenia solium* in the saliva from patients with neurocysticercosis. J Clin Lab Anal 4: 90–44
92. Correa D, Sandoval MA, Harrison LJS, et al (1989) Human neurocysticercosis: comparison of enzyme immunoassay capture techniques based on monoclonal and polyclonal antibod-ies for the detection of parasite products in cerebrospinal fluid. Trans Roy Soc Trop Med Hyg 83: 814–816
93. Choromanski L Estrada JJ, Kuhn RE (1990) Detection of antigens of larval *Taenia solium* in the cerebrospinal fluid of patients with the use of HPLC and ELISA. J Parasitol 76: 69–73
94. Rishi AK, McManus DP (1987) DNA probes which unambiguously distinguish *Taenia solium* from Taenia saginata (Letter). Lancet 1275–1276
95. Flisser A, Reid A, Garcia-Zepeda E, McManus DP (1988) Specific detection of *Taenia saginata* eggs by DNA hybridization (Letter). Lancet 1429–1430

96. Flisser A, Plancarte A, Correa D, et al (1990) New approaches in the diagnosis of *Taenia solium* cysticercosis and taeniasis. Ann Parasitol Hum Comp 65 [Suppl 1]: 95–98
97. Escobedo F, Penagos P, Rodriguez J, Sotelo J (1987) Albendazole therapy for neurocysticercosis. Arch Intern Med 147: 738–741
98. Escobedo F, Sotelo J, Penagos P, Rodriguez J, Del Brutto O (1989) Albendazole therapy for human neurocysticercosis, a controlled study with computerized tomography and magnetic resonance. Acta Leidensia 57: 247–254
99. Sotelo J, Penagos P, Escobedo F, Del Brutto OH (1988) Short course of albendazole therapy for neurocysticercosis. Arch Neurol 45: 1130–1133
100. Carpio A, Santiillan F, Leon P, Borreo A, Tinoco (1988) New treatment of brain cysticercosis with albendazole (Abstract). Ann Neurol 24: 144
101. Agapejev S, Meira DA, Barraviera B, et al (1988) Neurocysticercosis: treatment with albendazole and dextrochlorpheniramine (preliminary report). Rev Inst Med Trop Sao Paulo 30: 387–389
102. Gupta R, Yupta NV (1990) Failure of praziquantel and albendazole in neurocysticercosis. JAPI 38: 313–314
103. Del Brutto OH, Sotelo J (1990) Albendazole therapy for subarachnoid and ventricular cysticercosis. J Neurosurg 72: 816–817
104. Jung H, Hurtado M, Medina MT, Sanchez M, Sotelo J (1990) Dexamethasone increases plasma levels of albendazole. J Neurol 237: 279–280
105. Quintero-Rodriquez E (1989) Praziquantel vs. albendazole for cysticercosis (Letter). Neurosurgery 23: 128
106. Johnson KS, Harrison GB, Lightowlers MW, et al (1989) Vaccination against ovine cysticercosis using a defined recombinant antigen (Letter). Nature 338: 585–587
107. Mitchell GH (1989) A vaccine for ovine cysticercosis (Editorial). Vaccine 7: 379
108. Richards FO, Schantz PM, Ruiz-Tiben E, Sorvillo FJ (1985) Cysticercosis in Los Angeles County. JAMA 254: 3444–3448
109. Sorvillo FJ, Waterman SH, Richards FO, Schantz PM (1992) Cysticercosis surveillance: locally acquired and travel-related infections and detection of intestinal tapeworm carriers in Los Angeles county. Am J Trop Med Hyg (in press)
110. Centers for Disease Control (1992) Locally acquired neurocysticercosis – North Carolina, Massachusetts, and South Carolina, 1989–1991. MMWR 41: 1–4
111. Mata L (1982) Sociocultural factors in the control and prevention of parasitic diseases. Rev Infect Dis 4: 871–879

Antigenic Variation in Borrelial Diseases of Humans

Alan G. Barbour

Departments of Medicine and Microbiology, The University of Texas Health Science Center, San Antonio, Texas , U.S.A.

Introduction

Relapsing fever and Lyme disease are human infections caused by different members of the spirochetal genus *Borrelia* (1). In both diseases a spirochetemia in the vertebrate is the source of infection for the arthropod. One presumes that a bacterium persisting in the blood of the vertebrate longer than another bacterium would have a selective advantage over its more short-lived siblings. It is not surprising, therefore, to find that one of the strategies used by borrelias to achieve this persistence in the host is antigenic variation.

Antigenic variation has been a well-known feature of the pathogenesis of relapsing fever for decades. More recently it has been recognized that *Borrelia burgdorferi*, the agent of Lyme disease, also can vary its surface antigens. In this chapter the biology and molecular biology of antigenic variation of the pathogens in relapsing fever and Lyme disease are compared.

Ecology and Epidemiology

Spirochetes constitute a separate division of eubacteria and are no closer to Gram-negative bacteria than they are to Gram-positive bacteria and cyanobacteria in the taxonomy based on ribosomal RNA sequences (2). Spirochetes are characterized morphologically by a helical shape, two membranes, and flagella that extend longitudinally between the membranes (3). The genus *Borrelia* was originally distinguished from other spirochetes by their arthropod-association. All members of this genus are transmitted from vertebrate to vertebrate by arthropods (1).

The existence of relapsing fever was noted by Hippocrates, who included this form of fever in a group of fevers he called "typhus" (4). It was not until Obermeier in 1873 in Berlin identified spirochetes in the blood of patients with relapsing fever, though, that relapsing fever was clearly distinguished from other louse-borne infections called typhus (5). At first the etiologic agent of relapsing fever was named "*Spirochaeta recurrentis*". Later it was given the genus name *Borrelia* in honor of A. Borrel of France (6). Presently the term *Borrelia recurrentis* is used to describe borrelias causing louse-borne or epidemic relapsing fever (7). There are several species that cause tick-borne or endemic relapsing fever. The tick-associated species have, up to recently, been distinguished primarily on the basis of host and vector specificity (1).

Whereas relapsing fever was known to the ancients, another borrelial infection of humans and animals, Lyme disease, has only within the last century been noted in the medical literature. Lyme disease, or, as it is also known, Lyme borreliosis, is a common tick-borne disease of humans and domestic animals in the temperate regions of the Northern hemisphere. In the United States and much of Europe, Lyme disease is now the most common arthropod-borne disease (8). This zoonotic spirochetal infection may be brief and mild or chronic and severely disabling. The skin, joints, nervous system, heart, eye, and muscles may be affected. Like syphilis, Lyme disease may resemble several other diseases.

The major features of this infection, including its tick-borne nature, were recognized by physicians in Europe and Russia several decades ago. Although the occurrence of the infection in North America appears to be more recent, the disease derives its name from a town in Connecticut. In 1975, Steere and colleagues described an epidemic of arthritis in residents of Lyme, Connecticut (9). The illness, which was called "Lyme arthritis", was soon recognized to be similar to the tick-borne diseases, erythema migrans and Bannwarth's syndrome, described in the European and Russian medical literature. The primary vectors for these syndromes are members of the *Ixodes* genus of ticks: *I. ricinus* in Europe and Russia, *I. persulcatus* in Russia and Asia, and *I. dammini* in North America.

Until 1981, the etiology of Lyme disease was unknown. In that year a new spirochete was discovered in *Ixodes dammini* ticks, cultivated in the laboratory, and shown to be the likely agent of Lyme disease (10). Subsequently, it was isolated from patients, reservoir mammals, and ill domestic animals (11). DNA hybridization studies indicated that the newly discovered agent was in the genus *Borrelia* but different from all other known borrelial species. This hitherto unknown borrelia was given the species name *B. burgdorferi* in honor of Willy Burgdorfer, one of the discoverers of the agent.

Pathogenesis and Immunity

Antigenic Variation in Relapsing Fever

After the discovery of the etiologic agent of relapsing fever, turn-of-the-century microbiologists and immunologists, including Paul Ehrlich, were attracted to a pathogen that seemed to be the match for the newly-described immune system (12). In relapsing fever the etiologic spirochetes avoid complete clearance from the host's bloodstream; consequently, the disease may persist for several weeks (13). This persistent illness is uniquely characterized by a periodic rise and fall of the body temperature about every 4 to 7 days. The periodicity is a function of multiphasic antigenic variation: one antigen is replaced by one of a repertoire of different antigens during the course of an infection.

Although the chemical identity of the variable antigens was unknown at the time, early investigators of this phenomenon did have antisera that were specific for different relapse variants (14, 15). With a set of variant-specific antisera, the changes in a relapsing fever species of *Borrelia* could be tracked in experimental animals. In a typical experiment of this kind, a laboratory mouse is infected with a single borrelia (16). After the initial mouse suffers a relapse of spirochetemia, a second, immunologically naive animal is inoculated with the relapse variant. The experimenters found that an organism identical to the one that was inoculated into the first animal could be recovered from the second animal during one of the latter animal's relapses of illness. In other words, if the original isolate was serotype X and the first animal's relapse isolate was serotype Y, serotype X could be recovered from the second animal after it had been eliminated from the blood of the first animal. To put it even more succinctly: the hereditary information for making the antigen that specified serotype X was not lost from the cells, even when they displayed features of another serotype, such as Y.

This experimental finding indicated that antigenic variation was not the result of stepwise mutations accumulating within the host animal. Instead the results suggested that there were different alleles of the genes determining serotype-specificity. The borreliae were polymorphic in their surface coats in the same way that Mendel's sweetpeas were polymorphic with respect to color or petal shape.

If a gene that specifies one serotype is retained in a borrelia displaying different serotypic determinants, there must be a mechanism for activating a new gene without losing in the process the information necessary to express the original serotypic determinant. To understand this mechanism, we have studied the antigenic variation of a North American agent of relapsing fever, *Borrelia hermsii*. We started from the base provided by Herbert Stoenner (16). Over several years, Dr. Stoenner painstakingly isolated 24 different isogeneic serotypes of *B. hermsii* strain HS1 and produced the serospecific-antisera for each one of them.

Using this collection of microorganisms and antibodies, we identified the serotype-specific antigens of *B. hermsii*. They are abundant lipoproteins anchored in the outer membrane of the borreliae and exposed at the surface (17–20). These lipoproteins were entitled Variable Major Proteins, or Vmp's and further identified with the number or letter of serotype, as in the example "Vmp7" of serotype 7.

Subsequent studies of two particular serotypes 7 and 21, gave further details of the mechanism of antigen switching (21). In these serotypes the respective genes for each Vmp lipoprotein, that is *vmp*7 for Vmp7 and *vmp*21 for Vmp21, could be found in two different "environments": silent and ac-

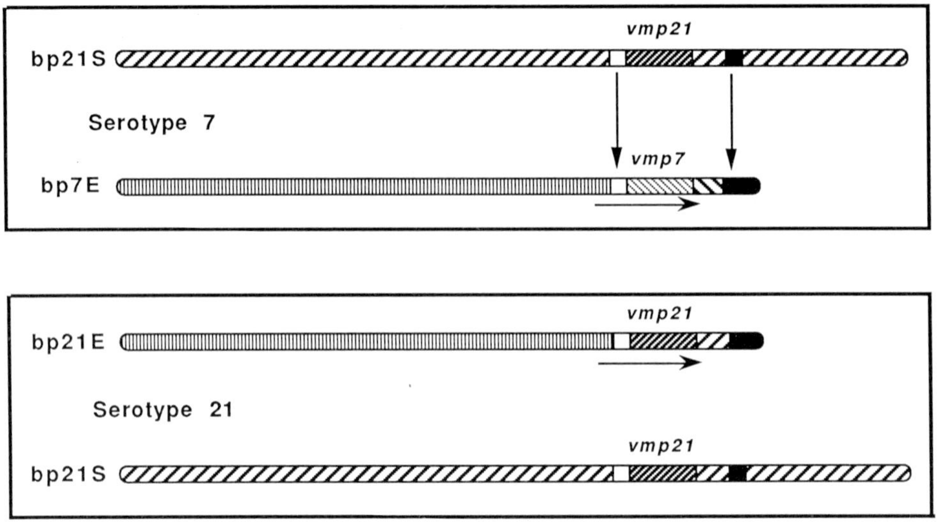

Fig. 1. An antigenic switch from serotype 7 to 21 by a cell of *Borrelia hermsii.* In the gene conversion, a silent *vmp*21 gene (dark cross-hatched pattern from bottom left to top right) and its 3' flanking region, which are located on the silent plasmid bp21S, replaces an active *vmp*7 gene (light cross-hatched pattern from bottom right to top left) on the expression plasmid bp7E. In the process, the expression plasmid bp21E is created and bp21S is retained. The switch is unidirectional and nonreciprocal. The boundaries of the recombination are two regions of homology upstream and downstream of the gene and, respectively, represented by white and black boxes.

tive. In cells of serotype 7, there was one genomic environment for *vmp*21 and two environments for the *vmp*7 gene; these environments were revealed in southern blot analysis. In cells of serotype 21 the opposite situation was found: one environment for *vmp7* and two for *vmp*21. These experiments showed that there were expression-linked copies of the *vmp* genes. Whatever *vmp* gene was found at the expression locus was the active one.

The switch itself is effectively nonreciprocal and unidirectional (21, 22). It occurs between two linear plasmids, one of which carries the silent *vmp* gene and the other carries the active gene (22). The active gene is near the end, or telomere, of the linear plasmid (23). In contrast, the silent genes that have been examined to date are located several kilobases away from the telomeres of the plasmids that bear them.

The recombination has the features of gene conversion, more specifically, telomere conversion. According to this model, the incoming silent *vmp* sequence "converts" the locus at the active telomeric site. In the process the old *vmp* gene copy at expression site appears to be destroyed. To provide for expression of the original active *vmp* gene in future generations of the population, the silent version of that gene is retained in each cell. The figure shows a simple version of how this model operates. In the switch illustrated, a single cell of *B. hermsii* changes from serotype 7 to serotype 21. The expression plasmids bp7E (serotype 7) and bp21E (serotype 21) and another plasmid bearing the silent *vmp*21 gene (both serotype 7 and 21) are shown. Not shown in the schematic representation is a third plasmid bearing the silent *vmp*7 gene. This third plasmid does not participate in the recombination, but it does serve as the repository of the hereditary information for the population to produce serotype 7 cells in the future.

The boundaries for the recombination are two homology blocks on either side of the *vmp* genes at their silent and active sites (23, 24). These are shown in the figure as the white and black boxes upstream and downstream of the *vmp*. The downstream homology block, represented by the black box, extends to within 50 bases of the telomere of the expression plasmid (23).

The expression site itself contains a *vmp* gene promoter that is lacking at the silent sites (24). Thus, the method of *vmp* gene activation in *B. hermsii* is promoter addition rather than removal of *vmp* gene from cis-acting repression on a silent plasmid. The initiating event in the activation remains to be defined, but it most likely is a single- or double-strand break of the expression-linked plasmid in the region of the *vmp* gene (25) Tandemly-arrayed insertion sequence-like elements have been found just upstream of active *vmp* genes on the expression plasmids (26). These elements are possibly the determinants of strand breakage on the expression plasmid.

Antigenic Variation in Lyme Disease

Noting the genetic relatedness between *B. burgdorferi* and the relapsing fever borreliae, one could reasonably ask whether a comparable degree of antigenic variation occurs in infections caused by *B. burgdorferi.* Studies to date suggest that if antigenic variation does occur during the course of *B. burgdorferi* infections it is of different type and magnitude than that of relapsing fever.

During *B. burgdorferi* infections in different mammals, including humans, spirochete numbers in the blood are orders of magnitude lower than what is found in relapsing fever (11). Nevertheless, these numbers may rise and fall in a pattern similar to what is seen in relapsing fever. In studies of infections of rabbits, cotton rats, gerbils, and mice, there has been evidence of fluctuation of spirochete numbers in the blood during the course of infections measured in weeks (27–29). Evidence that antigenic variation occurs during more chronic infections comes from a study of Lyme disease patients. Craft et al. found that some patients with Lyme disease exhibited the new appearance of OspB-specific immunoglobulin M antibodies a year or more after infection (30).

Strictly speaking, the phrase "antigenic variation" should only be applied to clonal populations of organisms that manifest antigenic changes during multiplication. This variation of the antigens may or may not be the consequence of alterations in the DNA. If the antigen switch is at the level of transcription, the genetic alteration may or may not be reversible. In any case, the variation in antigens occurs *de novo* in either an animal host or in culture medium. The ability to switch or otherwise regulate surface antigen expression would seem to confer selective advantage to pathogenic microorganisms against which animals can direct a very specific immune response.

The majority of studies looking at the heterogeneity of antigens of *B. burgdorferi* have been of large and small collections of strains from different geographic locations. In these studies differences in the antigenic makeup of the strains have been noted. But, inasmuch as this is not antigenic variation as defined above, a review of all these findings is beyond the scope of the present survey. Instead this chapter will focus on two major outer membrane lipoproteins, named OspA and OspB (31–34). These proteins are analogous to the Vmp proteins of *B. hermsii* and to the variable surface antigens of African trypanosomes, which also use the strategy of antigenic variation (20). We made the assumption that these outer membrane proteins would have a featured if not preeminent role in antigenic variation of *B. burgdorferi.*

Other evidence that leads us to suspect a role for OspA and/or OspB in antigenic variation are the aforementioned surveys of polymorphisms in the OspA and OspB proteins among different strains from different geographic locations. Differences in the molecular sizes and antibody reactivities of both OspA and OspB were demonstrated in these studies (35–44). In some strains either OspA or OspB appeared not to be produced at all.

The next level of examination of the phenomenon of Osp lipoprotein differences was that of individual strains that had been passed in vitro for various times. We had noted a change in the monoclonal reactivity of the original isolate of *B. burgdorferi,* B31 (35). This isolate was designated strain B31. Whereas the low passage isolate of B31 reacted with OspB-specific monoclonal antibody H5TS, a later passage of this strain did not. This change in antibody reactivity was associated with a difference in the relative migration of the OspB in polyacrylamide gels between the two isolates of B31. In subsequent studies Wilske et al. found that a European isolate had decreased production of both OspB and OspA during serial passage in the laboratory (38). Schwan et al. later found that white-footed field mice (*Peromyscus leukopus*) inoculated with a high-passage strain had a diminished antibody response to the OspA protein when compared with field mice infected with a low-passage strain (45).

Schwan and Burgdorfer and Schwan et al. expanded upon these observations and sampled populations of North American isolates over time during serial passages in broth medium (46, 47). These investigators demonstrated alterations in the OspB as well as in a lower molecular weight protein of *B. burgdorferi.* Although the original inoculum for these studies was obtained directly from a tick and hence may not have been clonal, these investigators confirmed that certain phenotypes of Osp proteins can be selected for during *in vitro* growth.

When truly clonal populations of *B. burgdorferi* were examined, the phenomenon of OspB antigenic variation was observed *in vitro* (48). Clones of a *B. burgdorferi* strain isolated from human blood differed in the size and antibody reactivity of their OspB proteins and also in lower molecular weight proteins which shared antigenic epitopes with full-length OspB proteins. There was one clone that phenotypically resembled one of the variants described by Schwan et al. in completely lacking a full-length OspB protein (47).

In these studies OspA was unchanged among all the clonal populations. There is evidence from other sources, though, that this protein also can be polymorphic. Bissett and Hill isolated from a California tick a strain of *B. burgdorferi* that did not express an immunoreactive OspA after passage in the laboratory (40). The OspA variant produced instead a lower molecular weight protein that did not bind OspA-specific monoclonal antibodies. Wilske et al. reported a European isolate of *B. burgdorferi* that was observed to express an OspA-type protein after losing this ability during *in vitro* cultivation (39). In this latter study, all of the isolates produced a protein of approximately 20–24 kDa, which had been designated "pC" (38). There seemed to be a relationship between OspA and pC: when OspA was being produced by the population of borreliae there was less pC detectable. Interestingly, Luft et al. reported a 22 kDa protein of a North American strain of *B. burgdorferi* that has an N-terminal amino acid sequence similar to that of OspA of strain B31 (49). Whether this low-molecular weight protein of North American isolates of *B. burgdorferi* is related to the pC protein of European strains remains to be determined.

In our own studies of North American and European isolates of *B. burgdorferi*, we found that even those isolates that did not express an OspA-type protein had DNA sequences highly similar to those of the genes for OspA proteins (36, 50). Among those isolates that do produce an OspA-type protein, there is considerable antigenic cross-reactivity between OspA proteins and similarity between *ospA* genes (36, 39, 50–52).

The mechanisms for the confirmed antigenic variation in OspB and the possible antigenic variation of OspA are beginning to be understood. In contrast to the circumstance in *B. hermsii*, there appears to be only one environment for major outer membrane protein genes, *ospA* and *ospB* (36, 48, 53, 54). When restriction digests of *B. burgdorferi* DNA were probed with either *ospB* or *ospA* sequences, only the locus at which expression occurs was hybridized by the probes. There appeared to be no silent versions of *ospA* and *ospB* elsewhere in the genomes of North American strains of *B. burgdorferi*. This may not be the case, though, with other antigens of this microorganism. Hindersson et al. found evidence of restriction fragment length polymorphisms and duplications of a sequence encoding another antigen of *B. burgdorferi* (55).

The clonal variants in OspB described above did not have large deletions, insertion sequences, or rearrangements in the osp operon or its flanking regions (48). Moreover, the variant cells produced full-length mRNA for OspA and OspB even when OspB was truncated or not detectable. A similar type of variation has been noted in expression of the gene for flagellin, the major structural component of *B. burgdorferi* flagella (56). These variants in OspB and flagellin expression may be the consequence of nonsense or frameshift mutations occurring in the coding region for OspB.

Other types of mutations that possibly could decrease OspB or flagellin expression after transcription are changes in the ribosome-binding sites, modification of tRNA to the point that codon usage is altered, and increased production of an anti-sense RNA to specific transcripts.

There is another difference between *B. hermsii* and *B. burgdorferi* in regard to the genes for their major outer membrane lipoproteins. Like *B. hermsii*, *B. burgdorferi* has its genes for outer membrane lipoproteins arrayed on linear plasmids (53). However, in contrast to the situation in *B. hermsii* (23), the active outer membrane protein genes of *B. burgdorferi* are located several kilobases away from the plasmid's telomere (54, 57). The significance of this difference is unknown.

Comparison of Relapsing Fever and Lyme Disease

Given the current knowledge of the processes of antigenic variation in relapsing fever and Lyme disease, can conclusions be drawn on how the etiologic agents of these disease differ in this regard? Although much more obviously remains to be determined, distinctions between *B. hermsii* and *B. burgdorferi* in the biology and molecular biology of antigenic variation are emerging.

Antigenic variation in the relapsing fever species *B. hermsii* has the following distinguishing features: (i) Numerous organisms are found in the blood of infected animals during relapses. (ii) There is a large repertoire of variable antigens with little cross-reactivity among them. (iii) A gene switch for a different variable antigen is accomplished by a recombination that is effectively telomere conversion; the formerly silent gene is activated by being placed downstream from a promoter. In its biology, immunology, and molecular biology, relapsing fever is remarkably similar to African trypanosomiasis, which is caused by an organism in another kingdom (23).

Antigenic variation observed to date in *B. burgdorferi* appears not to have any of these characteristics, or at least not to the same degree of development as found in B. *hermsii*. For one thing there are substantially fewer borreliae detectable in the blood during all stages of Lyme disease than what is seen in relapsing fever (14, 29). As a consequence there may not be the need for a large collection of antigenically distinct surface proteins in *B. burgdorferi*. *B. burgdorferi* appears to make do with two or perhaps three major surface proteins: OspA, OspB, and pC or other lower-molecular weight protein of 20–22 kDa.

With its lower total cellular mass in the blood during infection, a population of *B. burgdorferi* may escape immune recognition for a longer period of time than *B. hermsii*, which is highly populous in the blood during the acute illness. Moreover, the Lyme disease agent may employ a different mechanism from that of the relapsing fever borrelia. Instead of switching between different antigen genes, *B. burgdorferi* may at times not express at all a gene for major outer membrane protein. This has been observed in vitro. During animal and human infections, this would be an effective strategy to evade antibody-mediated neutralization. Whatever its form, variation of the major surface antigens of *B. burgdorferi* appears to be achieved not by major DNA rearrangements but by more subtle alterations in the genome.

If relapsing fever can be compared with African trypanosomiasis, one may reasonable compare Lyme disease with another trypanosomal disease, one of New World heritage. In chronic Chagas' disease, like Lyme disease, there are few if any organisms detected in the blood of the patient. Furthermore, the disorders in chronic Chagas' disease are more attributable to tissue invasion and the consequent immune response than directly to parasites circulating in the blood. This also seems to be the case in Lyme disease. Indeed, it is conceivable that antigenic variation of *B. burgdorferi* not only serves the pathogen in its goal of avoiding the host's immune response but also leads to exacerbations in inflammation when the patient responds to the appearance of a new variant in a tissue, such as the joint synovium.

Prospects for Control by Immunization

Relapsing fever in North America and most other continents is a low-incidence, endemic disease that humans acquire from contact with ticks (1). There are several different strains and species of *Borrelia* that cause tick-borne relapsing fever throughout the world. It is likely that each species has a different repertoire of surface antigens. There is not a pressing public health need for a vaccine against tick-borne relapsing fever, and vaccine developers would have to choose among the several species to focus on.

In contrast, the epidemic form of relapsing fever, which is transmitted among humans by lice, is caused by a single species, *B. recurrentis*, and has in the past caused morbidity and death to millions of people. Consequently, if a vaccine against relapsing fever were to be developed, the highest priority would be a vaccine against the epidemic, louse-borne form of the disease. Not only would such a vaccine likely provide the most benefit to humankind, but also the developers could concentrate on a single species.

Nevertheless, investigators with ambitions in this area are still faced with several problems. Foremost is the inability to cultivate *B. recurrentis in vitro* or even in experimental animals (11). Humans, and perhaps other primates, appear to be the only hosts capable of supporting growth of this borrelia. Because of this considerable technical impediment, little is known about the antigens of *B. recurrentis*. Furthermore, even if one knew more about the surface antigens of this species, this organism, like *B. hermsii*, probably has the ability to express any number of different antigens on its surface. Wouldbe vaccine developers would either have to provide a multivalent vaccine or identify another antigen that is capable of eliciting immunity but does not undergo antigenic variation.

The situation appears somewhat more hopeful with regard to a vaccine against Lyme disease. Although, as discussed above, *B. burgdorferi* shows evidence of antigenic variation, it seems of a different order of magnitude than what is observed in relapsing fever. Thus, the number of different antigens that many need to be included in a Lyme disease vaccine would predictably be a manageable number.

A compelling case can be made for a vaccine to prevent *B. burgdorferi* infection in persons in geographic areas, such as the northeast United States, with a high incidence of Lyme disease. Although the early form of Lyme disease responds well to antibiotic therapy, many patients with the late form of the disease, during which morbidity can be considerable, are helped little or, at best, very slowly by antibiotics. Moreover, the long-term consequences of latent *B. burgdorferi* infection are only now being revealed.

While the future prospects for a Lyme disease vaccine are greater than for a vaccine against relapsing fever, there are other considerations that may slow final application of such a vaccine, even if it is successful in small trials. First is the concern about the elicitation of autoimmune reactions by a vaccine. Because so much of the pathology in Lyme disease appears attributable to the host's immune response to the organisms, there is reason to suspect that some vaccinees may experience arthritic or neurologic disease in response to one or more vaccine components. For protection against a disease with an extremely low case-fatality rate, as has Lyme disease, such untoward vaccine reactions, even if at a low frequency, would be unacceptable. The answer to this potential problem is use of single components, preferably recombinant in origin, which had been thoroughly investigated and tested to minimize induction of deleterious immune responses. Single component vaccines may not be as effective as vaccines based upon whole cells or multiple components, though.

The other difficulty for developers of Lyme disease vaccines would be the assessment of vaccine efficacy in field trials. One of the biggest present problems in Lyme disease patient care and epidemiologic research is verification of infection. Generally, the diagnostic measures that are widely used to provide evidence for infection are not satisfactory at this time. If this condition holds, it will not be easy to evaluate whether the vaccine is effective or not. The vaccine trials may need to use large numbers of volunteers and to follow them for several years before we can conclude whether it will provide greater benefit than its costs.

References

1. Barbour AG, Hayes SF (1986) Biology of *Borrelia* species. Microbiol Rev 50: 381–400
2. Woese CR (1987) Bacterial evolution. Microbiol Rev 51: 221–271
3. Holt SC (1978) Anatomy and chemistry of spirochetes. Microbiol Rev 42: 114–160
4. Saint Giron I, Barbour AG (1991) Antigenic variation in Borrelia. Res Microbiol 142: 114–160
5. Obermeier O (1873) Vorkommen feinster eine Eigenbewegung zeigender Faden im Blute von Rekurrenskranken. Zentralbl Med Wiss 11: 145–155
6. Swellengrebel NH (1907) Sur la cytologie compare des spirochetes et des spirilles. Ann Inst Pasteur 21: 562–586
7. Nicolle C, Blaizot L, Conseil E (1913) Etiologie de la fievre recurrente. Son mode de transmission par les poux. Ann Inst Pasteur 27: 204–225
8. Schmid GP (1985) The global distribution of Lyme disease. Rev Infect Dis 7: 41–50

9. Steere AC, Malawista SE, Syndman DR (1977) Lyme arthritis: an epidemic of oligo-articular arthritis in children and adults in three Connecticut communities. Arthritis Rheum 20: 7–17
10. Burgdorfer W, Barbour AG, Hayes SF, Benach JL, Grunwaldt E, Davis JP (1982) Lyme disease – a tick-borne spirochetosis? Science 216: 1317–1319
11. Barbour AG (1988a) Laboratory aspects of Lyme disease. Clin Microbiol Rev 1: 399–414
12. Barbour AG (1987) Immunobiology of relapsing fever. Contrib Microbiol Immmunol 8: 125–137
13. Barbour AG (1990) Antigenic variation of a relapsing fever *Borrelia* species. Ann Rev Microbiol 44: 155–171
14. Goldsmid JM, Mahomed K(1972) The use of the microhematocrit technique for the recovery of *Borrelia duttonii* from the blood. Am J Clin Pathol 58: 165–169
15. Coffey EM, Evelund WC (1967) Experimental relapsing fever initiated by *Borrelia hermsii.* II. Sequential appearance of major serotypes in the rat. J Infect Dis 117: 29–34
16. Stoenner HG, Todd T, Larsen C (1982) Antigenic variation of *Borrelia hermsii.* J Exp Med 156: 1297–1311
17. Barbour AG, Barrera O, Judd RC (1983) Structural analysis of the variable major proteins of *Borrelia hermsii.* J Exp Med 158: 2127–2140
18. Barbour AG, Tessier SL, Stoenner HG (1982) Variable major proteins of *Borrelia hermsii.* J Exp Med 156: 1312–1324
19. Barstad PA, Coligan JE, Raum MG, Barbour AG (1985) Variable major proteins of *Borrelia hermsii:* epitope mapping and partial sequence analysis of CNBr peptides. J Exp Med 161: 1302–1314
20. Burman NS, Bergström S, Restrepo BI, Barbour AG (1990) The variable antigens Vmp7 and Vmp21 of the relapsing fever bacterium *Borrelia hermsii* are structurally analogous to the VSG proteins of the African trypanosome. Mol Microbiol 4: 1715–1726
21. Meier JT, Simon MI, Barbour AG (1985) Antigenic variation is associated with DNA rearrangements in a relapsing fever *Borrelia* sp. Cell 41: 403–409
22. Plasterk RHA, Simon MI, Barbour AG (1985) Transposition of structural genes to an expression sequence on a linear plasmid causes antigenic variation in *Borrelia hermsii.* Nature (London) 318: 257–263
23. Kitten T, Barbour AG (1990) Juxtaposition of expressed variable antigen genes with a conserved telomere in the bacterium *Borrelia hermsii.* Proc Natl Acad Sci (USA) 87: 6077–6081
24. Barbour AG, Burman N, Carter CJ, Kitten T, Bergström S (1991a) Variable antigen genes of the relapsing fever agent *Borrelia hermsii* are activated by promoter addition. Mol Microbiol 5: 489–493
25. Barbour AG (1989) Antigenic variation in a relapsing fever Borrelia: genetic aspects. In: Berg De, Howe MM (eds) Mobile DNA. Washington, American Society for Microbiology, 783–789
26. Barbour AG, Carter CJ, Burman N, Freitag CS, Garon CF, Bergström S (1991b) Tandem insertion sequence-like elements define the expression site for variable antigen genes of *Borrelia hermsii.* Infect Immun 59: 390–397
27. Burgdorfer W, Gage KL (1986) Susceptibility of the black-legged tick, *Ixodes scapularis,* to the Lyme disease spirochete, *Borrelia burgdorferi.* Zentralbl Bakteriol Parasitenkd Infektionskr Hyg Abt 1 Orig Reihe A 263: 15–20
28. Burgdorfer W, Gage KL (1987) Susceptibility of the hispid cotton rat (*Sigmodon hispidus*) to the Lyme disease spirochete (*Borrelia burgdorferi*). Am J Trop Med Hyg 37: 624–628
29. Stanek G, Burger I, Hirschl A, Wewalka G, Radda A (1986) Borrelia transfer by ticks during their life cycle. Studies of laboratory animals. Zentralbl Bakteriol Parasitenkd Infektionskr Hyg Abt 1 Orig Reihe A 263: 29–33
30. Craft JE, Fischer DK, Shimamoto GT, Steere AC (1986) Antigens of *Borrelia burgdorferi* recognized during Lyme disease. Appearance of a new IgM response and expansion of the IgG response late in illness. J Clin Invest 78: 934–939
31. Howe TR, Mayer LW, Barbour AG (1985) A single recombinant plasmid expressing two major outer surface proteins of the Lyme disease spirochete. Science 227: 645–646

32. Howe TR, LaQuier FW, Barbour AG (1986) Organization of genes encoding two outer membrane proteins of the Lyme disease agent *Borrelia burgdorferi* within a single transcriptional unit. Infect Immun 54: 207–212
33. Bergström S, Bundoc VG, Barbour AG (1989) Molecular analysis of linear plasmid-encoded major proteins, OspA and OspB, of the Lyme disease spirochete, *Borrelia burgdorferi*. Mol Microbiol 3: 479–486
34. Brandt ME, Riley BS, Radolf JD, Norgard MV (1990) Immunogenic integral membrane proteins of *Borrelia burgdorferi* are lipoproteins. Infect Immun 58: 983–989
35. Barbour AG, Tessier SL, Hayes SF (1984) Variation in a major surface protein of Lyme disease spirochetes. Infect Immun 45: 94–100
36. Barbour AG, Heiland RA, Howe TR (1985) Heterogeneity of major proteins in Lyme disease borreliae: a molecular analysis of North American and European isolates. J Infect Dis 152: 478–484
37. Barbour AG, Schrumpf ME (1986) Polymorphisms of major surface proteins of *Borrelia burgdorferi*. Zentralbl Bakteriol Hyg A 263: 83–91
38. Wilske B, Preac-Mursic V, Schierz G, Busch KV (1986) Immunochemical and immunological analysis of European *Borrelia burgdorferi* strains. Zentralbl Bakteriol Mikrobiol Hyg [A] 263: 92–102
39. Wilske B, Preac-Mursic V, Schier G, Kuhbeck R, Barbour AG, Kramer M (1988) Antigenic variability of *Borrelia burgdorferi*. Ann NY Acad Sci 539: 126–143
40. Bissett ML, Hill W (1987) Characterization of *Borrelia burgdorferi* strains isolated from *Ixodes pacificus* ticks in California. J Clin Microbiol 25: 2296–2301
41. Kryuchechnikov VN, Korenberg EI, Scherbakov SV, Yovalesky YuV, Levin ML (1988) Identification of Borrelia isolated in the USSR from *Ixodes persulcatus* schulze ticks. J Microbiol Epidemiol Immunobiol 12: 41–44
42. Anderson JF, Magnarelli LA, McAninch JB (1988) *Borrelia burgdorferi* antigenic variant isolated from *Ixodes dammini* from upstate New York. J Clin Microbiol 26: 2209–2212
43. Anderson JF, Magnarelli LA, LeFebvre RB, Andreadis TG, McAninch JB, Perng G-C, Johnson RC (1989) Antigenically variable *Borrelia burgdorferi* isolated from cotton-tail rabbits and *Ixodes dentatus* in rural and urban areas. J Clin Microbiol 27: 13–20
44. Lane RS, Pascocello JA (1989) Antigenic characteristics of *Borrelia burgdorferi* isolates from ixodid ticks in California. J Clin Microbiol 27: 2344–2349
45. Schwan TG, Kime KK, Schrumpf ME, Coe JE, Simpson WJ (1989) Antibody response in white-footed mice (*Peromyscus leukopus*) experimentally infected with the Lyme disease spirochete (*Borrelia burgdorferi*). Infect Immun 57: 3445–3451
46. Schwan TG, Burgdorfer W (1987) Antigenic changes of *Borrelia burgdorferi* as a result of *in vitro* cultivation. J Infect Dis 156: 852–853
47. Schwan TG, Burgdorfer W, Garon CF (1988) Changes in infectivity and plasmid profile of the Lyme disease spirochete *Borrelia burgdorferi* as a result of *in vitro* cultivation. Infect Immun 56: 1831–1836
48. Bundoc VG, Barbour AG (1989) Clonal polymorphisms of outer membrane protein OspB of *Borrelia burgdorferi*. Infect Immun 57: 2733–2741
49. Luft BJ, Jiang W, Munoz P, Dattwyler RJ, Gorevic PD (1989) Biochemical and immunological characterization of the surface proteins of *Borrelia burgdorferi*. Infect Immun 57: 3637–3645
50. Barbour AG (1988b) Plasmid analysis of *Borrelia burgdorferi*, the Lyme disease agent. J Clin Microbiol 26: 475–478
51. Barbour AG, Tessier SL, Todd WJ (1983) Lyme disease spirochetes and Ixodid tick spirochetes share a common surface antigenic determinant defined by a monoclonal antibody. Infect Immun 41: 795–804
52. Milch LJ, Barbour AG (1989) Analysis of North American and European isolates of *Borrelia burgdorferi* with antiserum to a recombinant antigen. J Infect Dis 160: 351–353
53. Barbour AG, Garon CF (1987) Linear plasmids of the bacterium *Borrelia burgdorferi* have covalently-closed ends. Science 237: 409–411
54. Barbour AG, Garon CF (1988) The genes encoding major surface proteins of *Borrelia burgdorferi* are located on a plasmid. Ann NY Acad Sci 539: 144–153

55. Hindersson P, Hansen K, Fjordvang H, Pallesen L (1990) Abstract #D-136. American Society for Microbiology Annual Meeting
56. Sadziene A, Thomas DD, Bundoc VG, Holt SC, Barbour AG (1991) A flagella-less mutant of *Borrelia burgdorferi:* structural, molecular, and in vitro functional characterization. J Clin Invest 88: 82–92
57. Hinnebusch J, Bergstrom S, Barbour AG (1990) Cloning and sequence analysis of linear plasmid telomeres of the bacterium *Borrelia burgdorferi*. Mol Microbiol 4: 811–820

Perspectives on Chagas Disease in Latin America and the United States

Louis V. Kirchhoff

Department of Internal Medicine, University of Iowa, and Department of Veterans Affairs Medical Center, Iowa City, Iowa, U.S.A.

Life Cycle of Trypanosoma Cruzi

A brief review of the life cycle of *T. cruzi* and the clinical manifestations and epidemiology of Chagas disease will facilitate an understanding of the public health problem caused by this organism. *T. cruzi* is a protozoan hemoflagellate that has a complex life cycle involving several parasite stages in hematophagous reduviid bugs and mammalian hosts (1, 2). Epimastigotes multiply in the midgut of the insect vector and transform to infective insect-derived metacyclic trypomastigotes in the hindgut. Transmission to humans occurs when metacyclic trypomastigotes in bug feces contaminate mucous membranes, conjunctivae or breaks in the skin and enter host macrophages and other cells. There, insect-derived metacyclic trypomastigotes transform into amastigotes, the proliferating form in the mammalian host. After several cycles of intracellular multiplication, amastigotes differentiate into bloodform trypomastigotes, which are then released as the host cell ruptures. Bloodform trypomastigotes penetrate adjacent cells and also spread hematogenously to distant tissues, especially cardiac muscle. After the acute phase of the infection is controlled by immune mechanisms, the parasite persists in low numbers for the life of the host, alternating asynchronously between intracellular amastigotes and circulating bloodform trypomastigotes. The cycle is completed when reduviids ingest blood containing trypomastigotes, which then differentiate into epimastigotes. All these parasite forms can be produced in the laboratory, and the occasional occurrence of laboratory accidents resulting in transmission is a persistent problem (3, 4). Vector-borne transmission of *T. cruzi* accounts for most new infections, but transmission by blood transfusion is common in some endemic countries (5, 6), and congenital transmission also occurs (7, 8).

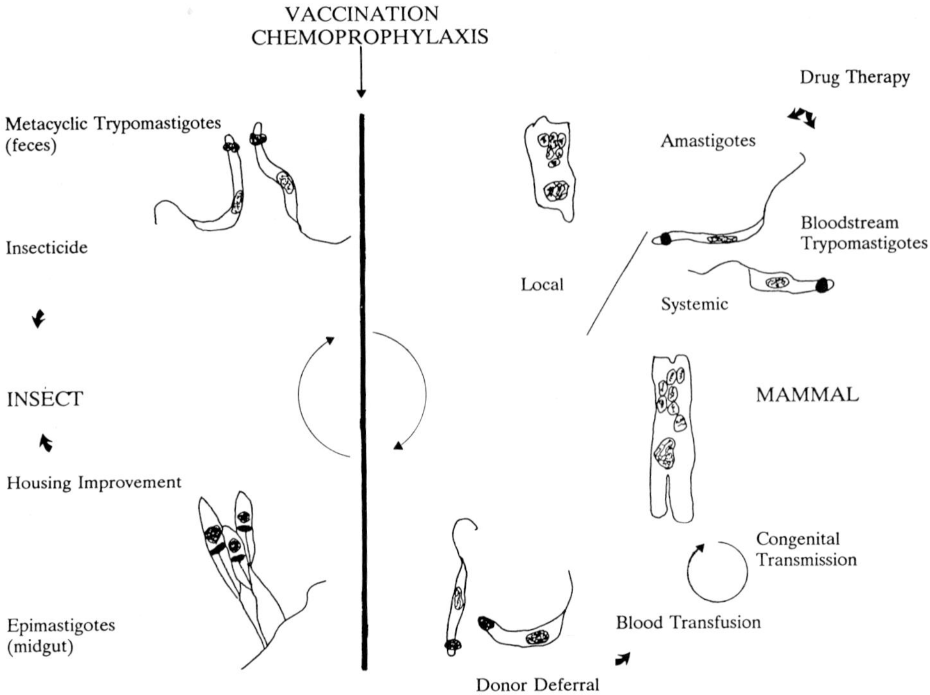

Fig. 1. Life cycle of *Trypanosoma cruzi*. Peripheral arrows indicate possible points of intervention to break the cycle of transmission

Clinical Manifestations and Pathology of Chagas Disease (American Trypanosomiasis)

Both acute and chronic Chagas disease can involve serious morbidity and death. Acute Chagas disease is usually a mild, febrile illness, but life-threatening heart failure, due to severe myocarditis, or meningo-encephalitis develops in a small proportion of patients (9, 10). In nearly all patients acute *T. cruzi* infection resolves over six to eight weeks as specific humoral and cellular responses to the parasite develop and control proliferation. Patients then enter the indeterminate phase of *T. cruzi* infection which is characterized by subpatent, life-long parasitemias and antibodies to a variety of parasite antigens. The persistence of *T. cruzi* in mammalian hosts may result in part because of immunosuppression induced by the parasite (reviewed in ref. 11). *In vitro* studies in which *T. cruzi* and lymphocytes from uninfected mice were cocultured have indicated that interleukin-2 (IL-2) production and expression of the IL-2 receptor are both suppressed (12–14). In other in vitro studies, expression of CD3, CD4, and CD8 markers on lymphocytes as well as the transferrin receptor were noted to be reduced in the presence of *T. cruzi* (15, 16). These findings provide initial perspectives on the complex interaction between *T. cruzi* and mammalian immune systems, and their relevance to chronic rather than acute disease and to humans instead of mice remain to be determined.

The symptoms of chronic Chagas disease become apparent years or even decades after the initial infection with *T. cruzi*. The heart is the organ most commonly involved, and sudden death due to arrhythmias often occurs (17) Cardiomyopathy may also develop, resulting in heart failure, thromboembolism and cerebrovascular accidents (18, 19). Megadisease (megaesophagus and/or megacolon) also occurs in infected patients and may cause life-threatening malnutrition and intractable constipation.

The development of symptomatic chronic Chagas disease is not the result of a reactivation of the persistent *T. cruzi* infection. From a parasitologic perspective patients with cardiac and/or gastrointestinal impairment associated with chronic *T. cruzi* infection are indistinguishable from those in the indeterminate phase. The pathogenesis of the lesions of chronic Chagas disease has been the object of considerable research for many years, and over the decades basically two schools of thought have developed. Köberle suggested that neuronal damage occurring during acute Chagas disease constitutes the fundamental pathogenic insult that years later results in the lesions of the chronic phase (20). In the second view, initially proposed by Cossio et al. (21) and Santos-Buch and Teixeira (22), autoimmunity is thought to play a major role. The role of autoimmunity in Chagas disease continues to be studied experimentally (23, 24) and debated (25–27).

Epidemiology

Infection with *T. cruzi* is a zoonosis, and the involvement of humans in the life cycle is not necessary for perpetuation of the organism in nature. *T. cruzi* exhibits little host specificity and is harbored by many species of reduviid bugs, as well as by a large number of non-human mammalian species such as armadillos and opossums (28). It is found in these hosts in all Latin American countries outside the Caribbean. Moreover, the existence of the sylvatic cycle of *T. cruzi* in western and southern areas of the United States has been well documented, and articles describing isolation of the parasite from vertebrate and non-vertebrate hosts in these areas continue to appear occasionally (29, 30).

The ability of *T. cruzi* to adapt to such a wide variety of animals, coupled with its life-long persistence in infected hosts, results in the existence of an enormous reservoir of parasites in enzootic regions. Humans typically become involved in the cycle of transmission when they build primitive houses in areas where the sylvatic cycle exists. Infected insects become domiciliary, taking up residence in the nooks and cracks of mud-walled houses that are common in poor, rural areas in much of Latin America. Humans are then exposed to *T. cruzi* as the insects fed upon them at night.

Chagas disease continues to be a major public health problem in Latin America. The World Health Organization recently estimated that 16 million persons harbor *T. cruzi* and that more than 50,000 people die each year of Chagas disease, for the most part due to the dysrhythmias and cardiomyopathies associated with chronic *T. cruzi* infection. Efforts to reduce transmission of *T. cruzi* to humans are primarily directed at reducing contact with vectors by spraying insecticides, installing screens, and plastering walls. Since the sylvatic reservoirs of *T. cruzi* are widespread and cannot be reasonably eliminated, control programs directed at reducing contact with vectors must remain active on a long-term basis as long as marginal housing conditions exist. Furthermore, identification of infected donors in blood banks by serologic screening is important in controlling transmission of *T. cruzi* (31–33). These two approaches currently offer the best hope for the control of Chagas disease, since no effective chemo- or immunoprophylactic agents are available.

In recent years large numbers of people have entered the United States from Central America, where the prevalence of *T. cruzi* infection is high, and the results of a recent study suggest that there may be 50,000–100,000 infected individuals now living in the United States (34). The presence of these infected immigrants here poses the risk of transfusion-associated transmission of *T. cruzi*, and three such cases have occurred recently (35–38). Moreover, immunosuppression of patients who harbor *T. cruzi* can lead to reactivation of the infection with serious consequences (39–41). As the population of *T. cruzi*-infected immigrants in the United States ages, increasing numbers of cases of severe reactivated Chagas disease caused by iatrogenic immunosuppression will occur.

Diagnosis

The diagnosis of acute Chagas disease is usually made by detection of parasites. Bloodform trypomastigotes can often be seen in wet preparations and stained smears of blood from patients with acute *T. cruzi* infection. In patients with acute Chagas disease but without patent parasitemias, xenodiagnosis is almost always positive. This procedure involves feeding fresh blood from the patient to laboratory-reared reduviid bugs, followed 30–40 days later by examination of their intestinal contents for the presence of flagellates. A possible role in the diagnosis of acute Chagas disease for an assay based on polymerase chain reaction (PCR) amplification of repetitive DNA sequences of *T. cruzi* is being investigated (unpublished data).

In contrast, the diagnosis of chronic *T. cruzi* infection is usually based on the detection of antibodies that bind to *T. cruzi* antigens. A number of highly sensitive serologic assays based on binding of antibodies to native *T. cruzi* antigens are used widely, but false-positive reactions have been a persistent problem (42). Some progress has been made in developing highly specific assays based on native antigens (43, 44), and recently several laboratories have focused on developing serodiagnostic tests in which recombinant *T. cruzi* proteins are used as target antigens (45, 46). Research is also underway that has as its goal the development of a PCR-based assay for direct detection of parasites circulating in the blood of chronically infected persons (47, 48).

Treatment

Unfortunately, *T. cruzi* is not susceptible to most of the large number of drugs tested for activity during the past several decades, including those effective against the African trypanosomes and other protozoans. Benznidazole (Radamil®, Roche 7-1051) and nifurtimox (Lampit®, Bayer 2502), the two drugs available for treatment of *T. cruzi*, are effective in reducing the severity of acute Chagas disease but have no role in the therapy of chronic infections (49, 50). Both must be taken for extended periods and often cause severe side effects. Moreover, many patients given full courses of treatment are not cured parasitologically. Additional concern relating to these drugs is raised by studies reported by Teixeira et al. (51, 52) in which 42% of rabbits receiving benznidazole and 33% of those treated with nifurtimox developed widely-invasive, mixed-cell type lymphomas, whereas none of the control animals developed tumors. Although these findings should be a source of concern, they should be viewed from the perspective that both drugs have both been used widely for decades in Latin America and no reports of increased frequency of lymphomas in treated patients have appeared.

An additional recent article relating to the treatment of *T. cruzi* is the report by Gallerano and coworkers (53) on the use of allopurinol in patients with Chagas disease. Allopurinol is a pyrazolopyrimidine analogue of hypoxanthine that was found in early studies to be active against *T. cruzi* in tissue culture and in mice (54). Gallerano et al. found that allopurinol was as effective in suppressing *T. cruzi* parasitemias, as measured by xenodiagnosis, and in causing conventional serologic tests to become negative, as were benznidazole and nifurtimox given in standard doses. The purported advantage of allopurinol, then, would be its relatively fewer side effects. However, the open, nonrandomized study structure employed in this trial and the lack of clearly-defined criteria for cure of *T. cruzi* infection make interpretation of the results difficult.

Efforts at developing new drugs for treating *T. cruzi* continue in a small number of laboratories. Gonzales-Perdomo and coworkers in Brazil assessed the *in vivo* anti-*T. cruzi* activity of several inhibitors of bacterial topoisomerases. Marked inhibition of parasite proliferation and differentiation was caused by these drugs, suggesting that *T. cruzi* has a enzyme similar to topoisomerase II of bacteria, thus opening a new avenue in the search for an effective agent for treating the parasite.

Possible Approaches to the Control of Chagas Disease

It has been demonstrated that reduction of transmission of *T. cruzi* can be achieved through vector control by spraying of insecticides and through improvement of housing conditions. Effective programs that use these approaches to limiting the spread of *T. cruzi* infection are lacking in many endemic areas, and their development should be given high priority by the health ministries of the affected countries. Similarly, programs for identification of blood donors infected with *T. cruzi* by serologic screening need to be refined and expanded in endemic countries. Although no vaccine is available for preventing transmission of *T. cruzi*, the development of a vaccine remains a viable but distant goal and research in this area is being performed in a handful of laboratories. Moreover, as noted above, drug therapy is unsatisfactory, and the two agents currently available for treating patients infected with *T. cruzi* are unlikely to play a significant role in the overall control of Chagas disease. In this context there is a pressing need for better drugs for Chagas disease. It is hoped that basic knowledge of the molecular biology of *T. cruzi* (55–59) and of the immunology of the host-parasite relationship (60, 61) will be applied in rational drug design projects that will provide the next generation of agents for treating this parasite.

References

1. Brener Z (1973) Biology of *Trypanosoma cruzi*. Ann Rev Microbiol 27: 347–382
2. Kirchhoff LV (1990) Trypanosoma species (American Trypanosomiasis, Chagas Disease): Biology of trypanosomes. In: Mandell GL, Douglas RG Jr Bennett JE (eds) Principles and practice of infectious diseases. New York, John Wiley & Sons, pp 2077–2084
3. Brener Z (1984) Laboratory-acquired Chagas' disease: An endemic disease among parasitologists? In: Morel CM (ed) Genes and antigens of parasites: A laboratory manual. Rio de Janeiro, Oswaldo Cruz, pp 3–9
4. Hofflin JM, Sadler RH, Araujo FG (1987) Laboratory-acquired Chagas' disease. Trans R Soc Trop Med Hyg 81: 437–440
5. Schmunis GA (1991) *Trypanosoma cruzi*, the etiologic agent of Chagas' disease: Status in the blood supply in endemic and nonendemic countries. Transfusion 31: 547–557
6. Carrasco R, Miguez H, Camacho C, Echalar L, Revollo S, Ampuero T, Dedet J-P (1990) Prevalence of *Trypanosoma cruzi* infection in blood banks of seven departments of Bolivia. Mem Inst Oswaldo Cruz 85: 69–73
7. Azogue E, La Fuente C, Darras CH (1985) Congenital Chagas' disease in Bolivia: Epidemiological aspects and pathological findings. Trans R Soc Trop Med Hyg 79: 176–180
8. Bettencourt AL (1976) Congenital Chagas' disease. Am J Dis Child 130: 97–103
9. Laranja FS, Dias E, Nobrega G, Miranda A (1956) Chagas' disease: A clinical, epidemiologic, and pathologic study. Circulation 14: 1035–1060
10. Spina-Franca A, Mattosinho LC (1988) South American Trypanosomiasis (Chagas' Disease) In: Vinken PJ, Bruyn GW, Klawans HL (eds) Handbook of clinical neurology. New York, Elsevier Science Publishing Co, pp 345–349
11. Kierszenbaum F, Sztein MB (1990) Mechanisms underlying immunosuppression induced by *Trypanosoma cruzi*. Parasitol Today 6: 261–264
12. Reed SG, Inverso JA, Roters SB (1984) Heterologous antibody responses in mice with chronic *Trypanosoma cruzi* infection: Depressed T helper function restored with supernatants containing interleukin 2. J Immunol 133: 1558–1563
13. Tarleton RL (1988) *Trypanosoma cruzi*-induced suppression of IL-2 production: I. Evidence for the presence of IL-2-producing cells. J Immunol 140: 2763–2768
14. Beltz LA, Kierszenbaum F, Sztein MB (1990) *Trypanosoma cruzi*-induced suppression of human peripheral blood lymphocytes activated via the alternative (CD2) pathway. Infect Immun 58: 1114–1116

15. Sztein MB, Cuna WR, Kierszenbaum F (1990) *Trypanosoma cruzi* inhibits the expression of CD3, CD4, CD8, and IL-2R by mitogen-activated helper and cytotoxic human lymphocytes. J Immunol 144: 3558–3562
16. Beltz LA, Kierszenbaum F, Sztein MB (1989) Selective suppressive effects of *Trypanosoma cruzi* on activated human lymphocytes. Infect Immun 57: 2301–2305
17. Amorim DS. Chagas' disease (1979) Prog Cardiol 1979; 8: 235–279
18. Kirchhoff LV, Neva FA (1985) Chagas' disease in Latin American immigrants. JAMA 254: 3058–3060
19. Hagar JM, Rahimtoola SH (1991) Chagas' heart disease in the United States. N Engl J Med 325: 763–768
20. Köberle F (1968) Chagas' disease and Chagas' syndromes: The pathology of American trypanosomiasis. Adv Parasitol 6: 63–116
21. Cossio PM, Diez C, Szarfman A (1974) Chagasic cardiopathy-demonstration of a serum gamma globulin factor which reacts with endocardium and vascular structures. Circulation 49: 13–21
22. Santos-Buch CA, Teixeira ARL (1974) The immunology of experimental Chagas' disease. III. Rejection of allogeneic heart cells in vitro. J Exp Med 140: 38–53
23. Van Voorhis WC, Schlekewy L, Trong HL (1991) Molecular mimicry by *Trypanosoma cruzi:* The F1-160 epitope that mimics mammalian nerve can be mapped to a 12-amino acid peptide. Proc Natl Acad Sci USA 88: 5993–5997
24. Ternynck T, Bleux C, Gregoire J, Avrameas S, Kanellopoulos-Langevin C (1990) Comparison between autoantibodies arising during *Trypanosoma cruzi* infection in mice and natural autoantibodies. J Immunol 144: 1504–1511
25. Kierszenbaum F (1985) Is there autoimmunity in Chagas' disease? Parasitol Today 1: 4–6
26. Petry K, Eisen H (1989) Chagas disease: A model for the study of autoimmune diseases. Parasitol Today 5: 111–116
27. Davila DF, Rossell RO, Donis JH (1989) Cardiac parasympathetic abnormalities: Cause or consequence of Chagas heart disease? Parasitol Today 5: 327–329
28. Goble FC. South American Trypanosomes (1970) In: Jackson GJ, Herman R, Singer I (eds) Immunity to parasitic diseases in animals. New York, Appleton-Century-Crofts, pp 597–689
29. Beard CB, Young DG, Butler JF, Evans DA (1988) First isolation of *Trypanosoma cruzi* from a wild-caught *Triatoma sanguisuga* (LeConte) (Hemiptera: Triatominae) in Florida, U.S.A. J Parasitol 74: 343–344
30. Yaeger RG (1988) The prevalence of *Trypanosoma cruzi* infection in armadillos collected at a site near New Orleans, Louisiana. Am J Trop Med Hyg 38: 323–326
31. Dias JCP (1987) Control of Chagas' disease in Brazil. Parasitol Today 3: 336–341
32. Acquatella H, Catalioti F, Gomez-Mancebo JR, Davalos V, Villalobos L (1987) Long-term control of Chagas' disease in Venezuela: Effects on serologic findings, electrocardiographic abnormalities, and clinical outcome. Circulation 76: 556–562
33. Mota EA, Guimaraes AC, Santana OO, Sherlock I, Hoff R, Weller TH (1990) A nine year prospective study of Chagas' disease in a defined rural population in Northeast Brazil. Am J Trop Med Hyg 42: 429–440
34. Kirchhoff LV, Gam AA, Gilliam FC (1987) American trypanosomiasis (Chagas' disease) in Central American immigrants. Am J Med 82: 915–920
35. Kirchhoff LV (1989) Is *Trypanosoma cruzi* a new threat to our blood supply? Ann Intern Med 111: 773–775
36. Grant IH, Gold JWM, Wittner M, Tanowitz HB, Nathan C, Mayer K, Reich L, Wollner N, Steinherz L Ghavimi F, O'Reilly RJ, Armstrong D (1989) Transfusion-associated acute Chagas disease acquired in the United States. Ann Intern Med 111: 849–851
37. Nickerson P, Orr P, Schroeder M-L, Sekla L, Johnston JB (1989) Transfusion-associated *Trypanosoma cruzi* infection in a non-endemic area. Ann Intern Med 111: 851–853
38. Kirchhoff LV (1991) American trypanosomiasis (Chagas' disease) – a persistent problem in Latin America now affects the United States. N Engl J Med
39. Rivero I, Moravenik M, Morales J, Gomez M, De Rosas JM (1974) Chagas' disease – another hazard in acute leukemia. N Engl J Med 290: 285–285

40. Stolf NAG, Higushi L, Bocchi E, Bellotti G, Costa Auler JO, Uip D, Amato Neto V, Pileggi F, Jatene AD (1987) Heart transplantation in patients with Chagas' disease cardiomyopathy. Heart Transplantation 6: 307–312
41. Libow LF, Beltrani VP, Silvers DN, Grossman ME (1991) Post-cardiac transplant reactivation of Chagas' disease diagnosed by skin biopsy. Cutis 48: 37–40
42. Camargo ME (1988) American Trypanosomiasis (Chagas' Disease). In: Balows A, Hausler WJ Jr, Lennette EH (eds) Laboratory diagnosis of infectious diseases – principles and practice. New York, Springer, pp 744–753
43. Kirchhoff LV, Gam AA, Gusmao Rd'A, Goldsmith RS, Rezende JM, Rassi A (1987) Increased specificity of serodiagnosis of Chagas' disease by detection of antibody to the 72- and 90-kilodalton glycoproteins of *Trypanosoma cruzi*. J Infect Dis 155: 561–564
44. Schechter M, Luquetti AO, Rezende JM, Rassi A, Miles MA (1985) Further evaluation of lectin affinity purified glycoprotein (GP90) in the enzyme linked immunosorbent assay (ELISA) for diagnosis of *Trypanosoma cruzi* infection. Trans R Soc Trop Med Hyg 79: 637–640
45. Cotrim PC, Paranhos GS, Mortara RA, Wanderley J, Rassi A, Camargo ME, da Silveira JF (1990) Expression in *Escherichia coli* of a dominant immunogen of *Trypanosoma* C171Zi recognized by human chagasic sera. J Clin Microbiol 28: 519–524
46. Luquetti AO (1990) Use of *Trypanosoma cruzi* defined proteins for diagnosis-multicentre trial: Serological and technical aspects. Mem Inst Oswaldo Cruz 85: 497–505
47. Moser DR, Kirchhoff LV, Donelson JE (1989) Detection of *Trypanosoma cruzi* by polymerase chain reaction gene amplification. J Clin Microbiol 27: 1744–1749
48. Sturm NR, Degrave W, Morel C, Simpson L (1989) Sensitive detection and schizodeme classification of *Trypanosoma cruzi* cells by amplification of kinetoplast minicircle DNA sequences: use in diagnosis of Chagas' disease. Mol Biochem Parasitol 33: 205–214
49. Brener Z (1979) Present status of chemotherapy and chemoprophylaxis of human trypanosomes in the western hemisphere. Pharmacol Ther 7: 71–90
50. Marr JJ, Docampo R (1986) Chemotherapy for Chagas' disease: A perspective of current therapy and considerations for future research. Rev Infect Dis 8: 884–903
51. Teixeira ARL Silva R, Cunha Neto E, Santana JM, Rizzo LV (1990) Malignant, non-Hodgkin's lymphomas in *Trypanosoma cruzi*-infected rabbits treated with nitroarenes. J Comp Path 103: 37–48
52. Teixeira ARL, Cordova JC, Souto Maior I, Solorzano E (1990) Chagas' disease: Lymphoma growth in rabbits treated with benznidazole. Am J Trop Med Hyg 43: 146–158
53. Gallerano RH, Marr JJ, Sosa RR (1990) Therapeutic efficacy of allopurinol in patients with chronic Chagas' disease. Am J Trop Med Hyg 43: 159–166
54. Avila JL, Avila A (1981) *Trypanosoma cruzi:* Allopurinol in the treatment of mice with experimental acute Chagas disease. Exp Parasitol 51: 204–208
55. Feagin JE (1990) RNA editing in kinetoplastid mitochondria. J Biol Chem 265: 19373–19376
56. Sartorius C, Franklin RM (1991) The use of antisense oligonucleotides as chemotherapeutic agents for parasites. Parasitol Today 7: 90–93
57. Buck GA, Lu H-Y (1991) Expression of an exogenous gene in *Trypanosoma cruzi* epimastigotes. Mol Biochem Parasitol 44: 109–114.
58. Eid J, Sollner-Webb B (1991) Stable integrative transformation of *Trypanosoma brucei* that occurs exclusively by homologous recombination. Proc Natl Acad Sci USA 88: 2118–2121
59. Smith DF (1990) Trypanosomatid transfection: stable introduction of DNA into protozoa. Parasitol Today 6: 245–247
60. Reed SG (1988) In vivo administration of recombinant IFN-gamma induces macrophage activation and prevents acute disease, immune suppression, and death in experimental *Trypanosoma cruzi* infections. J Immunol 140: 4342–4347
61. Tarleton RL (1990) Depletion of CD8+ T cells increases susceptibility and reverses vaccine-induced immunity in mice infected with *Trypanosoma cruzi*. J Immunol 144: 717–724

Strategies for the Twenty-First Century – Control or Eradication?*

D. A. Henderson

Associate Director for Life Sciences, Office of Science and Technology Policy, Executive Office of the President, Washington, D.C.

Abstract

The eradication of smallpox has renewed a once dormant debate about the feasibility and desirability of undertaking eradication campaigns against other infectious agents. In their enthusiasm for such programs, protagonists for eradication overlook a regrettable history of program failures which ultimately called into question the credibility of public health professionals. Characteristically, failed programs have not been scientifically well-grounded nor have they had effective surveillance or research components. The present global polio program bears certain of these attributes. Rather than to agonize over policy issues of what to eradicate or to control, it would make more practical sense to develop an effective international research infrastructure, especially in the tropics and in third world countries. With qualified staff *in situ*, the difficult questions are more likely to be asked – and answered – than they are at present.

Introduction

In the field of tropical medicine, it is especially critical that we look ahead to the next century. Recent advances in biomedical sciences offer undreamed of vistas for prevention, diagnosis and treatment of that incredible array of tropical diseases which plague the third world. Once, not so long ago, those who specialized in the communicable diseases, were regarded as occupying a niche in a medical backwater. Today, research on the immune system, if not yet on all the pathogens which assault it, is at the cutting edge of biomedical science. A magnificent future beckons which

* Presented at the Centennial Symposium on Tropical Medicine at the University of Texas Medical Branch at Galveston, Texas, on May 31, 1991

should not be distracted by all too futile policy debates about eradication and control or by evangelists who preach a gospel of eradication without comprehending it. Let me try to offer a perspective on future strategies and some directions for the future.

Eradication, as the ultimate objective for a disease control program, is not a recent development. The concept that it might be possible to eradicate a disease, at least regionally, dates back just a century – to 1884 (1). That year Congress created a Bureau of Animal Industries whose sole, stated objective was to eradicate a disease of cows – bovine contagious pleuropneumonia – which had been imported from Europe 40 years before and had spread across the country. The Bureau was given a 5 year target and, surprisingly, it succeeded. Soon, other animal diseases and vectors began to be targeted (2). By and large, the programs relied on isolation or slaughter of infected herds – an approach not well-suited for dealing with human disease.

These experiences generated the belief that there might be a substantial number of microorganisms or vectors which clung so tenuously to an ecological niche that simple measures, thoroughly applied, could upset the balance of nature. Disease eradication programs soon became a familiar concept to the veterinary community.

Eradication programs for human diseases, however, were not discussed until early this century. This is somewhat surprising because smallpox until recently was a disease of major international concern; vaccination was widely employed, at least in Europe and North America; and quarantine measures were widely applied to keep the disease out of smallpox-free areas. But no one spoke of smallpox eradication as a concept or objective until the 1950's. Meanwhile the first eradication programs were launched, respectively, for hookworm in 1907 and yellow fever in 1910 (3, 4). The basis for these campaigns was more firmly based in visionary belief than in a scientific understanding of the diseases and their ecology. Both were products of the philanthropy John D. Rockefeller.

The magnitude of the efforts was extraordinary, even by contemporary standards. Hookworm programs eventually extended over 52 countries on 6 continents; yellow fever programs and laboratories were developed throughout the Americas and some African countries. The programs were highly centralized and quasi-military in nature with rigidly prescribed activities to be applied everywhere. Innovation was discouraged. Progress was measured by inputs – for hookworm, it was the numbers of treatments administered and the number of privies constructed; for yellow fever, it was the number of dwellings inspected and treated to destroy *Aedes aegypti* mosquitoes. Neither program sought to measure the numbers of cases of the disease in question and their decline in incidence – or lack thereof. Neither had a program for research. The belief quite simply was that the tools were available. The problem was solely an administrative one – to apply them.

Not until 10 years after the hookworm campaign began was an effort made to assess the impact (5). When this was done, it was discovered that, even with an optimum program, the prevalence of infection was unchanged. However, those infected did have fewer worms, on average, and thus fewer symptoms. For the yellow fever program, more than 15 years were to elapse before the jungle reservoir of the disease was detected (6). When it was, the target was shifted from yellow fever eradication to *Aedes aegypti* eradication with little consideration given to either the cost or practicability of hemisphere-wide extermination of a mosquito species (7). That program in various guises extended for another 30 years before finally being abandoned as impractical.

With the discovery of DDT, malaria eradication became the next campaign to emerge – in 1955 – and this was not a regional but a global commitment (8). Its genesis rested more on evangelistic commitment than upon sound science. In fact, although billed as global in scope, it was recognized that existing methods then offered no hope for the whole of sub-Saharan Africa (9). Nevertheless, a research program was not high on anyone's agenda. Conversely, many existing research centers were closed in the conviction that the necessary tools were available. All that was thought to be required were sound administration, rigidly applied methods, national commitment and money. Jeffery, a senior statesman, ruefully pointed out: "The *science* of malaria control ... was almost overnight converted to the rather simplistic *technology* of malaria eradication, which basically required that one know how to deliver 2 grams of something to every square meter of a sometime elusive wall." (10) McGregor lamented the diminishing number of "malariologists" and the proliferation of "eradicationists" (11).

The same quasi-military, highly structured methods were used as with yellow fever eradication. Seventeen years later and after an expenditure of more than $2 billion, it was apparent that eradication was nowhere in sight. And the program gradually began to be phased down. Efforts began to be made to reconstruct a once-robust research activity, but there was little left to build upon.

In 1965, about the time it was becoming apparent that malaria eradication was not a viable concept, Rene Dubos published his book, *Man Adapting*. In the book, he reflected the views of many in the science community when he wrote: "Public health administrators, like social planners, have to compromise with the limitations of human nature. For this reason, and many others, eradication programs will eventually become a curiosity item on library shelves, just as have all social utopias." (12)

Clearly, there was widespread disillusionment with eradication programs as public health policy. The year of my arrival in Geneva – 1966 – was not an auspicious time for a neophyte eradicator to assume direction of a budding smallpox eradication effort. It was discouraging but not surprising to find that antipathy towards smallpox eradication extended from the Director General throughout the Organization and indeed to many national health administrators as well. Even the initial WHO smallpox budget of $2.4 million had been controversial. That budget provided just $50,000 per year for each country where a program was needed but it passed by only

2 votes with 12 nations abstaining (13). No WHO budget, before or since, has proved to be so divisive as that one. Contributions were sparse. During the first *seven years* of the program, the *combined* cash contribution of all donors amounted to less that $200,000 per year. UNICEF, a major supporter of malaria eradication refused to support the program as did many bilateral contributors. Indeed, smallpox eradication, as other categorical programs, was considered suspect and derisively labelled a "vertical" program to be discouraged if not abandoned. I will not further dwell on the issue and the manifestations. The important point is to appreciate how damaging unrealistic eradication programs had been to public health credibility.

Two features, in particular, distinguished smallpox eradication from previous eradication efforts. These proved critical to its success: surveillance and research. The goal, as we saw it, was a simple and specific one – zero cases of smallpox. To measure progress we needed a reporting system and this was given priority. Systems were established to assure weekly reporting of cases from all health units in all endemic countries. Through the data which flowed in, we learned that the distribution of smallpox and its manner of spread was quite different from our original planning assumptions. We learned that vaccine immunity was far more durable than any had believed and we discovered that little of the vaccine in use met accepted standards. With this continuing flow of surveillance information, program strategy continually evolved in an on-going effort to bring to bear the maximum of resources where the problems were greatest. No two national programs were identical. Innovation and change were welcomed.

A plea for research funds was initially denied by WHO on the grounds that a good vaccine was available; that the epidemiology of smallpox had been thoroughly studied; and that the sole problem was an administrative one – to vaccinate everyone. After a year, a $40,000 research budget was reluctantly agreed upon, and with this we were able to leverage a broad scale cooperative research program. This resulted in changes in the smallpox vaccine strain, in the methods of vaccine production, in the basic vaccination instrument, in the discovery and characterization of monkeypox and, finally, in the sequencing of the virus – a development which resolved some very disturbing and contentious issues related to a possible animal reservoir.

Neither disease surveillance nor research were important components of earlier eradication efforts. Those programs were driven more by evangelism than by science, by emotion more than reason, by the belief that answers lay primarily in diligent administration, by the belief that it was better to try and fail than not to try at all. By the time smallpox eradication was decided upon, the most feasible of all programs, public credibility was at a low ebb. We have now recaptured some of that credibility.

Today, proposals are regularly being advanced to undertake a host of new eradication campaigns – measles, poliomyelitis, even tuberculosis, leprosy, yaws, urban rabies, hunger and many others (14–16). However, as public health professionals, our credibility simply cannot tolerate another debacle comparable to those of the past with all the attendant repercussions.

Have we learned from these experiences of the past? With notable exceptions, the answer has to be – not well. The clarion cry to eradication is regularly sounded by some as an attention-getting, fund-raising initiative albeit with little expectation of achievement of the objective. The stated rationale is that it is better to try and fail than not to try at all. Such scientific misrepresentation is to be deplored. Regrettably often such advocates continue to receive an undeserved hearing and respect.

There are three specific programs, however, which deserve comment – two are stated global objectives – for Guinea worm and polio; one, for measles, is widely regarded as perhaps the next target. The Guinea worm campaign, whose champion and guiding spirit is Don Hopkins, is proceeding exceptionally well. When it began, it readily passed the primary acid test of having already been demonstrably effective in some developing countries. Adequate methods were available to interrupt transmission and, through research, these have been steadily improved. Surveillance, conducted primarily by area-wide search, has proven its worth and is steadily improving. And, finally, its strategy has steadily evolved based on empirical experience. If adequate resources and national commitment can be sustained, it should be successful. The biggest problem is that it is a disease of the rural poor, a group not high on the priority list of governments or donors.

The experience with measles has been quite the converse. Many have argued – and passionately – that global eradication is vitally important because of the severity of the disease. None can argue with this premise, but because eradication is desirable doesn't mean it is feasible. To be noted is the fact that no industrialized country, let alone a developing one, has yet succeeded in stopping transmission for more than a matter of a few months. A more antigenic vaccine, one which could be given at or near birth, conceivably could provide the necessary opening to eradication – and there are lines of research which might open the way to such a vaccine. However, few are being explored and these in a more casual than deliberate effort.

The saga of global polio eradication is more encouraging but only so in its launching. A brief recapitulation of events illustrates the problem. In 1985, the Director of PAHO called together a small group to advise on the feasibility of a regional eradication effort (17). WHO's expanded program on immunization had been operative for a decade and polio incidence in the Americas had fallen dramatically even in the tropical areas where the oral vaccine was known to be generally less effective. After due deliberation, we concluded that eradication was a conceivable objective with the caveat that due attention be paid to the development of surveillance and to research. Funds were promised from UNICEF, AID, the IADB and Rotary. A major stumbling block, however, was that none saw the need for research and only one agreed to make such funds available – and then only with great reluctance.

The director of that program, Dr. Ciro de Quadros, has proved to be an impresario of uncommon skill. Within a year after the program began, surveillance revealed distressingly large numbers of type III cases among well-immunized children. Field studies were immediately undertaken which showed the need to double the type III component of the vaccine, the first modification of the vaccine in 20 years. Quite promptly, the type III problem disappeared. The surveillance program called for reporting of all cases of acute flaccid paralysis in young children, once considered to be all but pathognomonic of polio. To everyone's surprise, acute flaccid paralysis in young children, even in polio free areas, was far more prevalent than any had expected. Rates of 1 to 2 cases per 100,000 children under 15 years of age were common. A range of clinical studies were needed to help refine diagnostic criteria. A network of laboratories was established, and stool specimens were collected. With support from program funds, Kew and his CDC colleagues sequenced the virus strains which were isolated. They discovered distinct regional variations in strains. They showed also that the variations were sustained overtime. This suggested that polio did not spread easily or frequently over long distances. Surveillance data complemented this observation in showing that the epidemiology of the disease most closely resembled smallpox, i.e., it was widely prevalent over a country during peak seasons but retreated to crowded urban settings during the interseasonal low. DeQuadros utilized these findings to develop a strategy which called for intensive house-to-house vaccination campaigns in crowded, lower socio-economic areas during interseasonal periods. Polio incidence dropped precipitously. In brief, the program rapidly changed and adapted in response to a good surveillance and research program. Today, a network of 10,000 health posts report cases of acute flaccid paralysis every week, 80% of which are detected within 2 weeks of onset and from 80% of them, stool specimens are obtained. During the period of December 1990 to May 1991, only two cases of poliomyelitis have been detected in the whole of the western hemisphere.

In 1988, WHO decided that the progress in the Americas justified launching a global eradication program (18). In candor, its feasibility had to be questioned if for no other reason than that the vaccine is so heat sensitive as to require refrigeration up to the point of administration. It is of such poor antigenicity in tropical areas that seroconversion cannot be assured with as many as 5 doses. It is, at best, marginally satisfactory for Latin America. For Africa and most of Asia, a far less developed infrastructure of services makes it a doubtful commodity indeed. Those who expressed reservations about a global program were assured by WHO that a research program would be vigorously pursued. Three years have elapsed, few funds have been found for needed research and little progress has been made. Surveillance programs are still vestigial; reporting is more often monthly than weekly; and most countries depend on information from only a few sentinel sites. The dominant theme which extends through all discussions is that we have a protective vaccine; and that the problem is basically an administrative one.

Polio eradication is inevitably a far more difficult proposition than smallpox eradication, given the problems of surveillance and accurate diagnosis. Even with a vaccine which is thermostable at ambient temperatures for a month or more and which is fully protective with one or at most two doses, the task will be difficult. We must recall that smallpox eradication succeeded but by only the narrowest of margins and that the basic infrastructure of services in many developing countries has changed very little over the past 15 years.

Eradication of a disease is a difficult, complex task for which we need far sharper tools than we now have. Thus you will understand my gloomy appraisal that, on entry into the 21st century, I foresee, at present, little prospect of even being able to contemplate global disease eradication except possibly for Guinea worm. The current problems in eradication exemplify to me a far more basic and serious problem which pertains to all tropical diseases. That, quite simply, is the lack of resources for research. This derives, in part, from limited understanding on the part of program managers of the potential created by progress in biomedical research especially over the past decade. At the same time, there is a lack of comprehension by so many who are doing basic research as to the practical needs of those in the field. The case for research is simply not being made and development agencies, in consequence, are funding precious little. A schism has been permitted to grow – and perhaps has been encouraged – between administrators of health programs and those in the research laboratories. In part, the fault lies with a generally traditional administrative cadre who are most comfortable with what they know than with the unknown and uncertain. In part, the fault lies with those in basic research, the majority of whom reside in industrialized countries far removed from the tropics and who assert little interest in the application of what they discover or in learning about diseases and their manifestations under natural settings.

It seems to me that one fundamental approach to begin to cope with this problem rests in the development of a network of multidisciplinary centers firmly anchored in the countries which daily must cope with tropical infections. Where better to decide priorities, where better to link presently insoluble disease problems with the biomedical research which might provide the answers?

Much has been written and said by the development community over recent years regarding the need for capacity building both of institutions and people. So far, there has been little but rhetoric in the health field. There are those who would argue that our philanthropy has been extended quite far enough and that unless such a program could be defined in terms of a national interest, it is a non-starter. Happily, Lederberg, Morse and their colleagues are now providing an all too obvious raison d'etre in calling attention to the potentially devastating problems posed by new and emerging viruses and other microbial agents (19, 20). As they have pointed out, if we are to have any hope of dealing with a newly emergent microorganism, an HIV-like infection, for example, a contemporary swine flu or who knows what other agents, early detection and an accelerated research agenda are the only possible answers. To achieve this, there is absolutely no choice but to have a network of effective multidisciplinary research centers in countries around the world, especially in the tropics and near densely populated lower socio-economic areas of third world countries. It is in our own interests as well as theirs. In fact, our very survival could be at stake. It would seem to me that this is a rationale for an investment worthy of as much attention as, for example, a super-conducting supercollider.

Let me conclude by suggesting that debates over what or whether we eradicate or contain are idle exercises. Without far better tools and a far better understanding of diseases in the tropics, satisfactory disease control, let alone eradication, is simply not in the cards. Rather, the thrust of our policy should be to staff and support a research infrastructure working in optimal locations to ask the right questions.

References

1. Hinman EH (1966) World Eradication of Infectious Diseases. Springfield, Thomas
2. Hagan WA (1958) The control and eradication of animal diseases in the United States. Ann Rev Microbiol 12: 127–144
3. Fosdick RB (1952) The story of the Rockefeller Foundation. New York, Harper and Brothers
4. Strode GK (1951) Yellow Fever. New York, McGraw-Hill
5. Smillie WG (1922) The results of hookworm disease prophylaxis in Brazil. Am J Hyg 2: 77–95
6. Soper FL (1936) Jungle yellow fever: new epidemiological entity in South America. Rev Higiene Saude Pub 10: 107–144
7. Duffy J (1977) Ventures in world health. The memoirs of Fred Lowe Soper. Washington, Pan American Health Organization
8. Pampana EJ (1963) A textbook of malaria eradication. London, Oxford University Press
9. Downs WG (1981) A new look at yellow fever and malaria. Am J Trop Med Hyg 30: 516–522
10. Jeffery GM (1976) Malaria control in the twentieth century. Am J Trop Med Hyg 25: 361–371
11. McGregor I (1984) Malaria-recollections and observations. Trans R Soc Trop Med Hyg 78: 1–8
12. Dubos R (1965) Man adapting. New Haven, Yale University Press
13. Fenner F, Henderson DA, Arita I, Jezek Z, Ladnyi I (1988) Smallpox and its eradication. Geneva, World Health Organization
14. Stetten D Jr (1980) Eradication. Science 210: 1203
15. Hopkins DR, Hinman AR, Koplan JP, Lane JM (1982) The case for global measles eradication. Lancet 1: 1396–1398
16. Hopkins DR (1976) After smallpox eradication: yaws? Am J Trop Med Hyg 25: 860–865
17. de Quadros C (1990) Polio eradication: fulfilling the first EPI promise. In: Protecting the world's children: An agenda for the 1990's. Atlanta, Task force for child survival, pp 79–102
18. World Health Organization (1984) Global eradication of poliomyelitis in the year 2000. Geneva, World Health Organization (Resolution WHA 41.28)
19. Lederberg J (1990) Medical science, infectious disease and the unity of humankind. JAMA 260: 684–685
20. Morse SS, Schleuderberg A (1990) Emerging viruses: the evolution of viruses and viral diseases. J Infect Dis 162: 1–7

ISSN 0304-8608
Title No. 705

Archives of Virology

Official Journal of the Virology Division of the International Union of Microbiological Societies

Archives of Virology publishes original contributions from all branches of research on viruses, viruslike agents, and virus infections of humans, animals, plants, insects, and bacteria. Coverage includes the broadest spectrum of topics, from initial descriptions of newly discovered viruses, to studies of virus structure, composition, and genetics, to studies of virus interactions with host cells, host organisms, and host populations. Multidisciplinary studies are particularly welcome, as are studies employing molecular biologic, molecular genetic, and modern immunologic and epidemiologic approaches. For example, studies on the molecular pathogenesis, pathophysiology, and genetics of virus infections in individual hosts, and studies on the molecular epidemiology of virus infections in populations, are encouraged. Studies involving applied research, such as diagnostic technology, development, monoclonal antibody panel development, vaccine development, and antiviral drug development, are also encouraged. However, such studies are often better presented in the context of a specific application or as they bear upon general principles of interest to many virologists. In all cases, it is the quality of the research work, its significance, and its originally which will decide acceptability.

As a new opportunity for publication of proceedings of meetings, treatises, and large reviews the series of Special Issues of *Archives of Virology* was initiated in 1990. Individuals who are organizing a meeting, symposium, conference, or congress, and individuals who would like to organize a treatise or large review are invited to communicate directly with one of the Special Issues Editors for further information: Dr. C. H. Calisher, Fort Collins, Colorado, or Dr. H.-D. Klenk, Marburg, FRG.

Subscription Information:
1992. Vols. 122–127 (4 issues each):
DM 1.908,–, öS 13.356,–, plus carriage charges

Springer-Verlag Wien New York

C. de Bac, W. H. Gerlich, G. Taliani (eds.)

Chronically Evolving Viral Hepatitis

(Archives of Virology, Supplementum 4)

1992. Approx. 250 pages.
Soft cover approx. DM 180,–, öS 1.260,–
10% price reduction for subscribers to
"Archives of Virology"
ISBN 3-211-82350-6

Prices are subject to change without notice

The volume deals with chronic viral hepatitis in a multidisciplinary approach. The main goal of the editors was to assemble contributions from clinicians, laboratory physicians, epidemiologists, pathologists and molecular biologists to provide a synopsis of all important aspects of this disease. A key element in the chronic evolution of viral hepatitis is the persistent coexistence of a cytotoxic immune response and viral gene expression which is discussed in eleven articles on immune pathogenesis. Oncogenicity of hepatitis B virus at the molecular level and of hepatitis C virus at the epidemiological level are discussed in two chapters. Application of PCR for the detection of hepatitis viruses and their variants is a major topic of both practical and theoretical interest. The clinical significance of newly developed serological assays for diagnosis and prevention is discussed in depth by specialists from clinics, transfusion centers and virological laboratories. Therapy of chronic viral hepatitis is still unsatisfactory, but some slow progress is described in several articles. Furthermore, the volume has a special chapter on the often neglected topic of chronic hepatitis in childhood.

Springer-Verlag Wien New York

Charles H. Calisher (ed.)

Hemorrhagic Fever with Renal Syndrome, Tick- and Mosquito-Borne Viruses

(Archives of Virology/Supplementum 1)

1991. 75 figures. VII, 347 pages.
Soft cover DM 258,–, öS 1800,–
Reduced price for subscribers to "Archives of Virology":
Soft cover DM 232,20, öS 1625,–
ISBN 3-211-82217-8

Prices are subject to change without notice

This book summarizes selected papers presented at two symposia convened in the fall of 1989. The papers include information on the molecular biology, antigenicity, diagnosis, epidemiology, clinical aspects, pathogenesis, vaccines, and other aspects of hemorrhagic fever with renal syndrome and tick- (tick-borne encephalitis, Congo-Crimean hemorrhagic fever, Dugbe, orbiviruses, orthomyxoviruses) and mosquito-borne (California serogroup, alphaviruses from Mongolia, sandfly fevers in Central Asia and Afghanistan) viruses. Although covering a wide range of subjects and perspectives, the issue is intended to provide readers with an integrated view of the geographical distribution, properties and effects, recognition, and prevention of infections with these and other viruses. Included are papers describing newly recognized viruses, newly recognized virus diseases, newly recognized foci, new techniques for detection and diagnosis, and new vaccines. Many of the papers contain information never before available to readers of English-language scientific literature.

Springer-Verlag Wien New York